Basics of Respiratory Mechanics and Artificial Ventilation

Springer
Milano
Berlin
Heidelberg
New York
Barcelona
Hong Kong
London
Paris
Singapore
Tokyo

J. Milic-Emili
U. Lucangelo
A. Pesenti
W.A. Zin (Eds)

Basics of Respiratory Mechanics and Artificial Ventilation

Series edited by
Antonino Gullo

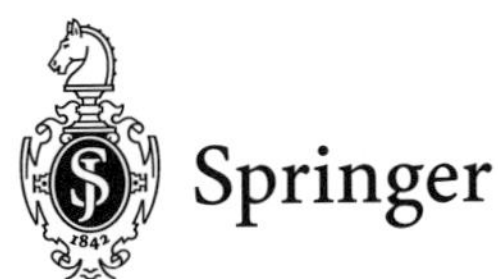

Springer

J. MILIC-EMILI, MD
Meakins-Christie Laboratories
McGill University, Montreal, Canada

U. LUCANGELO, MD
Department of Anaesthesia, Intensive Care and Pain Therapy,
University of Trieste, Cattinara Hospital, Italy

A. PESENTI, MD
Department of Anaesthesia and Intensive Care
New S. Gerardo Hospital, Monza, Italy

W.A. ZIN, MD
Department of Biophysic "Carlos Chagas Filho"
Laboratory of Respiratory Physiology
Federal University of Rio de Janeiro, Brazil

Series of Topics in Anaesthesia and Critical Care edited by
A. GULLO, MD
Department of Anaesthesia, Intensive Care and Pain Therapy
University of Trieste, Cattinara Hospital, Italy

ISBN 88-470-0046-7

Cover design: Simona Colombo, Milan
Typesetting: Graphostudio, Milan
Printing and binding: Staroffset, Cernusco S/N (Milan)

SPIN 10697841

Foreword

Management of the intensive care patient afflicted by respiratory dysfunction requires knowledge of the pathophysiological basis for altered respiratory functions. The etiology and therapy of pulmonary diseases, such as acute respiratory distress syndrome (ARDS) and chronic obstructive pulmonary disease (COPD), are highly complex. While physiologists and pathophysiologists work prevalently with theoretical models, clinicians employ sophisticated ventilation support technologies in the attempt to understand the pathophysiological mechanisms of these pulmonary diseases which can present with varying grades of severity from mild to "poumon dépassé". Despite the availability of advanced technologies, it is a common practice to personalize the treatment protocol according to the patient's "physiologic" structure. Generally speaking, artificial ventilation cannot fully replace the patient's own physiology, and in certain situations can actually cause severe lung damage (i.e. barotrauma).

Given the complexity and difficulties of treating respiratory diseases, a strong cooperation between clinicians and physiologists is of fundamental importance. Such interdisciplinary approaches are imperative in the study of the resistive and viscoelastic properties of the respiratory system, and in the study of the diaphragm, especially regarding the evaluations of muscle fatigue and work breathing in both physiological conditions secondary to respiratory or systemic illness.

Beside monitoring of patients sustained by artificial respiration requires evaluation of the intrinsic positive end-expiratory pressure (PEEP) and of the pulmonary gas exchange. Variations in respiratory mechanics during anaesthesia represent an important study model. Clinical guidelines are available to assist in the implementation of artificial ventilation or alternative strategies such as high frequency ventilation. Controversial techniques such as servocontrolled mechanical ventilation and proportional assisted ventilation (PAV) supposedly adapt to the actual physiological needs of the patient based upon sophisticated monitoring of respiratory parameters. These technologies represent the future directions for clinical research and applications in the treatment of patients with respiratory dysfunction due to ARDS or COPD.

November 1998 *Antonino Gullo, MD*

Contents

Contributors

Andreose U.
Department of Anaesthesia, Conselve Rehabilitation Centre, Padova, Italy.

Brandolese R.
Department of Anaesthesia, Conselve Rehabilitation Centre, Padova, Italy.

Braschi A.
Department of Anaesthesia and Intensive Care, Laboratory of Biomedical Techniques, IRCCS S. Matteo Hospital, Pavia, Italy.

Brazzi L.
Department of Anaesthesia and Reanimation, University of Milan, IRCCS Maggiore Hospital, Milan, Italy.

Cereda M.
Department of Anaesthesia and Intensive Care, New S. Gerardo Hospital, Monza, Italy.

D'Angelo E.
Department of Human Physiology I, University of Milan, Milan, Italy.

Galbusera C.
Department of Anaesthesia and Intensive Care, Laboratory of Biomedical Techniques, IRCCS S. Matteo Hospital, Pavia, Italy.

Gattinoni L.
Department of Anaesthesia and Reanimation, University of Milan, IRCCS Maggiore Hospital, Milan, Italy.

Gomes R.F.M.
Department of Biophysics "Carlos Chagas Filho", Laboratory of Respiratory Physiology, Federal University of Rio de Janeiro, Rio de Janeiro, Brazil

Hantos Z.
Department of Medical Informatics and Engineering, Albert Szent-Györgyi Medical University, Szeged, Hungary

Hedenstierna G.
Department of Medical Sciences, Clinical Physiology, University Hospital, Uppsala, Sweden.

Iotti G.
Department of Anaesthesia and Intensive Care, Laboratory of Biomedical Techniques, IRCCS S. Matteo Hospital, Pavia, Italy.

Lucangelo U.
Department of Anaesthesia, Intensive Care and Pain Therapy, University of Trieste, Cattinara Hospital, Italy.

Ludwig M.S.
Meakins-Christie Laboratories, Royal Victoria Hospital, McGill University, Montreal, Quebec, Canada.

Milic-Emili J.
Meakins-Christie Laboratories, McGill University, Montreal, Canada.

Olivei M.C.
Department of Anaesthesia and Intensive Care, Laboratory of Biomedical Techniques, IRCCS S. Matteo Hospital, Pavia, Italy.

Pelosi P.
Department of Anaesthesia and Reanimation, University of Milan, IRCCS Maggiore Hospital, Milan, Italy.

Pesenti A.
Department of Anaesthesia and Intensive Care, New S. Gerardo Hospital, Monza, Italy.

Peslin R.
Respiratory Physiopathology, Unit 14, National Institute of Health and Medical Research, Vandoeuvre-les-Nancy, France.

Pride N.B.
Thoracic Medicine, NHLI, Imperial College School of Medicine, London, UK.

Resta M.
Department of Anaesthesia and Reanimation, University of Milan, IRCCS Maggiore Hospital, Milan, Italy

Roca J.
Department of Pneumology, Clinical Hospital of Barcelona, Villanoel, Barcelona, Spain.

Rocca E.
Department of Human Physiology I, University of Milan, Milan, Italy.

Romero P.V.
Experimental Pneumology Unit, Pneumology Service, Ciutat Sanitaria i Universitaria de Bellvitge, L'Hospitalet de Llobregat, Barcelona, Spain.

Rossi A.
Department of Respiratory Pathophysiology, Maggiore Hospital, Borgo Trento (VR), Italy.

Zanierato M.
Department of Anaesthesia and Intensive Care, Laboratory of Biomedical Techniques, IRCCS S. Matteo Hospital, Pavia, Italy.

Zin W.A.
Department of Biophysics "Carlos Chagas Filho", Laboratory of Respiratory Physiology, Federal University of Rio de Janeiro, Rio de Janeiro, Brazil.

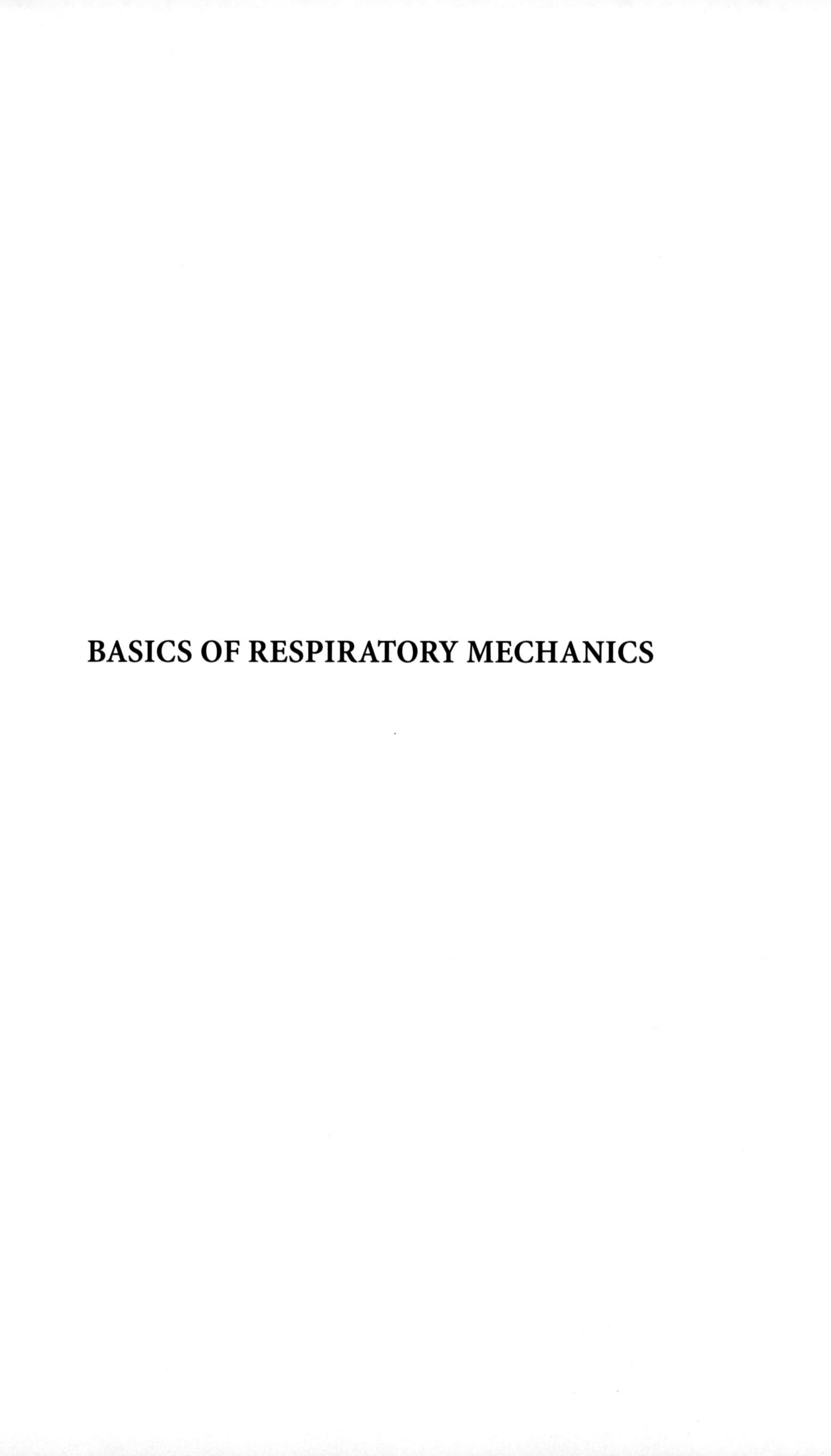

BASICS OF RESPIRATORY MECHANICS

Chapter 1

Principles of measurement of respiratory mechanics

W.A. Zin

Facing a patient presenting respiratory functional impairment, the physician is left with the task of running tests to determine whether there is a mechanical component to the illness. At this point he must be qualified to extract the desired information from a given measurement. Although not difficult to accomplish, the precise interpretation of the results demands awareness of exact methodological and theoretical concepts.

Fundamental aspects of measurements

Frequency response of measuring instruments

Dynamic characteristics of measuring instruments are usefully described by their frequency responses [1]. Consider a signal represented by a square wave. An overdamped recording device smoothes out the sharp corners and delays the rise and fall of the input wave, providing a somewhat rounded output signal. On the other hand, for the same input signal an underdamped apparatus generates an output wave that oscillates after each transient [2]. Of course, the ideally damped apparatus would provide a true "copy" of the original curve.

Compliance and resistance of the experimental circuit

Letting alone the frequency response aspect, compliance and resistance of the experimental circuit may distort the measurements to a great extent. For instance, a very compliant piece of rubber tubing added in series to the airways of a mechanically ventilated patient will reduce the amount of gas injected into the lungs by retaining part of the tidal volume delivered by the ventilator. The resistance of the circuit (Req) will add to the patient's, thus leading to an overestimation of the latter, if not taken into account. Furthermore, if turbulence occurs, the relationship between equipment resistive pressure (Pres, eq) and flow ($\dot{V}$):

$$\text{Pres,eq} = \text{Req} \cdot \dot{V} \tag{1}$$

will be adequately expressed either by Rohrer's equation:

$$\text{Pres,eq} = K_1 \cdot \dot{V} + K_2 \cdot \dot{V}^2 \tag{2}$$

where K_1 and K_2 are constants, or by the power function:

$$\text{Pres, eq} = a \cdot \dot{V}^b \tag{3}$$

where a represents the pressure when $\dot{V}$ equals 1 l/s, and ^{b} is a dimensionless index of the shape of the curve.

Tracheal tubes

Within the physiological range of airflows, tracheal tubes always add a flow-dependent resistance (Eqs. 2 and 3) to the system [3]. As a consequence, for the same driving pressure, the tidal volume achieved will be smaller than in the non-intubated condition. Naturally, the lost volume increases with diminishing tube diameter [4].

Sampling frequency

Analogue information is data that correspond to a physical measurement, which is usually provided electronically as a change in either voltage or current. With the aid of an analogue-to-digital converter the continuous electrical signal can be converted to discrete digital format in order to be processed by a computer. Ideally, the interval between each sample should be as minute as possible so that the digital data points would closely approximate the analogue signal. The faster the changes in the input signal, the higher the sampling frequency should be [5].

Oesophageal pressure measurement

Pleural pressure measurement is essential for splitting respiratory system mechanical properties into their pulmonary and chest wall components. Because of the risks involved in direct pleural pressure determination, oesophageal pressure (Poes) has been registered instead. The most widely used method for recording Poes employs air-containing latex balloons sealed over catheters which in turn transmit balloon pressures to transducers. Although this approach was proposed more than a century ago by Luciani, its precise standardization occurred not earlier than 1964 [6]. Poes measurements should be validated in all instances. For such purposes, static Valsalva and Mueller manoeuvres or the dynamic "occlusion test" can be used [7].

A comprehensive description of oesophageal pressure measurement has recently been published [8].

Theories and interpretation of respiratory mechanics

Parameters

The respiratory system is composed of a multitude of structural elements both at microscopic as well as at macroscopic levels. For practical purposes the system ought to be represented by simple models able to describe as accurately as possible its mechanical behaviour.

Linear one-compartment model

The simplest model of the respiratory system incorporates two lumped elements [9]: one single compartment of constant elastance (E) served by a pathway of constant resistance (R), as portrayed in Figure 1a. It is based on the assumption that the mechanical properties of the respiratory system are independent of V and $\dot{V}$, and that inertial forces are negligible. The latter assertion is probably acceptable for breathing frequencies smaller than 2 Hz [10].

Figure 1b also illustrates that from the mechanical standpoint the deformation of the respiratory system (i.e. volume change V) results from the movement of a Voigt body (one dashpot R and a spring E, arranged in parallel, constitute a Voigt body). One should always bear in mind that dashpots dissipate energy as heat, whereas springs store potential energy which will be returned to the system.

The linear one-comparment model can be represented by a single first order differential equation:

$$P(t) = EV(t) + R\dot{V}(t) \tag{4}$$

where P is the driving pressure.

The values of E and R can be determined during continuous breathing by fitting Eq. 4 to P, V and $\dot{V}$ using multiple linear regression [11, 12] or by the electrical subtraction method [13]. Alternatively, E and R can be obtained during relaxed expiration [14].

However, the linear one-compartment model cannot describe a few mechanical phenomena presented by the respiratory system, such as: 1) the slow decay in pressure observed after sustained airway occlusion at end inspiration [15-17]; 2) the frequency dependence of elastance and resistance [12, 18-20]; and 3)

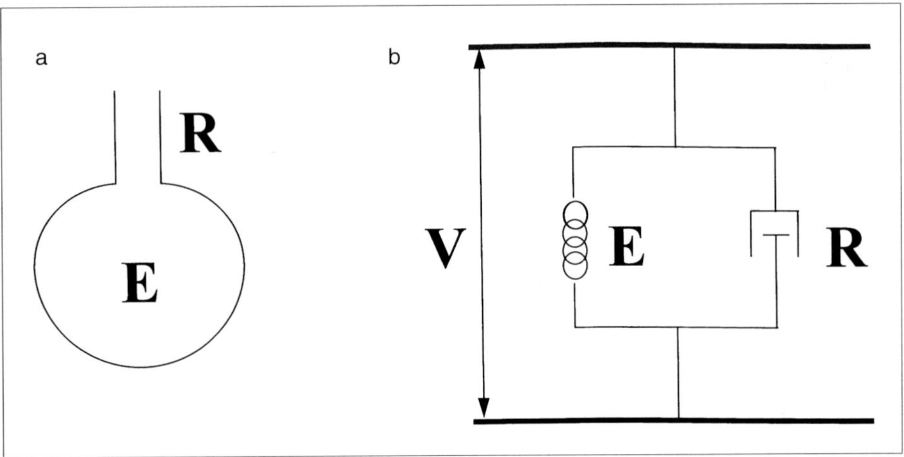

Fig. 1a,b. Linear one-compartment model. (a) Anatomic representation; (b) rheological representation by a Voigt body. *R*, respiratory system resistance; *E*, respiratory system elastance; *V*, changes in lung volume

the quasi-static pressure-volume hysteresis in isolated lungs. Therefore, in order to better describe the respiratory system mechanical profile more complex approaches are required.

Linear viscoelastic model

The linear viscoelastic model is a rheological two-compartment model that explains frequency dependence of respiratory parameters and stress adaptation. In fact, this approach extends the one-compartment model by incorporating a viscoelastic element in parallel to the latter [21, 22].

Furthermore, it does not consider the existence of uneven distribution of ventilation. Indeed, supporting this postulate no inhomogeneous gas distribution could be detected under normal conditions [23, 24].

The viscoelastic model of the respiratory system considers that stress adaptation originates from lung or chest wall tissues and surfactant (E_2 and R_2, Fig. 2a). The deformation of the Maxwell body (E_2, R_2) shown in Figure 2b is the sum of the individual distortions of its elastic and resistive components, and its slow time constant (τ_2=R_2/E_2) might account for tissue stress adaptation. Currently, the precise structural basis of the viscoelastic parameters in Figure 2 is poorly understood.

As a result of viscoelastic pressure dissipations, the effective resistance of the respiratory system (and its pulmonary and chest wall components as well) is higher at low respiratory frequencies *f* (or long inspiratory durations) than during elevated *f* [25-28]. Indeed, at high *f* spring E_2 (Fig. 2) will oscillate so quickly that no time will be allowed for the dissipation of its energy through dashpot R_2, Conversely, at low *f* R_2 will be given time to move and dissipate the applied energy or the energy stored in E_2. Therefore, it can be easily foreseen that according to the values of E_2, R_2, and *f* the respiratory system will display a broad range of lumped elastance and resistance values, as originally proposed by Mount [21].

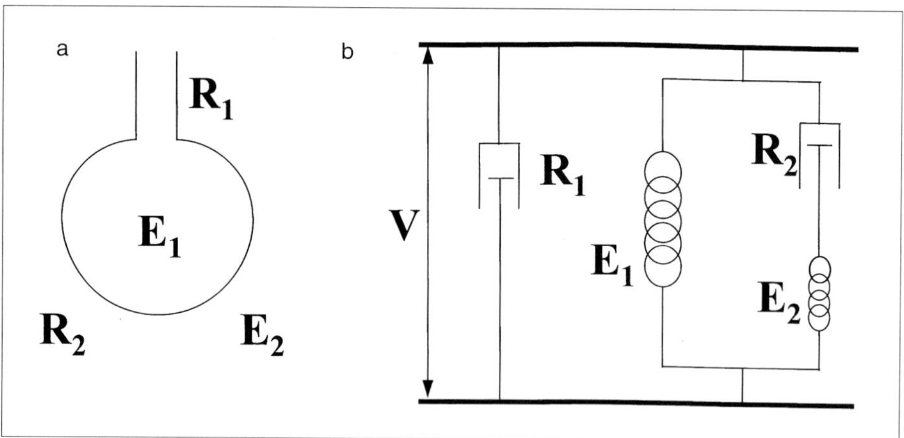

Fig. 2a,b. Linear viscoelastic compartment model. (a) Anatomic representation; (b) rheological representation by a dashpot. (R_1) associated in parallel with a spring (E_1) coupled in parallel with a Maxwell body (R_2, E_2)

Other models

Time dependency of elastance and resistance can also be caused by time constant inequalities within the system. Thus, parallel [28] and serial [29] two-compartment gas redistribution models have been proposed, together with multi-compartment models [30-32]. The existence of various time constants is implicit in the latter group.

The plastoelastic model could account for the quasi-static pressure-volume hysteresis in isolated lungs. However, it is rarely used in vivo under small volume excursions because its parameters have been found difficult to be mechanically interpreted [33, 34].

Finally, nonlinear viscoelasticity is also capable of accounting for the amplitude and frequency-dependent properties of lung tissue [35], and of generating a response similar to that of the plastoelastic model [32].

References

1. Fry DL (1960) Physiologic recording by modern instruments with particular reference to pressure recording. Physiol Rev 40:753-788
2. Butler JP, Leith DE, Jackson AC (1986) Principles of measurement: applications to pressure, volume, and flow. In: Macklem PT, Mead J (eds) The respiratory system. Mechanics of breathing. Handbook of physiology. Vol III. American Physiological Society, Bethesda, pp 15-33
3. Behrakis PK, Higgs BD, Baydur A et al (1983) Respiratory mechanics during halothane anesthesia and anesthesia-paralysis in humans. J Appl Physiol 55:1085-1092
4. Rocco PRM, Zin WA (1985) Modelling the mechanical effects of tracheal tubes on normal subjects. Eur Respir J 8:121-126
5. Fessler HE, Shade D (1997) Measurement of vascular pressure. In: Tobin MJ (ed) Principles and practice of intensive care monitoring. McGraw-Hill, New York, pp 91-106
6. Milic-Emili J, Mead J, Turner JM et al (1964) Improved technique for estimating pleural pressure from esophageal balloons. J Appl Physiol 19:207-211
7. Baydur A, Behrakis PK, Zin WA et al (1982) A simple method for assessing the validity of the esophageal balloon technique. Am Rev Respir Dis 126:788-791
8. Zin WA, Milic-Emili J (1998) Esophageal pressure measurement. In: Tobin MJ (ed) Principles and practice of intensive care monitoring. McGraw-Hill, New York, pp 545-552
9. Otis AB, Fenn WO, Rahn H (1950) The mechanics of breathing in man. J Appl Physiol 2:592-607
10. Sharp JT, Henry JP, Sweany SK et al (1964) Total respiratory inertance and its gas and tissue components in normal and obese men. J Appl Physiol 43:503-509
11. Hantos Z, Daróczy B, Klebniczki J et al (1982) Parameter estimation of transpulmonary mechanics by a nonlinear inertive model. J Appl Physiol 52:955-963
12. Bates JHT, Shardonofsky F, Stewart DE (1989) The low-frequency dependence of respiratory system resistance and elastance in normal dogs. Respir Physiol 78:369-382
13. Mead J, Whittenberger JL (1953) Physical properties of human lungs measured during spontaneous respiration. J Appl Physiol 5:779-796
14. Zin WA, Pengelly LD, Milic-Emili J (1982) Single-breath method for measurement of respiratory mechanics in anesthetized animals. J Appl Physiol 52:1266-1271

15. Hughes R, May AJ, Widdicombe JG (1959) Stress relaxation in rabbits' lungs. J Physiol 146:85-97
16. Don HF, Robson JG (1965) The mechanics of the respiratory system during anesthesia. Anesthesiol 26:168-178
17. Bates JHT, Rossi A, Milic-Emili J (1985) Analysis of the behavior of the respiratory system with constant inspiratory flow. J Appl Physiol 58:1840-1848
18. Barnas GM, Yoshino K, Loring SH et al (1987) Impedance and relative displacements of relaxed chest wall up to 4 Hz. J Appl Physiol 62:71-81
19. Brusasco V, Warner DO, Beck KC et al (1989) Partitioning of pulmonary resistance in dogs: effects of tidal volume and frequency. J Appl Physiol 66:1190-1197
20. Hantos Z, Daróczy B, Suki B et al (1986) Forced oscillatory impedance of the respiratory system at low frequencies. J Appl Physiol 60:123-132
21. Mount LE (1955) The ventilation flow-resistance and compliance of rat lungs. J Physiol 127:157-167
22. Bates JHT, Brown KA, Kochi T (1989) Respiratory mechanics in the normal dog determined by expiratory flow interruption. J Appl Physiol 67:2276-2285
23. Bates JHT, Ludwig MS, Sly PD et al (1988) Interrupter resistance elucidated by alveolar pressure measurements in open-chest normal dogs. J Appl Physiol 65:408-414
24. Saldiva PHN, Zin WA, Santos RLB et al (1992) Alveolar pressure measurement in open-chest rats. J Appl Physiol 72:302-306
25. Kochi T, Okubo S, Zin WA et al (1988) Flow and volume dependence of pulmonary mechanics in anesthetized cats. J Appl Physiol 64:441-450
26. Similovski T, Levy P, Corbeil C et al (1989) Viscoelastic behavior of lung and chest wall in dogs determined by flow interruption. J Appl Physiol 67:2219-2229
27. D'Angelo E, Calderini E, Torri G et al (1989) Respiratory mechanics in anesthetized-paralyzed humans: effects of flow, volume, and time. J Appl Physiol 67:2556-2564
28. Otis AB, McKerrow CB, Bartlett RA et al (1956) Mechanical factors in distribution of pulmonary ventilation. J Appl Physiol 8:427-443
29. Mead J (1969) Contribution of compliance of airways to frequency-dependent behavior of lung. J Appl Physiol 26:670-673
30. Hildebrandt J (1969) Dynamic properties of air-filled excised cat lung determined by liquid plethysmography. J Appl Physiol 27:246-250
31. Hildebrandt J (1969) Comparison of mathematical models for cat lung and viscoelastic balloon derived by Laplace transform methods from pressure-volume data. Bull Math Biophys 31:651-667
32. Hildebrandt J (1970) Pressure-volume data of cat lung interpreted by a plastoelastic, linear viscoelastic model. J Appl Physiol 28:365-372
33. Navajas D, Farré R, Cannet J et al (1990) Respiratory input impedance in anesthetized paralyzed patients. J Appl Physiol 69:1372-1379
34. Shardonofsky F, Sato J, Bates JHT (1990) Quasi-static pressure-volume hysteresis in the canine respiratory system in vivo. J Appl Physiol 68:2230-2236
35. Suki B, Bates JHT (1991) A nonlinear viscoelastic model of lung tissue mechanics. J Appl Physiol 71:826-833

Chapter 2

Statics of the respiratory system

E. D'ANGELO

The statics of the respiratory system and its component parts are studied by determining and analyzing the corresponding volume-pressure relationships. These relationships are usually represented as single lines, implying that: a) static pressures depend on volume alone; and b) pressure across any respiratory structure can be dealt with as a single value. Neither of these assumptions is, however, correct. In fact, static pressures differ depending on the volume and time history of the respiratory system. For example, static curves obtained as volume is changed in progressive steps from residual volume to total lung capacity and back again are loops, called "hysteresis loops". Static or quasi-static (i.e. long-term) elastic hysteresis is a common phenomenon exhibited by the various tissues of the body [1]. In the respiratory system it is attributed to both viscoelasticity, such as stress adaptation, i.e. a rate-dependent phenomenon, and plasticity, i.e. a rate-independent phenomenon. This relates partly to the definition chosen to qualify static conditions, and partly to the technical difficulties encountered in order to satisfy that definition, particularly in in vivo studies. Indeed only plasticity should be held responsible for hysteresis which, in a mechanical analogue, would occur only in the presence of dry friction. There is no information concerning pressure related to tissue plasticity in humans; however, it has been suggested that this pressure component should be very small in the tidal volume range [2]. Moreover the static pressure across the lung and chest wall varies at different sites because of the effects of gravity on the lung and the chest wall and because of the different shapes of these two structures [3]. It is therefore important to keep in mind that the balance between the lung and the chest wall under physiological conditions results from a wide distribution of pressures. The static pressure across the respiratory system may become nonuniform under conditions involving airway closure. Nevertheless, for analytical purposes, the static volume-pressure relationships will be hereafter considered as single functions. Moreover, in the following description of the mechanical properties of the respiratory system under static conditions reference will be made to normal subjects only.

Respiratory system

During relaxation of the respiratory muscles the net pressure developed by the respiratory system under static conditions (Prs) results from the forces exerted by its elastic elements and equals the difference between alveolar pressure (PA) with airway openings closed, or mouth pressure with the glottis open, and body surface pressure (Pbs). Conversely, Prs indicates the pressure that the respiratory muscles must exert to maintain that lung volume with open airways. This applies, however, only if the shape of the respiratory system is the same whether the respiratory muscles are active or not. For a given volume, the elastic energy, and hence the elastic pressure, is minimum for the configuration occurring during relaxation, and is increased whenever that configuration is changed.

The volume-pressure curve of the relaxed respiratory system is sigmoidal. In the middle volume range, the relation is almost linear with a slope, the compliance of the respiratory system (Crs), that is 2% of the vital capacity (VC) per 1 cm H_2O, or 0.1 l/cm H_2O. Above 85% and below 15% VC, Crs rapidly decreases. The volume at PA=0 is the resting volume of the respiratory system: during quiet breathing it usually corresponds to the lung volume at the end of a spontaneous expiration, which is the definition of the functional residual capacity (FRC). Measurements of lung volume and mouth pressure do not pose any major technical problem; however, voluntary relaxation is difficult to obtain. The assumption by Heaf and Prime [4] that muscles are relaxed at the end of expiration during spontaneous breathing at atmospheric and moderately increased airway pressures may not be valid. Indeed, recent evidence suggests that tonic respiratory muscle activity is often present in awake subjects [5]. Certainly the volume-pressure relation obtained in paralyzed subject reflects only the elastic forces that develop in the respiratory system. Its comparison with that in the awake subject requires, however, some caution (see below).

Lung and chest wall

Because the chest wall (W) and lung (L) are placed pneumatically in series, the volume changes of the chest wall (ΔVW) and the lung (ΔVL) should be the same (except for shifts of blood) and equal to that of the respiratory system (ΔVrs), whereas, under static conditions during relaxation, the algebraic sum of the pressure exerted by each part equals the pressure of the respiratory system (Prs=PA=PW+PL). It follows that the reciprocal of the compliance of the respiratory system equals the sum of the reciprocals of lung and chest wall compliance. Because Pw indicates pressures exerted by the relaxed chest wall, it follows that when the respiratory muscles contract at fixed lung volumes PA= PW+PL+Pmus.

The pressure exerted by the lung is the difference between alveolar and pleural surface pressure PL=PA-Ppl; that exerted by the chest wall is the difference between pleural surface and body surface pressure PW=Ppl-Pbs. Thus, during relaxation PW=Ppl; when the muscles contract at constant lung volume Ppl=PW+Pmus and Ppl=PA-PL; when the subject actively holds a given lung volume with airway and glottis open Ppl=-PL. In man, Ppl is usually obtained from esophageal pressure measurements; the interpretation of these measures requires, however, some caution [6, 7].

The volume-pressure relations of the lung and chest wall are curvilinear: the former increases its curvature with increasing lung volume, the opposite being true for the latter. The fall in Crs at high lung volumes is therefore due to the decrease of C_L, that at low lung volume to the decrease of C_W. In the tidal volume range the volume-pressure relations of both the lung and chest wall are nearly linear and C_L and C_W are about the same, amounting to 4% VC per 1 cm H_2O, or 0.2 l/cm H_2O. In normal young subjects the resting volume of the lung (P_L=Pbs) is close to RV and the lung recoils inward over nearly all the VC. Hence, the resting volume of the respiratory system is reached when the inward recoil of the lung is balanced by the outward recoil of the chest wall, i.e. $P_W+P_L=0$. This volume depends on posture (see below).

Rib cage, diaphragm and abdominal wall

Lung volume changes occur because of the displacement of the rib cage facing the lung (rc,L) and of the diaphragm-abdomen (di-ab). From this viewpoint, these two structures may be considered to operate in parallel: hence $P_W=P_{rc,L}$ $=P_{di\text{-}ab}$ and $\Delta V_W=\Delta V_{rc,L}+\Delta V_{di\text{-}ab}$. These volumes were obtained by Wade [8] from measurements of the changes in rib cage circumference and of the displacements of the dome of the diaphragm relative to its insertion on the rib cage over the inspiratory capacity and the expiratory reserve volume in the supine and standing posture. Agostoni et al. [9] used a geometric approach to estimate roughly the volume contributed by the change in the dimensions of the pulmonary part of the rib cage as a function of lung volume in the standing, sitting and supine postures, the volume contributed by the diaphragm displacement being obtained by subtraction from the lung volume change. Both approaches invoke questionable assumptions; because the results were similar while the assumptions differed, it seems possible that the errors involved are not marked. These results indicate that:

a. the volume contributed by the diaphragm-abdomen displacement is greater than that contributed by the displacement of the pulmonary part of the rib cage;
b. the volume contributed by the pulmonary part of the rib cage at FRC is about the same in supine and erect postures, changes in FRC with posture being therefore essentially due to displacement of the diaphragm-abdomen (see below);
c. at any given lung volume, that contributed by the pulmonary part of the rib cage is larger in the supine than in the erect posture, indicating a volume displacement from the rib cage to the diaphragm-abdomen;
d. the compliance of the pulmonary part of the rib cage and of the diaphragm-abdomen decreases progressively below FRC, whilst $C_{rc,L}$ increases more than $C_{di\text{-}ab}$ with increasing the lung volume above FRC;
e. the volume-pressure curve of the pulmonary part of the rib cage does not change its shape with posture, whereas that of the diaphragm-abdomen

becomes markedly more concave in the erect posture. This latter effect is probably because of postural tonus of the abdominal muscles [10] and greater distortion of the abdominal wall due to the greater top-to-bottom difference of abdominal pressure in the erect than supine posture.

Konno and Mead [11] showed that partitioning of chest wall volume could be made avoiding any assumption when the two parallel pathways were represented by the rib cage (rc) and the abdominal wall (ab,w): hence $\Delta Vw=\Delta Vrc+\Delta Vab,w$. This approach is similar to those of Wade and Agostoni since it also implies a system with two moving parts operating in parallel. Whilst the pressure across the rib cage equals Pw in both models, that across the other pathway is abdominal pressure (Pab) and Pw in the former and latter approach, respectively. The data of Konno and Mead [11, 12] confirm, however, some conclusions reached with the approach of Agostoni et al. [9]: a) the volume of the rib cage or of its pulmonary part at FRC is nearly the same in all postures in spite of different lung volumes; b) the relationship between the volume contributed by the two parts over the VC shifts rightwards on turning from the supine to the erect posture. Because of the lifting and expansion of the rib cage, ΔVdi-ab (Wade and Agostoni approach) is shared partly by rib cage and partly by abdominal wall displacement (Konno and Mead approach); a comparison between the volume partitioning obtained by the two approaches suggests that the fraction of the volume displaced by the diaphragm not shared by the abominal wall is roughly 0.5 over of the VC.

Mead [13] redefined the pressure acting on the rib cage taking into account that: a) this structure is facing both the lungs and the abdominal contents, being affected partly by Ppl and partly by Pab; b) the diaphragm operates in series with the rib cage as a pressure generator tending in general to move the ribs out and up. Hence, in the Mead's model the pressure exerted by the passive rib cage should be given by $Prc=(1-f)Pw+fPab-kPdi$, where f is the fraction of the internal surface of the rib cage not facing the lung and k, which includes the pertinent geometrical features, is the fraction of transdiaphragmatic pressure acting on the rib cage. Moreover, considering that Pdi=Pw-Pab and setting $K=f+k$, $Prc=(1-K)Pw+KPab$. When Pdi=0 and, hence, Pw=Pab, as in the erect posture at or above FRC, Prc=Pw, which was the primitive definition of the pressure developed by the passive rib cage. On the other hand, when Pdi≠0 as in the erect posture below FRC or in the supine posture over most of the VC, Prc should be higher than Pw and closer to Pab the smaller the lung volume, since f increases with decreasing lung volume. Indeed, it appears that Prc=Pab when $K=1$, as it could be the case near RV owing to the cranial position of the diaphragm. Unfortunately, the values of K and their dependence on lung volume are not known with precision, particularly in the supine posture. However, assuming that K changes linearly from 0.9 to 0.2 between RV and TLC, both in the standing and supine postures, it appears that with decreasing the lung volume no progressive decrease of rib cage compliance occurs in Mead's model, implying that the increasing stiffness of the chest wall below FRC should not be due to both the rib cage and the diaphragm, but essentially to the latter, particularly in the supine posture. On the other hand, like in the previous models, there is a rightwards displacement of the curve on turning from the erect to the supine posture.

Other models of the chest wall [14-16] have been proposed in addition to those mentioned above; yet it can be shown [16] that in all of them the same force balance equations apply for the rib cage and the abdominal compartment, respectively. Indeed common to all models are the assumptions that: a) the rib cage and the abdominal wall can move independently, i.e. ΔVab,w and ΔVrc are unique functions of Pab and ΔPrc, respectively, thus allowing the compliance to be obtained as the ratio between the changes in compartmental volume and pressure; b) the relaxed rib cage and abdomen move with one degree of freedom. While some results suggest that coupling between the rib cage and the abdominal wall can be ignored [17, 18], it is questionable whether forces acting on small areas of the rib cage surface, like diaphragmatic tension, should be considered to affect the rib cage motion (and hence the apparent volume-pressure relationship of the relaxed rib cage) in the same way as those acting on relatively large fractions of the rib cage surface, like (1-*f*)Pw or *f*Pab. In fact, distortion of the relaxed rib cage should be expected to take place whenever Pw≠Pab and hence Pdi≠0, as in the supine posture or in the erect posture below FRC. Indeed, rib cage distortion occurs with contraction of the diaphragm in tetraplegic subjects [19], with electrophrenic stimulation both in animals [20] and men [21], and also in normal subjects during voluntary and involuntary respiratory acts [22-24]. In the dog, the relationships between indices of pulmonary rib cage motion and Pw [20, 25] as well as between indices of abdominal wall motion and Pab [25], obtained during isolated diaphragm contractions, fall close to their respective relaxation lines, thus indicating high rib cage flexibility [26] and, hence, negligible mechanical coupling between pulmonary and abdominal rib cage compartments. If this were also the case for the human rib cage, volume-pressure relationships for the pulmonary and abdominal rib cage compartment could be readily obtained once satisfactory criteria for partitioning ΔVrc into ΔVrc,L and ΔVrc,ab are established. While the pattern of motion of the relaxed rib cage during immersion in seated subjects [27] suggests that rib cage flexibility is fairly large also in humans, Ward et al. [28] concluded that in men coupling between pulmonary and abdominal rib cage should ensure transmission to the pulmonary rib cage of a substantial fraction of the force acting on the abdominal rib cage. The authors, however, pointed out the several theoretical and technical limitations of their approach.

Effects of aging

The static behavior of the respiratory system, lungs and chest wall, changes throughout life. From young adulthood on, the vital capacity decreases almost linearly with age, the decrease being due to an increase of the residual volume [29-31], as total lung capacity remains essentially unchanged [30, 31]. The recoil of the lung decreases with age particularly at high lung volume, while its resting volume increases substantially [30-33]. On the other hand, the recoil of the chest wall increases and its resting volume decreases with age: hence, the volume-pressure curve of the chest wall becomes less steep, pivoting around a point at about mid-lung volume, where its recoil remains the same [31]. The increase of FRC with age is therefore mainly due to the decrease of lung recoil and is less marked than that of RV. Since in the mid-volume range the compliance of the lung increases while that of the chest wall decreases, the compliance of the respiratory sytem becomes only slightly smaller with age [31].

Effects of posture

The volume-pressure curve of the lung does not change appreciably with posture while that of the chest wall does, mainly because of the effect of gravity on the abdomen. Indeed, when the effect of gravity in the erect posture is simulated in the supine subject by applying negative pressure around the lower abdomen, the volume pressure curve of the respiratory system becomes almost equal to that in the sitting posture [19].

The relaxed abdomen can be likened to a container filled with liquid, in which part of the wall is distensible [34]. The level at which the abdominal pressure is equal to ambient pressure, the "zero level", depends on the equilibrium among the elastic forces of the abdominal wall, diaphragm, rib cage, lung and the gravitational force of the abdominal contents. The position of the zero level with respect to the lung height indicates whether gravity exerts inflationary or deflationary effects on the respiratory system. At the end of a normal expiration, i.e. at the resting volume of the respiratory system, the zero level of Pab is about 3-4 cm beneath the diaphragmatic dome in the erect posture, close to the ventral and dorsal wall of the abdomen in the supine and prone postures, respectively, midway between the two sides in the lateral decubitus [34]. As a consequence, the resting volume of both the chest wall and respiratory system decreases from the erect, to the lateral, prone and supine postures.

The zero level shifts, however, with lung volume and to a different degree in the upright and horizontal postures. The hydrostatic pressure applied on the abdominal surface of the diaphragm is about -20 cm H_2O at RV, nil at about 55% VC (the resting volume of the chest wall), while at higher volumes it is above atmospheric. In the supine position, like in the other horizontal postures, changes in Pab over the VC are nearly half those occurring in the upright posture, and shift of the zero level with lung volume is accordingly smaller, while ΔVab,w is larger in the erect posture. The reduced compliance of the abdominal wall in the latter posture should in turn be attributed to the larger average hydrostatic pressure applied to the abdominal wall. In the lateral posture the action of gravity on the abdomen-diaphragm is expiratory in the lower part and inspiratory in the upper part. Because the two lungs have different sizes, the volume-pressure relationships should therefore differ somewhat between the right and left lateral decubitus. Indeed when anesthetized paralyzed subjects were moved from the supine to the left or right lateral posture, FRC increased by 0.79 liters (15% VC) and 0.93 liters (17% VC), respectively [35].

Effects of anesthesia and paralysis

The most frequently reported effect of general anesthesia in normal supine subjects is a reduction of FRC: according to Rehder and Marsh [36] this decrease is given by ΔFRC=10.18-0.23 (age)-46.7 (weight/height), where ΔFRC is expressed as percent FRC while awake, and age, weight and height are in years, kilograms, and centimeters, respectively. Such a decrease also occurs in the prone posture, but not in the sitting position [37] and, probably, in the lateral decubitus too [35]. Several mechanisms have been invoked to explain the reduction of FRC in recumbent human subjects; the marked intersubject variability of this reduction suggests that this decrease depends on several factors, none of which consistently prevails.

Tonic activity of both inspiratory rib cage muscles and diaphragm has been suggested to augment the chest wall recoil in awake subjects [38-40]. However, this tone is minimal in the supine position when ΔFRC is larger, and larger in the erect posture when ΔFRC is absent; its presence in the diaphragm is controversial [39, 40]. Perhaps, tonic activity affects only the shape of the diaphragm. Indeed recent studies have documented changes in shape of the diaphragm not followed by any net cephalad displacement with induction of anesthesia and paralysis [40-42]. Expiratory activity that appears in abdominal muscles with anesthesia [43] does not seem a main factor in lowering FRC, since the latter does not further decrease with muscular paralysis [44]. The shape of the chest wall also changes with anesthesia: the anteroposterior diameters of both the rib cage and abdomen decrease, whilst the transverse diameters increase [45]. On the other hand, it is unclear whether the volume of the thoracic cavity is effectively reduced because of these dimensional changes [40, 46, 47].

Increases in intrathoracic blood volume up to 0.3 l have been reported to occur with anesthesia-paralysis [40, 46]. Although these changes could be large enough to account for the reported reductions in FRC, the lack of an established intrasubject relationship with the fall of FRC prevents any firm conclusion concerning their impact.

The decrease of FRC in supine or prone anesthetized subjects reflects the increase in the elastic recoil of the respiratory system that takes place at all lung volumes; this increase is independent of the depth of anesthesia and not affected by muscular paralysis [48], does not change with time and is not prevented by large, repeated lung inflations [44]. As for FRC changes, also those in the mechanical properties of the respiratory system presents large intersubject variability, suggesting that the same factors could be responsible for both changes. In this connection, the entity of the resting volume with anesthesia might be critical: indeed, no change in respiratory system compliance occurs in sitting subjects both with anesthesia, when FRC does not fall [37], and with submaximal muscular paralysis, when FRC decreases because of blood shift but remains still larger than that of awake, supine subjects [49].

The decrease of Crs is entirely due to changes in lung mechanical properties [44, 50]. Several mechanisms can lower CL, such as increased smooth muscle tone or stimulation of other contractile elements in the airways or lung parenchyma, atelectasis or small airway closure, and changes in surfactant function. It is at present impossible to tell which of these mechanisms is the main cause of the decrease in CL. Lung volume-pressure curves on inflation from FRC are often S-shaped [50], a fact which could be indicative of alveolar recruitment. In normal supine, anesthetized, paralyzed subjects, atelactasis developing at FRC is eliminated with positive end-expiratory pressure [51]. Such alveolar recruitment can quantitatively account for both the increase in CL and leftward shift of the static volume-pressure curve of the lung observed with positive end-expiratory pressure in some normal supine, anesthetized, paralyzed subjects [52]. However similar changes in lung mechanics have also been observed in normal seated subjects after maintained hyperinflation and have been attributed to changes in either pulmonary blood volume [53, 54] or airway muscle tone [55]. It also remains unclear whether the decrease in CL during anesthesia is primarily due to any of the mechanisms mentioned above. Westbrook et al. [44] suggested that changes in CL are in fact secondary to changes in chest wall function leading to volume reduction, as conditions where ventilation occurs at low lung volumes are eventually associated with increases in elastance probably due to higher surface tension [56]. This sequence of events contrasts, however, with the observation that in supine, anesthetized, paralyzed subjects CL, though increased with positive end-expiratory pressure, remains substantially lower [52] than that reported for awake supine subjects at comparable lung volumes [5].

The volume-pressure relationship of the chest wall seems to undergo only relatively minor changes with anesthesia and paralysis in the supine posture. Static compliance in the mid-volume range [44, 50, 52, 57] is similar to that reported for awake supine subjects during relaxation [5], but the static volume-pressure curve either shifts to the right or becomes less curved at low lung volumes [44]. Indeed, the increase in chest wall compliance with positive end-expiratory pressure in anesthetized paralyzed subjects [52] is only one-fourth of that occurring over the same range of lung volume during relaxation in awake supine subjects [5].

Changes in the elastic properties of lung and chest wall with anesthesia and paralysis should likely influence the distribution of inspired gas during mechanical ventilation. Only part of the differences in the distribution of ventilation observed in most postures between awake, spontaneously breathing and anesthetized, paralyzed subjects [58] can be attributed to differences in the distribution of force applied by the respiratory muscles and the ventilator. Indeed the direction of changes in regional ventilation with anesthesia-paralysis in the different postures is not always consistent with the known pattern of respiratory muscle activation in awake subjects; thus, no change in the distribution of inspired gas has been found in the prone posture [58]. Although several mechanisms, like mechanical interdependence of lung parenchyma, collateral ventilation, and lobar sliding, may limit the modification of regional ventilation, the changes in chest wall shape occurring with anesthesia should therefore influence regional lung expansion, and hence the distribution of regional lung compliance. Moreover, these changes, while implying relatively minor changes in the overall compliance, might reflect important changes in regional chest wall compliance, and thus, further influence the distribution of ventilation. Unfortunately, because of lack of the relevant information, these considerations are at present only speculative.

References

1. Remington JW (1955) Hysteresis loop behavior of the aorta and other extensible tissues. Am J Physiol 180:83-95
2. Jonson B, Beydon L, Brauer K, Manson C, Valid S, Grytzell H (1993) Mechanics of respiratory system in healthy anesthetized humans with emphasis on viscoelastic properties. J Appl Physiol 75:132-140
3. Agostoni E (1972) Mechanics of the pleural space. Physiol Rev 52:57-128
4. Heaf PJD, Prime FJ (1956) The compliance of the thorax in normal human subjects. Clin Sci 15:319-327
5. Agostoni E, Hyatt R (1986) Static behavior of the respiratory system. In: Macklem PT, Mead J (eds) Handbook of Physiology. The respiratory system. Mechanics of breathing. Vol III. American phisiological society, Bethesda, pp 113-130
6. D'Angelo E (1984) Techniques for studying the mechanics of the pleural space. In: Otis AB (ed) Techniques in life science. Vol. P415. Elsevier, Amsterdam, pp 1-32
7. Milic-Emili J (1984) Measurements of pressures in respiratory physiology. In: Otis AB (ed) Techniques in Life Science. Vol. P412. Elsevier, Amsterdam, pp 1-22
8. Wade OL (1954) Movements of the thoracic cage and diaphragm in respiration. J Physiol 124:193-212
9. Agostoni E, Mognoni P, Torri G, Saracino F (1965) Relation between changes of rib cage circumference and lung volume. J Appl Physiol 20:1179-1186
10. Strohl KP, Mead J, Banzett RB, Loring SH, Kosch PC (1981) Regional differences in abdominal muscle activity during various maneuvers in humans. J Appl Physiol 51:1471-1476
11. Konno K, Mead J (1967) Measurement of the separate volume changes of rib cage and abdomen during breathing. J Appl Physiol 22:407-422
12. Konno K, Mead J (1968) Static volume-pressure characteristics of the rib cage and abdomen. J Appl Physiol 24:544-548
13. Mead J (1981) Mechanics of the chest wall. In: Hutas I, Debreczeni LA (eds) Advances in physiological sciences. Vol 10. Pergamon Press, Oxford, pp 3-11
14. Macklem PT, Macklem DM, De Troyer A (1983) A model of inspiratory muscle mechanics. J Appl Physiol 55:547-557
15. Hillman DR, Markos J, Finucane K (1990) Effect of abdominal compression on maximum transdiaphragmatic pressure. J Appl Physiol 68:2296-2304
16. Boynton BR, Barnas GM, Dadmun JT, Fredberg JJ (1991) Mechanical coupling of the rib cage, abdomen, and diaphragm through their area of apposition. J Appl Physiol 70:1235-1244

17. Agostoni E, Gurtner G, Torri C, Rahn H (1966) Respiratory mechanics during submersion and negative-pressure breathing. J Appl Physiol 21:251-258
18. Deschamps C, Rodarte JR, Wilson TA (1988) Coupling between rib cage and abdominal compartments of the relaxed chest wall. J Appl Physiol 65:2265-2269
19. Zechman FW, Musgrave FS, Mains RC, Cohn JB (1967) Respiratory mechanics and pulmonary diffusing capacity with lower body negative pressure. J Appl Physiol 22:247-250
20. D'Angelo E, Sant'Ambrogio G (1974) Direct action of the contracting diaphragm on the rib cage in rabbits and dogs. J Appl Physiol 36:715-719
21. Danon J, Druz WS, Goldberg NB, Sharp JT (1979) Function of isolated paced diaphragm and cervical accessory muscles in C1 quadriplegics. Am Rev Respir Dis 119:909-919
22. D'Angelo E (1981) Cranio-caudal rib cage distortion with increasing inspiratory airflow in man. Respir Physiol 44:215-237
23. Crawford ABH, Dodd D, Engel LA (1983) Change in rib cage shape during quiet breathing, hyperventilation and single inspirations. Respir Physiol 54:197-209
24. Mc Cool FD, Loring SH, Mead J (1985) Rib cage distortion during voluntary and involuntary breathing acts. J Appl Physiol 58:1703-1712
25. Jiang J, Demedts M, Decramer M (1998) Mechanical coupling of upper and lower canine rib cages and its functional significance. J Appl Physiol 64:620-626
26. D'Angelo E, Michelini S, Miserocchi G (1973) Local motion of the chest wall during passive and active expansion. Respir Physiol 19:47-59
27. Reid MB, Loring SH, Banzett RB, Mead J (1986) Passive mechanics of upright human chest wall during immersion from hips to neck. J Appl Physiol 60:1561-1570
28. Ward ME, Ward JW, Macklem PT (1992) Analysis of human chest wall motion using a two-compartment rib cage model. J Appl Physiol 72:1338-1347
29. Needham CB, Rogan MC, McDonald I (1954) Normal standard for lung volumes, intrapulmonary gas mixing and maximum breathing capacity. Thorax 9:313-325
30. Pierce JA, Ebert RV (1958) The elastic properties of the lungs in the aged. J Lab Clin Med 51:63-71
31. Turner JM, Mead J, Wohl MB (1968) Elasticity of human lungs in relation to age. J Appl Physiol 25:664-671
32. Frank NR, Mead J, Ferris BC Jr (1957) The mechanical behaviour of the lungs in healthy elderly persons. J Clin Invest 36:1680-1687
33. Gibson CJ, Pride NB, O'Cain C, Quagliato R (1976) Sex and age differences in pulmonary mechanics in normal nonsmoking subjects. J Appl Physiol 41:20-25
34. Duomarco JL, Rimini R (1947) La presion intrabdominal en el hombre. El Ateneo, Buenos Aires
35. Hedenstierna C, Bindslev L, Santesson J, Norlander DP (1981) Airway closure in each lung of anesthetized human subjects. J Appl Physiol 50:55-64
36. Rehder K, Marsh M (1986) Respiratory mechanics during anesthesia and mechanical ventilation. In: Macklem PT, Mead J (eds) The respiratory system. Mechanics of breathing. Handbook of physiology. Vol III. American Physiological Society, Bethesda, pp 737-752
37. Rehder K, Sittipong R, Sessler AD (1972) The effects of thiopental-meperidine anesthesia with succinylcholine paralysis on functional residual capacity and dynamic lung compliance in normal sitting man. Anesthesiology 37:395-398
38. Muller N, Volgyesi G, Becker L, Bryan MH, Bryan AC (1979) Diaphragmatic muscle tone. J Appl Physiol 47:279-284
39. Druz WS, Sharp JT (1981) Activity of respiratory muscles in upright and recumbent humans. J Appl Physiol 51:1552-1561

40. Krayer S, Rehder K, Beck KC, Cameron PD, Didier EP, Hoffman EA (1987) Quantification of thoracic volumes by three-dimensional imaging. J Appl Physiol 62:591-598
41. Krayer S, Rehder K, Vettermann J, Didier EP, Ritman FL (1989) Position and motion of the human diaphragm during anesthesia-paralysis. Anesthesiology 70:891-898
42. Drummond GB, Allan PL, Logan MR (1986) Changes in diaphragmatic position in association with the induction of anaesthesia. Br J Anaesth 58:1246-1251
43. Freund F, Roos A, Dodd RB (1964) Expiratory activity of the abdominal muscles in man during general anesthesia. J Appl Physiol 19:693-697
44. Westbrook PR, Stubbs SE, Sessler AD, Rehder K, Hyatt RE (1973) Effects of anesthesia and muscle paralysis on respiratory mechanics in normal man. J Appl Physiol 34:81-86
45. Vellody VP, Nassery M, Dius WS, Sharp JT (1978) Effects of body position change on thoracoabdominal motion. J Appl Physiol 45:581-589
46. Hedenstierna G, Löfström B, Lundh R (1981) Thoracic gas volume and chest-abdomen dimensions during anesthesia and muscle paralysis. Anesthesiology 55:499-506
47. Hedenstierna G, Strandberg A, Brismar B,, Lundquist H, Svensson L, Tokics L (1985) Functional residual capacity, thoracoabdominal dimensions, and central blood volume during general anesthesia with muscle paralysis and mechanical ventilation. Anesthesiology 62:247-254
48. Rehder K, Mallow JE, Fibuch EE, Krabill DR, Sessler AD (1974) Effects of isoflurane anesthesia and muscle paralysis on respiratory mechanics in normal man. Anesthesiology 41:477-485
49. Kimball WR, Loring SH, Basta SJ, De Troyer A, Mead J (1985) Effects of paralysis with pancuronium on chest wall statics in awake humans. J Appl Physiol 58:l638-1645
50. D'Angelo E, Robatto F, Calderini E, Tavola M, Bono D, Milic-Emili J (1991) Pulmonary and chest wall mechanics in anesthetized paralyzed humans. J Appl Physiol 70:2602-2610
51. Brismar B, Hedenstierna G, Lundquist H, Strandberg A, Svensson L, Tokics L (1985) Pulmonary densities during anesthesia with muscular relaxation. A proposal of atelectasis. Anesthesiology 62:422-428
52. D'Angelo E, Calderini E, Tavola M, Bono D, Milic-Emili J (1992) Effect of PEEP on respiratory mechanics in anesthetized paralyzed humans. J Appl Physiol 73:1736-1742
53. Goldberg HS, Mitzner W, Adams K, Menkes H, Lichtenstein S, Permutt S (1975) Effect of intrathoracic pressure on pressure-volume characteristics of the lung in man. J Appl Physiol 38:411-417
54. Hillman DR, Finucane KE (1983) The effect of hyperinflation on lung elasticity in healthy subjects. Respir Physiol 54:295-305
55. Duggan CJ, Castle WD, Berend N (1990) Effects of continuous positive airway pressure breathing on lung volume and distensibility. J Appl Physiol 68:1121-1126
56. Young SL, Tierney DF, Clements JA (1970) Mechanism of compliance change in excised rat lungs at low transpulmonary pressure. J Appl Physiol 29:780-785
57. Sharp JT, Johnson FN, Goldberg NB, Van Lith P (1967) Hysteresis and stress adaptation in the human respiratory system. J Appl Physiol 23:487-497
58. Rehder K, Knopp TJ, Sessler AD (1978) Regional intrapulmonary gas distribution in awake and anesthetized-paralyzed prone man. J Appl Physiol 45:528-535

Chapter 3

Respiratory mechanics during general anaesthesia in healthy subjects

P. PELOSI, M. RESTA, L. BRAZZI

General anesthesia deeply influences the behavioral state, altering consciousness and sensation by the direct or indirect effects of various anesthetic drugs. However, these drugs may cause additional effects, sometimes undesirable on other organ systems. In particular, the effects on respiratory function seem to be significant. Although several studies investigated the effects of general anaesthesia on respiratory function, they were specifically performed in healthy young people, and did not include patients with different ages or anthropometric characteristics. Moreover, general anaesthesia may be performed in different positions or surgical conditions (i.e. during laparoscopy), which may further influence the respiratory function compared to the supine position. In this chapter we will discuss the effects of general anaesthesia on respiratory system mechanics in different categories of patients and surgical conditions, as well as the possible clinical implications of these findings and some therapeutic approaches.

Methods of measurement

Compliance and resistance

Airway pressure (P_{ao}) is usually measured proximal to the endotracheal tube or tracheostomy cannula by means of polyethylene tubing, connected to a pressure transducer. To partition the total respiratory system mechanics into its lung and chest wall components, the esophageal pressure (P_{es}) is usually measured with a balloon inflated with 0.5-1 ml of air. The validity of P_{es} is verified using the "occlusion test" of Baydur et al. [1], and the balloon is fixed in that position. Gas flow is recorded with a pneumotachograph and volume is obtained by integration of the flow signal.

The most popular method to measure compliance and resistance is that of rapid airway occlusion during constant flow [2]. This method, when applied together with the esophageal balloon technique, allows the partitioning of lung and chest wall components of the respiratory system [3]. The rapid airway occlusion technique is appealing both for its simplicity and because it provides a comprehensive on-line assessment of respiratory mechanics. As shown in Figure 1 at end-inspiratory phase, brief (3-7 s) airway occlusions are performed. Occlusion is maintained until both Pao and Pes decrease from a maximum value (P_{max}) to an apparent plateau (P_2). After the occlusion, an intermediate drop from P_{max} to a lower value (P_1), at flow 0, is appreciable in P_{ao} but not usually in P_{es} [3].

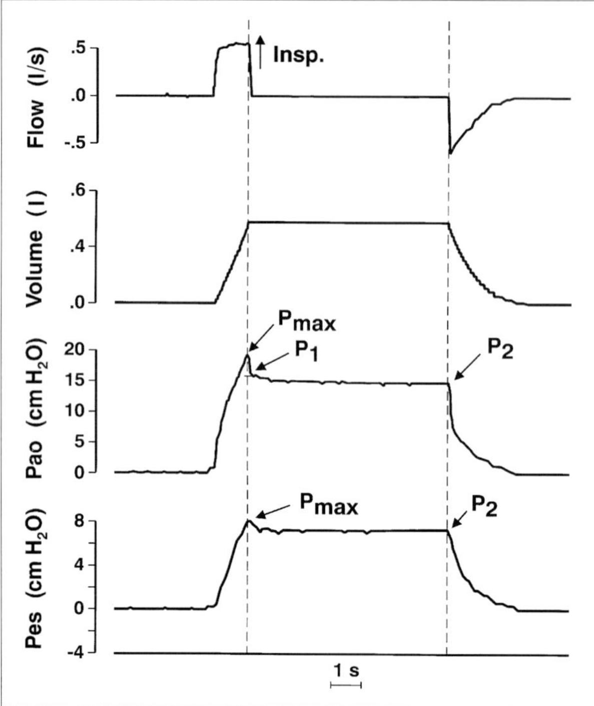

Fig. 1. Tracings (top to bottom) of Flow, Volume, Pressure at the airway opening (Pao) and Esophageal pressure (Pes) during rapid airway occlusion

The plateau pressures (P_2) of P_{ao} and P_{es} are taken to represent the static end-inspiratory recoil pressures of the respiratory system (Pst,rs) and chest wall (Pst,w), respectively.

The compliance of the static respiratory system (Cst,rs) or that of the chest wall (Cst,w) is obtained by dividing tidal volume (V_t) by the difference Pst,rs - P_{ao} or Pst,w-P_{es}, respectively, at end-expiratory phase. The static lung compliance (Cst,L) is obtained from Cst,rs and Cst,w according to the following equation:

$$\text{Cst,L} = \frac{\text{Cst,rs} \cdot \text{Cst,w}}{\text{Cst,w} - \text{Cst,rs}}$$

Total (R,rs) and interrupter (Rmin,rs) resistance of the respiratory system are computed from P_{ao} as (Pmax'-P_2)/V and (Pmax'-P_1)/V, where Pmax' represents the new Pmax' value obtained by correcting Pao for tube resistance. V is the flow immediately preceding the occlusion. Rmin,rs represents the "ohmic" resistive component of the respiratory resistance caused by stress relaxation or time constant inequalities within the respiratory system tissues. The difference between R,rs and Rmin,rs and is termed ΔR,rs. Since usually there is no appreciable drop in P_{es} (i.e. P_1 in the esophageal tracings is not identifiable), immediately following the occlusion Rmin,rs essentially reflects airway resistance (Rmin,L). Minimum chest wall resistance (Rmin,w) can be considered negligible. As a consequence, total chest wall resistance (R,w) is entirely due to the viscoelastic properties of the chest wall tissues (i.e. R,w=ΔR,w). Nevertheless in a recent study using a rapid airway shutter D'Angelo et al. [4] reported that the chest wall may account for approximately 27% of Rmin,rs in normal anesthetized subjects. "Additional" resistance of the lung (ΔR,L) is obtained as ΔR,rs-ΔR,w while the sum of Rmin,L+ΔR,L gives the total lung resistance (R,L). ΔR,L and ΔR,w (i.e. R,w) are due to stress relaxation or time constant inequalities within the lung and chest wall, respectively.

Functional residual capacity

Functional residual capacity (FRC) may be measured by different methods, of which the most common and easiest is the helium dilution method [5]. Briefly, an anaesthesia bag is filled with 1.5-2 l of a known gas mixture (13% helium in oxygen) and is connected to the airway opening at end-expiration; 15 deep manual breaths are made. The helium concentration in the anaesthesia bag is then measured with a common helium analyzer. The FRC is computed according to the following formula:

$$FRC = V_i \cdot [He]_i/[He]_f - V_i$$

where V_i is the initial gas volume in the anaesthesia bag, and $[He]_i$ and $[He]_f$ are the initial and final helium concentrations, respectively. This method of measurement may be also applied in infants. However some limitations should be discussed. FRC measurements may be affected by airway closure or bag shrinkage [6]. Airway closure may interfere with correct mixing of helium between the bag and lung according to three possibilities: 1) the closed airways do not open in any phase of bag ventilation; 2) at the first inflation the closed airways open, but during the next expiration they close and remain closed during further inflations, so part of the helium is stopped and not recollected into the bag; 3) at each inflation the airways open during inspiration and close during expiration. However using sufficient inflation lung volumes, we should reopen all the closed airways. Another technical problem derives from gas volume loss during rebreathing due to gas exchange. However, this loss should be counteracted by the increase in volume due to temperature and humidity changes, thus the total volume (bag+lung) probably remains constant.

Anaesthesia and respiratory functions

Anaesthesia and functional residual capacity

In the majority of recumbent human subjects, the induction of general anaesthesia in supine position reduces FRC [7]. The mean FRC awake is 2.7±0.07 (SE) l, whereas mean FRC during anaesthesia and during anaesthesia and paralysis is 2.15±0.06 l. This decrease occurs rapidly after induction [8, 9], and does not appear to change with time [10-12] or to be influenced by subsequent paralysis [11]. Most anesthetic drugs except ketamine, decrease FRC [13, 14].

The mechanisms causing the decrease in FRC remain unclear. Current hypotheses focus on a loss of tonic activity in chest wall muscles (both rib cage and diaphragm) and changes in blood volume in the thoracoabdominal cavity.

Some studies suggest that both inspiratory rib cage muscles and diaphragm possess tonic activities that contribute to normal chest wall recoil [15, 16] but this tone, at least in supine position, is minimal. Other studies documented changes in chest wall shape with induction of anaesthesia, with controversial results. Froese and Bryan [17], with Hedenstierna et al. [18], found a cephalic shift of the end-expiratory position of the dependent regions of the diaphragm. In contrast, other studies using high-speed three-dimensional computed tomography (CT) found consistent net cephalic shift of the diaphragm [19, 20]. However, the studies noted a consistent change in diaphragmatic shape, as dependent diaphragmatic regions tended to shift caudally. The resulting effect was atelectasis formation in the dependent lung regions (Fig. 2).

The shape of rib cage also changes with anaesthesia, with a reduction in the external anteroposterior diameter and an increase in the lateral diameter of the thorax and abdomen [11, 21, 22]. Increases in intrathoracic blood volume can decrease FRC [23]. Anaesthesia decreases total thoracic volume less than gas volume, suggesting an increase in intrathoracic tissue volume (approximately 0.3 l).

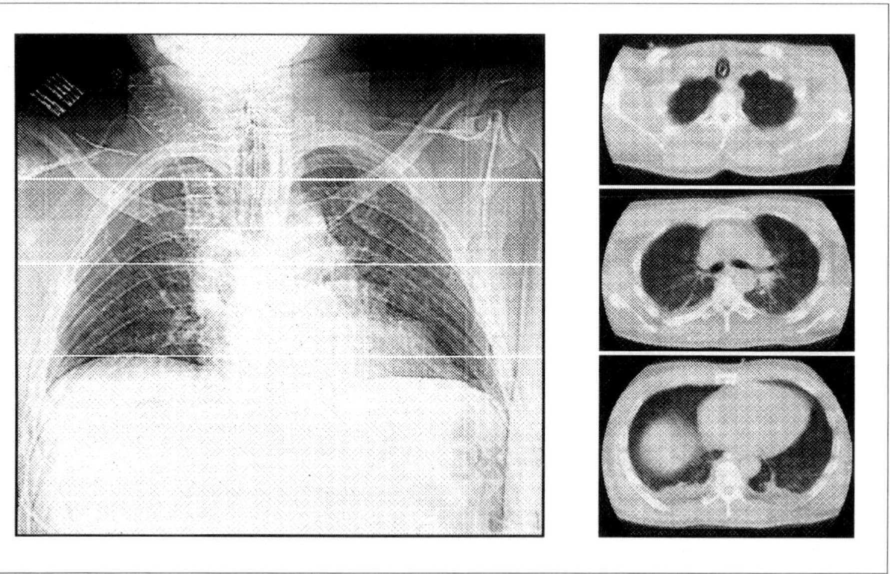

Fig. 2. Transverse section of the thorax during general anaesthesia and paralysis at end expiration in an healthy subject. Note the development of densities in the dependent lung regions, in supine position

Anaesthesia and respiratory mechanics

Anaesthesia changes the mechanical behavior of the lungs and the chest wall [7, 11, 24-31]. In general anaesthesia, respiratory compliance decreases with induction of anaesthesia. This primary source of decreased respiratory compliance is the lung. In fact, chest wall compliance appears to be little affected over most of the range of lung volumes. The mechanisms leading to decreased lung compliance during anaesthesia are unclear. The most likely is the reduction in lung volume, although other factors such as surfactant alterations, altered relationships with the chest wall, and changes in thoracic blood volume may be implied.

General anaesthesia also increases respiratory resistance [7, 30]. Respiratory resistance is composed of on airway resistance component and the "additional" resistance as previously discussed. In normal subjects, the main determinant of respiratory resistance is the "additional" one [2], being approximately 65% of the total resistance.

However, both airway and "additional" resistance behave differently according to inflated volumes and inspiratory flow. Infact increasing inspiratory flow airway resistance increases while additional resistance decreases.

On the contrary, increasing volume airways resistance decrease while additional resistance increases. The chest wall resistance is of minimal importance in determining total respiratory resistance [3]. The increase in respiratory resistance with the induction of general anaesthesia has been attributed to the reduction in lung volume. However, studies on airflow resistance during general anaesthesia are complicated by the use of varying anesthetics which may differently influences the bronchomotor tone [7].

Anesthesia and mechanical ventilation

During mechanical ventilation, chest wall motion is determined by the regional impedences (compliance and resistance) of the respiratory system. The relative contribution of the rib cage to tidal volume increases [32, 33], while the anteroposterior diameter of both rib cage and abdomen increases during tidal breathing and the lateral diameters decrease. The pattern of diaphragmatic motion during mechanical ventilation in supine position predominates in the nondependent regions, as does that of inflated gas distribution [17, 19].

Effects of age

Aging processes cause marked alterations on the different components of the respiratory system (i.e., compliance, resistance and lung volume) [34-40]. As discussed above, general anaesthesia itself modifies these parameters. However, the interaction between age and the effects of general anaesthesia on the respiratory system have seldomly been investigated. In awake patients, the aging process is reported to increase lung volume, lung compliance and resistance with the appearance of "emphysema-like" lesions characterized by an enlargement of the alveolar spaces [34-36, 41-43]. On the other hand, a reduction in chest wall compliance has been hypothesized but never measured [34, 36]. These anatomical alterations are paralleled by a gradual reduction in oxygenation (0.18-0.55 mm Hg/year) [37-39]. The induction of anaesthesia generally produces a greater reduction in FRC in elderly patients. However, Gunnarson et al. [40] found only a slight relationship between atelectasis formation and age. In a recent study [44], we investigated the influence of age on respiratory function in 38 normal-weighted patients (20 females and 18 males) free from previous cardiopulmonary disease during general anaesthesia in supine position. Respiratory compliance significantly decreased with age (Fig. 3).

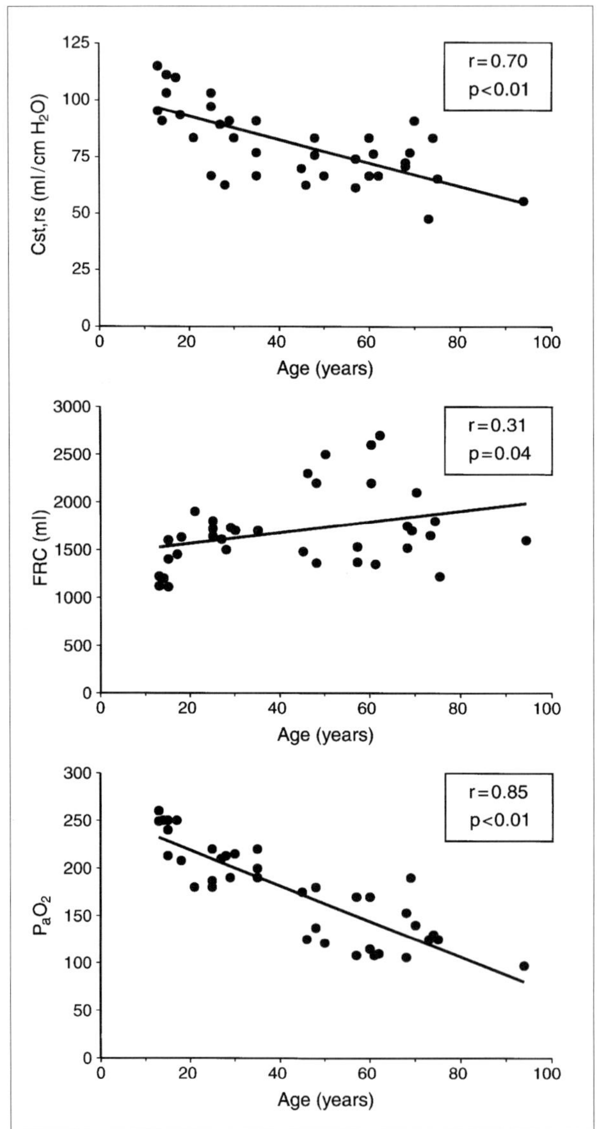

Fig. 3. Relationship between age and compliance of respiratory system (Cst,rs), functional residual capacity (FRC), and oxygenation (PaO_2)

This reduction was equally due to lung and chest wall components. Similarly, we found a considerable effect of age on respiratory and lung resistance. The effect on resistance was much greater than that on compliance. The reduction of lung compliance with age was not paralleled by a severe reduction in FRC (Fig. 3), contrary to what was expected from pulmonary functional data while awake. However, oxygenation deteriorated with age, suggesting that alterations in ventilation/perfusion mismatch more than true shunt ($V_A/Q=0$) are responsible for gas exchange abnormalities with age [37]. These findings imply that the altered gas-exchange in eldery patients cannot be presumably improved by application of high inspiratory pressure levels in the airways (inspiratory or expiratory pressures), but only by increasing the inspiratory oxygen fraction. Finally, respiratory mechanics measurements, especially in patients with lung disease, should always be standardized for age for correct interpretation of the data.

Effects of body weight

Body mass index (BMI) assesses excess body weight and is calculated as weight per height^2 (kg/m^2) [6]. BMI less than 24-25 kg/m^2 is considered normal; 25-30 kg/m^2 is considered overweight and more than 30 kg/m^2 is considered true obesity. Obesity is a serious social problem in North America since at least 33% of the population is overweight and almost 5% is morbidly obese. Body mass is known to deeply affect respiratory function while awake, due to the increased mass loading of the ventilatory system, particularly on the thoracic and abdominal components of the chest wall [45-47]. Anaesthesia may thus produce more adverse effects on respiratory function in overweight patients than in normal subjects [6, 48, 49]. We recently investigated the influence of body mass on lung volume, respiratory mechanics, and gas exchange during general anaesthesia in supine position in healthy patients [50]. The compliance of the respiratory system was found to decrease with BMI, and this decrease was paralleled by a reduction in FRC and oxygenation (Fig. 4). The reduction in compliance of the respiratory system was due to a reduction in compliance (i.e. the reciprocal of elastance) of both the lung and chest wall, although the former was prevalent (Fig. 5).

Alterations of respiratory system mechanics in overweight patients primarily derive from high intra-abdominal pressure [6]. This pressure, unopposed during general anaesthesia and paralysis, causes an increase of pleural pressure and reduction in chest wall compliance (Fig. 5). The consequent decrease of transmural pressure (i.e. alveolar-pleural pressure) is such as to lead to huge lung collapse. This sequence of events results in low lung volume, decreased lung compliance and hypoxemia, likely caused by shunt flow through the collapsed lung regions.

In general, body mass is an important determinant of lung volume, oxygenation and respiratory mechanics, mainly affecting the lung component. More

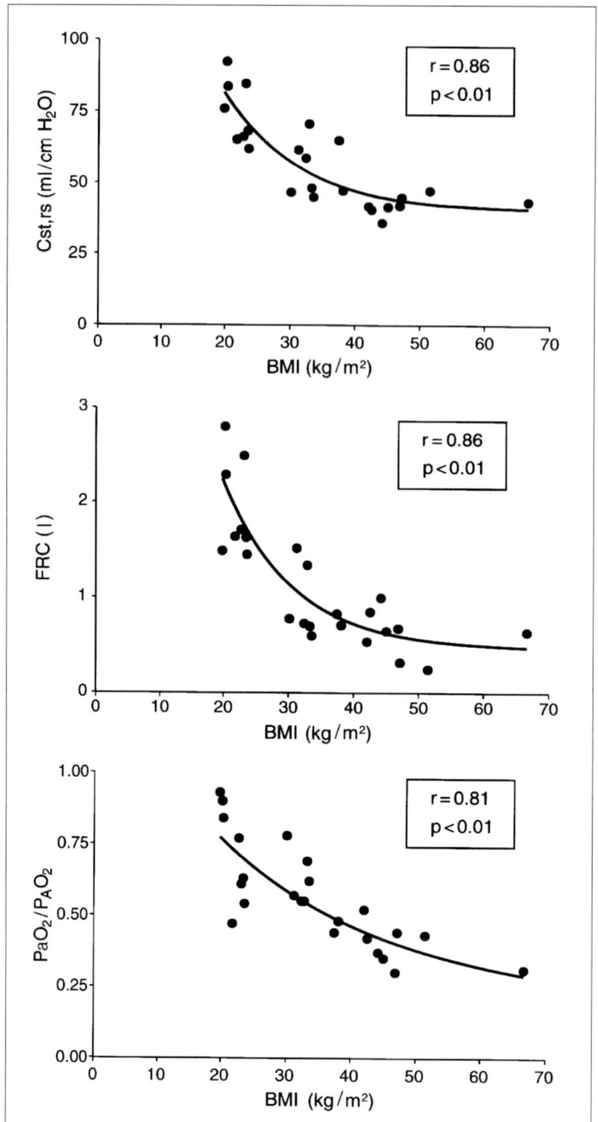

Fig. 4. Relationship between body mass index and compliance of respiratory system (Cst,rs), functional residual capacity (FRC), and oxygenation (PaO_2/PAO_2)

importantly, alterations in respiratory mechanics are present not only in patients with severe obesity, but also in patients with moderate obesity.

The results of these studies may have several clinical implications in the anesthesiological management of overweight patients and give new insights for the treatment of morbid obesity. First, we found that oxygenation, lung volume, and respiratory compliance decreased, while respiratory resistance increased, with increasing BMI. This reduction was evident not only in patients with severe obesity, as expected, but also in patients with an high degree of obesity,

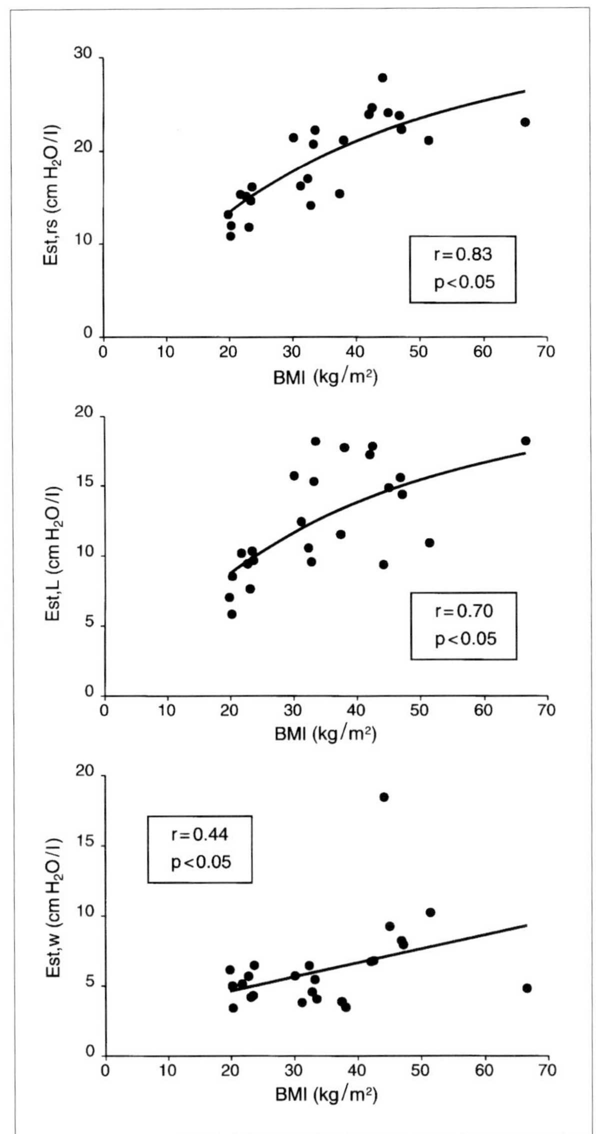

Fig. 5. Relationship between body mass index and elastance of respiratory system (Est,rs), elastance of lung (Est,L), elastance of chest wall (Est,w). Elastance is the reciprocal of compliance (i.e. Est = 1/Cst)

as expected, but also in patients with a moderate degree of obesity. Moreover, it is known that morphological alterations of the upper airways partly depend on BMI [51]. Thus, at the moment of anaesthesia induction, dramatic changes in mechanics of the upper and lower tracts of the respiratory system are supposed to occur depending on the BMI. We expected many more difficulties related to BMI while ventilating by mask and intubating the patients (lower compliance, higher resistance, morphological upper airway alterations); little time was allowed to perform these maneuvers due to the low compensatory times, i.e. marked and rapid reduction in oxygenation due to the severe fall in lung volume. From these considerations, great attention should be given at the moment of anaesthesia induction, not only in morbidly obese patients but also in patients with a moderate degree of obesity. Sometimes awake intubation, performed by different methods, should be considered to reduce the consequent risks produced by respiratory alterations observed after the induction of anaesthesia.

Second, since overweight patients present a greater risk of atelectasis and oxygenation impairment, they likely will benefit from application of higher airway pressures. Recently, we showed that the application of positive end-expiratory pressure (PEEP) in obese subjects improved respiratory mechanics (increasing respiratory system, lung and chest wall compliance, while reducing lung resistance) and oxygenation without deleterious effects on hemodynamics [52]. On the other hand, the use of periodical hyperinflations (sigh) may result beneficial.

Third, many reports describe an increase in FRC of about 25% and an increase in oxygenation of about 10 mm Hg in air and no changes in the mechanical characteristics of the respiratory system after a weight loss to maximum BMI of 35 kg/m^2 [53]. From our data, we may speculate that, contrary to previous beliefs, the major changes in oxygenation, lung volume, respiratory mechanics and work of breathing should be obtained by reducing the BMI to approximate threshold values equal to or lower than 30 kg/m^2.

Fourth, we found an increase in respiratory system work of breathing with increasing BMI. Moreover, we found that the majority of patients with a BMI higher than 30 kg/m^2 presented a work of breathing of the lung approximately 0.7-0.8 J/l, which is usually considered close to the level of respiratory muscle fatigue. This means that, at least in supine position, overweight patients may have a severe reduction in compensatory mechanisms, and if their need of work of breathing increases for whatever reason, respiratory fatigue may occur.

Effects of positioning

During surgery, the prone position is commonly used to expose the dorsal surface of the body for specific surgical indications. In general, prone position is considered to produce negative effects on the respiratory function during general anaesthesia. However, the modifications in respiratory mechanics and gas exchange during anaesthesia in the prone position have not been extensively investigated. Some authors found a reduction in minute ventilation and oxygenation during general anaesthesia and spontaneously breathing, while others found a reduction in respiratory compliance without using appropriate supports [54, 55]. We recently prospectively investigated the influence of prone position in normal subjects during general anaesthesia [56]. We showed that, if correctly performed to assure free abdominal movements, the prone position does not significantly alter either lung or chest wall mechanics, while it markedly improves lung volumes and oxygenation. Thus, it does not seem to have any adverse effects on the mechanics of breathing and gas exchange. Positive effects on respiratory function of prone position during general anaesthesia have been also reported in obese subjects [57]. Thus, we demonstrated that, contrary to a common notion, prone position during general anaesthesia is safe both in normal and obese subjects since it improves respiratory function without negative effects on hemodynamics.

Effects of laparoscopy

Laparoscopic cholecystectomy is an important and increasingly used surgical technique, mainly due to claims of minimal postoperative morbidity and markedly reduced hospital stays [58]. It is well recognized that abdominal insufflation with carbon dioxide and the Trendelenburg's position, during pelvic laparoscopy can cause serious physiological changes in respiratory mechanics, lung volume and gas exchange with consequent risk for the patient [59-61]. We recently made a systemic investigation of the changes in lung volume, gas exchange and mechanical properties of the respiratory system, lung and chest wall, during laparoscopic cholecystectomy in healthy adults [62]. We found that the abdominal insufflation (15 mm Hg max) markedly reduced static compliance of the respiratory system, lung, and chest wall, reduced the lung volume to a lesser amount, increased the resistance of the respiratory system and did not affect oxygenation. On the contrary, arterial carbon dioxide (P_aCO_2) was increased, which closely correlated with the end-expiratory carbon dioxide (P_ECO_2). The duration of anaesthesia did not affect respiratory system, lung and chest wall mechanics, lung volume, oxygenation or P_{a-E} CO_2 gradient. These results may have some clinical implications. First, laparoscopy should be performed with careful respiratory and hemodynamic monitoring, especially in patients with previous lung or chest wall diseases. Since the reduction in FRC and oxygenation appear to be clinically irrelevant (i.e. no additional atelectasis formation), the use of positive end-expiratory pressure should not be generally suggested at least in normal subjects. Second, the effects of laparoscopy are only present during the abdominal insufflation phase but have no consequences after the abdominal desufflation. Third, the noninvasive monitoring of P_ECO_2 during the surgical procedure is precise and accurate at least in healthy subjects.

Conclusions

General anaesthesia deeply modifies the respiratory function, influencing respiratory mechanics, lung volume and gas exchange. However, the effects of general anaesthesia depend on the age and body weight of the patients, even if free from previous cardiorespiratory diseases. Moreover, positioning and specific surgical operations (i.e. laparoscopy) may further influence the effects of general anaesthesia on the respiratory function. The thorough knowledge of these physiological modifications is important to optimize ventilatory settings during general anaesthesia.

References

1. Baydur A, Sassoon SH, Stiles CM (1987) Partitioning of respiratory mechanics in young adults. Effects of duration of anaesthesia. Am Rev Respir Dis 135:165-172
2. D'Angelo E, Calderini E, Torri G, Robatto FM, Bono D, Milic-Emili J (1989) Respiratory mechanics in anesthetized paralyzed humans: effects of flow, volume, and time. J Appl Physiol 67:2556-2564
3. D'Angelo E, Robatto FM, Calderini E, Tavola M, Bono D, Torri G, Milic-Emili J (1991) Pulmonary and chest wall mechanics in anesthetized paralyzed humans. J Appl Physiol 70(6):2602-2610
4. D'Angelo E, Prandi M, Tavola M, Calderini E, Milic-Emili J (1994) Chest wall interrupter resistance in anesthetized paralyzed humans. J Appl Physiol 77:883-887
5. Damia G, Mascheroni D, Croci M, Terenzi L (1988) Perioperative changes in the functional residual capacity in morbidly obese patients. Br J Anaesth 60:574-578
6. Pelosi P, Croci M, Ravagnan I, Cerisara M, Vicardi P, Lissoni A, Gattinoni L (1997) Respiratory system mechanics in sedated, paralyzed morbidly obese patients. J Appl Physiol 82:811-818
7. Rehder K, Marsh MH (1986) Respiratory mechanics during anaesthesia and mechanical ventilation. In: Macklem PT, Mead J (eds) Respiration. Handbook of physiology. Vol III. American Physiological Society, Bethesda, pp 737-752
8. Howell JB, Peckett BW (1957) Studies of the elastic properties of the thorax of supine anaesthetized paralyzed human subjects. J Physiol 136:1-19
9. Bergman NA (1982) Reduction in resting end-expiratory position of the respiratory system with induction of anaesthesia and neuromuscular paralysis. Anesthesiology 57:14-17
10. Don Hillary F, Wahba WM, Craig Douglas B (1972) Airway closure, gas trapping, and the functional residual capacity during anaesthesia. Anesthesiology 36:533-539
11. Westbrook PR, Stubbs SE, Sessler AD, Rehder K, Hyatt Robert E (1973) Effects of anaesthesia and muscle paralysis on respiratory mechanics in normal man. J Appl Physiol 34:81-85
12. Hewlett AM, Hulands GH, Nunn JF, Minty KB (1974) Functional residual capacity during anaesthesia: methodology. Br J Anaesth 46:479-503
13. Shulman D, Beardsmore CS, Aronson HB, Godfrey S (1985) The effect of ketamine on the functional residual capacity in young children. Anesthesiology 62:551-556
14. Mankikian B, Cantineau JP, Sartene R, Clergue F, Viars P (1986) Ventilatory pattern and chest wall mechanics during ketamine anaesthesia in humans. Anesthesiology 65:492-499
15. De Troyer A, Bastenier J, Delhez L (1980) Function of respiratory muscles during partial curarization in humans. J Appl Physiol 49:1049-1056
16. Drummond GB (1987) Reduction of tonic rib cage muscle activity by anaesthesia with thiopental. Anesthesiology 67:695-700
17. Froese AB, Bryan AC (1974) Effects of anaesthesia and paralysis on diaphragmatic mechanics in man. Anesthesiology 41:242-255
18. Hedenstierna G, Srandberg A, Brismar B, Lundquist H, Svensson L, Tokics L (1985) Functional residual capacity, thoracoabdominal dimension, and central blood volume during general anaesthesia with muscle paralysis and mechanical ventilation. Anesthesiology 62:247-254
19. Krayer S, Rehder K, Vettermann J, Didier EP, Ritman EL (1989) Position and motion of the human diaphragm during anaesthesia-paralysis. Anesthesiology 70:891-898

20. Warner DO, Warner MA, Ritman EL (1996) Atelectasis and chest wall shape during halothane anaesthesia. Anesthesiology 85:49-59
21. Freund F, Roos A, Dodd RB (1964) Expiratory activity of the abdominal muscles in man during general anaesthesia. J Appl Physiol 19:693-697
22. Kaul SU, Heath JR, Nunn JF (1973) Factors influencing the development of expiratory muscle activity during anaesthesia. Br J Anaesth 45:1013-1018
23. Kimball WR, Loring SH, Basta SJ, De Tryer A, Mead J (1985) Effects of paralysis with pancuronium on chest wall statics in awake humans. J Appl Physiol 58:1638-1645
24. Behrakis PK, Higgs BD, Baydur A, Zin WA, Milic-Emili J (1983) Respiratory mechanics during halothane anaesthesia and anaesthesia-paralysis in humans. J Appl Physiol 55:1085-1092
25. Fletcher ME, Stack C, Ewart M, Davies CJ, Ridley S, Hatch DJ, Stocks J (1991) Respiratory compliance during sedation, anaesthesia, and paralysis in infants and young children. J Appl Physiol 70(5):1977-1982
26. Gold MI, Helrich M (1965) Pulmonary compliance during anaesthesia. Anaesthesiology 26:281-288
27. Auler JOC, Saldiva PHN, Martins MA, Zin WA (1990) Flow and volume dependence of respiratory system mechanics during constant flow ventilation in normal subjects and in adult respiratory distress syndrome. Crit Care Med 18:1080-1086
28. Nims RG, Conner EH, Comroe JH (1955) The compliance of the human thorax in anesthetized patients. J Clin Invest 34:744-750
29. Hedenstierna G, McCarthy G (1975) Mechanics of breathing gas distribution and functional residual capacity at different frequencies of respiration during spontaneous and artificial ventilation. Br J Anaesth 47:706-712
30. Rehder K, Mallow JE, Fibuch EE, Krabill DR, Sessler AD (1974) Effects of isoflurane anaesthesia and muscle paralysis on respiratory mechanics in normal man. Anaesthesiology 41:477-485
31. Benameur M, Goldman MD, Ecoffey C, Gaultier C (1993) Ventilation and thoracoabdominal asynchrony during halothane anaesthesia in infants. J Appl Physiol 74:1591-1596
32. Grimby G, Hedenstierna G, Lofstrom B (1975) Chest wall mechanics during artificial ventilation. J Appl Physiol 38:576-580
33. Vellody VP, Nassery M, Druz WS, Sharp JT (1978) Effects of body position change on thoracoabdominal motion. J Appl Physiol 45:581-589
34. Agostoni E, Hyatt RE (1986) Static behavior of the respiratory system. In: Macklem PT, Mead J (eds) Respiration. Handabook of physiology. Vol III. American Physiological Society, Bethesda, pp 113-130
35. Knudson RJ, Clark DF, Kennedy TC, Knudson DE (1977) Effect of aging alone on mechanical properties of the normal adult human lung. J Appl Physiol 43:1054-1062
36. Pierce JA, Ebert RV (1958) The elastic properties of the lungs in the aged. J Lab and Clin Med 51:63-71
37. Marshall BE, Wyche MQ (1972) Hypoxemia during and after anaesthesia. Anaesthesiology 37:178-209
38. Cardus J, Burgos F, Diaz O, Roca J, Barberà JA, Marrades RM, Rodriguez-Roisin R, Wagner PD (1997) Increase in pulmonary ventilation-perfusion inequality with age in healthy individuals. Am J Respir Crit Care Med 156:648-653
39. Guenard H, Marthan H (1996) Pulmonary gas exchange in elderly subjects. Eur Respir J 9:2573-2577
40. Gunnarsson L, Tokics L, Gustavsson H, Hedestierna G (1991) Influence of age in

atelectasis formation and gas exchange impairment during general anaesthesia. Br J Anaesth 66:423-432
41. Verbeken EK, Cauberghs M, Mertens I, Clement J, Lauweryns JM, Van De Woestijne KP (1992) The senile lung. Comparison with normal and emphysematous lung. Functional aspects. Chest 101: 800-809
42. Gillooly M, Lamb D (1993) Airspace size in lungs of lifelong non-smokers: effect of age and sex. Thorax 48:39-43
43. De Mello, D Reid LM (1994) Development, growing and aging of the lung. In: Saldanan (ed) Pathology of pulmonary disease. JB Lippincott, Philadelphia, pp 15-24
44. Resta M, Allegritti E, Pelosi P, Brazzi L, Gattinoni L (1998) Effetti dell'età sulla funzionalità respiratoria durante anestesia generale in soggetti normali. In: Braschi A, Gattinoni L, Pesenti A et al (Eds) Proceeding of SMART. Springer-Verlag, Milan, p 34
45. Suratt PM, Wilhoit SC, Hsiao HS et al (1984) Compliance of chest wall in obese subjects. J Appl Physiol 57:403-407
46. Naimark A, Cherniack RM (1960) Compliance of respiratory system and its components in health and obesity. J Appl Physiol 15:377-382
47. Sharp JT, Henry JP, Sweany SK et al (1964) The total work of breathing in normal and obese man. J Clin Invest 43:728-739
48. Pelosi P, Croci M, Ravagnan I, Vicardi P, Gattinoni L (1996) Total respiratory system, lung, and chest wall mechanics in sedated-paralyzed postoperative morbidly obese patients. Chest 109:144-151
49. Hedenstierna G, Santesson J (1976) Breathing mechanics, dead space and gas-exchange in extremely obese, breathing spontaneously and during anaesthesia with intermittent positive pressure ventilation. Acta Anaesthesiol Scand 20:248-254
50. Pelosi P, Croci M, Ravagnan I, Tredici S, Pedoto A, Lissoni A, Gattinoni L (1998) The effects of body mass on lung volumes, respiratory mechanics, and gas exchange during general anaesthesia. Anesth Analg 87:654-660
51. Horner RL, Mohiaddin RH, Lowell DG, Shea SA, Burman ED, Longmore DB, Guz A (1989) Sites and sizes of fat deposits around the pharynx in obese patients with obstructive sleep apnea and weight matched controls. Eur Respir J 2:613-622
52. Pelosi P, Croci M, Ravagnan I, Pedoto A, Lissoni A, Gattinoni L (1998) Positive end-expiratory pressure improves respiratory function in sedated-paralyzed morbidly obese patients. Anesthesiology (in press)
53. Rochester DF (1995) Obesity and abdominal distention. In: Roussos C (ed) The thorax. Marcel Dekker, New York, pp 1951-1973
54. Lynch S, Brand L, Levy A (1959) Changes in lung-thorax compliance during orthopedic surgery. Anesthesiology 20:278-282
55. Safar P, Agusto-Escarraga L (1959) Compliance in apneic anesthetized adults. Anesthesiology 20:283-289
56. Pelosi P, Croci M, Calappi E, Cerisara M, Mulazzi D, Vicardi P, Gattinoni L (1995) The prone position during general anaesthesia minimally affects respiratory mechanics while improving functional residual capacity and increasing oxygen tension. Anaesth Analg 80:956-960
57. Pelosi P, Croci M, Calappi E, Mulazzi D, Cerisara M, Vercesi P, Vicardi P, Gattinoni L (1996) Prone positioning improves pulmonary function in obese patients during general anaesthesia. Anesth Analg 83:578-583
58. The southern surgeon club (1991) A prospective analysis of 1518 laparoscopic cholecystectomies. New Engl J Med 324:1073-1078
59. Cunningham AJ (1993) Laparoscopic cholecystectomy: anaesthetic implications. Anesth Analg 76:1120-1123

60. Drummond GB, Martin LVH (1978) Pressure-volume relationship in the lung during laparoscopy. Br J Anaesth 50:261-270
61. Puri GD, Singh H (1992) Ventilatory effects of laparoscopy under general anaesthesia. Br J Anaesth 68:211-213
62. Pelosi P, Foti G, Cereda M, Vicardi P, Gattinoni L (1996) Effects of carbon dioxide insufflation for laparoscopic cholecystectomy on the respiratory system. Anaesthesia 51:744-749

Chapter 4

Resistance measurements. Forced oscillations and plethysmography

R. PESLIN

Whether a subject breathes spontaneously or is artificially ventilated, the pressure which must be applied to the respiratory system to ventilate (Prs) includes two basic components: 1) a static or elastic component (Pel) to sustain the elastic recoil of the lung and chest wall, as described elsewhere in this book; 2) a dynamic or resistive component (Pres) to provide for energy losses by friction occurring in the airways and in the tissues. While Pel is essentially related to the volume (V) of the system, Pres is basically a function of the rate of change of volume, that is of the flow ($\dot{V}$=dV/dt). At frequencies one order of magnitude larger than normal breathing frequency, the rate of change of flow (acceleration $\ddot{V}=d^2V/dt^2$) becomes comparatively large and the pressure necessary to accelerate or decelerate the gas and the tissues is no longer negligible; then, Prs includes a third inertial component (Pin), related to $\ddot{V}$. A classic "equation of motion" of the respiratory system is therefore the following [1]:

$$Prs = Pel + Pres + Pin = f_1(V) + f_2(\dot{V}) + f_3(\ddot{V}) \qquad (1)$$

where f_1, f_2 and f_3 are functions describing the relationships of Pel, Pres and Pin to V, $\dot{V}$ and $\ddot{V}$, respectively. Even in healthy subjects, f_1 and f_2 are rather complex functions because elastic and resistive properties of the system are interdependent, frequency-dependent, time-dependent, and non-linear. They are even more complex in patients whose lungs are mechanically nonhomogeneous. However, over a limited range of V, $\dot{V}$ and $\ddot{V}$, the system is well described, as a useful approximation, by the following linear relationship:

$$Prs = Ers \cdot (V-Vo) + Rrs \cdot \dot{V} + Irs \cdot \ddot{V} \qquad (2)$$

where Vo is the volume at which elastic recoil pressure is zero, and where Ers (total respiratory elastance), Rrs (total respiratory resistance) and Irs (total respiratory inertance) are constants which describe the elastic, frictional and inertial properties of the respiratory system. Therefore, by definition, Rrs is the coefficient of proportionality between Pres and $\dot{V}$. Similar Euations may be written for the various parts of the respiratory system-airways, lung tissue, lung (airways+lung tissue) and chest wall-and form the basis for the measurement of the corresponding resistances: airway resistance (Raw), lung tissue resistance, lung resistance, chest wall resistance. The objective of this chapter and of the next is to describe methods which may be used to measure some of these resistances. In the present chapter, I deal with the measurement of Raw by body plethysmography, and of Rrs by forced oscillations.

Measurement of airway resistance by body plethysmography

Airway resistance originates from frictional and other pressure losses in the gas flowing in either direction between the alveoli and the airway opening. These pressure losses depend on the flow, the flow regime (laminar, turbulent), the physical properties of the gas (viscosity, density) and the geometry of the airways.

Principle

The pressure drop along the airways (Paw) is the difference between mouth (Pmo) and alveolar (PA) pressures. It is related to both airway resistance (Raw) and gas inertia in the airways (Iaw):

$$\mathrm{Paw} = \mathrm{Pmo} - \mathrm{P_A} = \mathrm{Raw} \cdot \dot{V} + \mathrm{Iaw} \cdot \ddot{V} \tag{3}$$

At frequencies below a few Hertz, inertial phenomena are negligible and Paw is almost entirely related to Raw. Pmo and $\dot{V}$ are easily measured, but PA cannot be directly sampled, except in experimental situations [2]. The measurement of Raw in humans therefore relies upon an indirect estimate of PA [3], based upon measuring the changes of alveolar gas volume (TGV) induced by changes in PA (ΔPA). Indeed, according to Boyle's law (pressure times volume equal constant for a given mass of gas at constant temperature), any change in alveolar pressure will result in a change of alveolar gas volume (ΔV) in the opposite direction:

$$\Delta V = -\mathrm{TGV} \cdot \Delta \mathrm{P_A}/(\mathrm{P_B}-\mathrm{P_{H_2O}}) \tag{4}$$

where PB is barometric pressure and $\mathrm{PH_2O}$ is water vapor pressure in the alveoli. Then, combining Eqs. 3 and 4 and neglecting inertial effects:

$$\mathrm{Raw} = (\Delta V/\dot{V}) \cdot ((\mathrm{P_B}-\mathrm{P_{H_2O}})/\mathrm{TGV}) - \mathrm{Req} \tag{5}$$

where Req ($=-\mathrm{Pmo}/\dot{V}$) is the resistance of the instruments (i.e., flowmeter) connected to the airway. ΔV may be measured by using a whole body plethysmograph in which the subject is enclosed and breathes [3]; the plethysmograph will detect any difference between the volume of gas entering or leaving the airways and the corresponding external volume change of the body. The main problem with the method is that such differences may also originate from other causes, mainly:

- changes in temperature and water vapor pressure of the inspired or expired gas in the airways (thermal factor) [3-5];
- instantaneous differences between O_2 uptake and CO_2 output (gas exchange factor) [3, 6].

The first of these factors is particularly worrisome because the change in volume occurring when a tidal volume of 0.6 l at 50% water vapor saturation is conditioned to BTPS (at body temperature and pressure, saturated with water vapor) in the airways amounts to about 57 ml. This is much more than the ΔV resulting from alveolar pressure variations in healthy subjects (about 8 ml for a ΔPA of 2 hPa and a TGV of 4 l). Fortunately, because thermal exchanges are fast in the airways, the thermal component of ΔV is largely in phase with V [4, 5] while Pres is (by definition) in phase with $\dot{V}$. Different methods may be used to minimize these unwanted components of ΔV, as described later.

For computing ΔPA from the measured ΔV according to Eq. 4, it is necessary to know TGV. The latter may also be measured in the plethysmograph [7] by occluding the airway and asking the subject to make inspiratory and expiratory efforts against the occlusion. In that situation there is almost no gas flow in the airway and the variations in mouth pressure (ΔPmo) should closely reflect ΔPA. Then TGV may be obtained by a variant of Eq. 4:

$$TGV = -\Delta V \cdot (PB\text{-}PH_2O)/\Delta Pmo \qquad (6)$$

Equipment

Plethysmographs exist in different types according to the principle used to measure ΔV. Detailed technical specifications of these instruments may be found in a number of reports [8-10]. In the constant volume or pressure-type plethysmograph (Fig. 1), the chamber (or "box") is completely closed, except for a small leak to avoid pressure build-up in relation to the heat released by the subject. Then ΔV will result in pressure changes in the chamber; the latter are expressed in terms of volume changes after proper calibration. In other instruments, the chamber is connected either to a flowmeter (flow-type plethysmo-

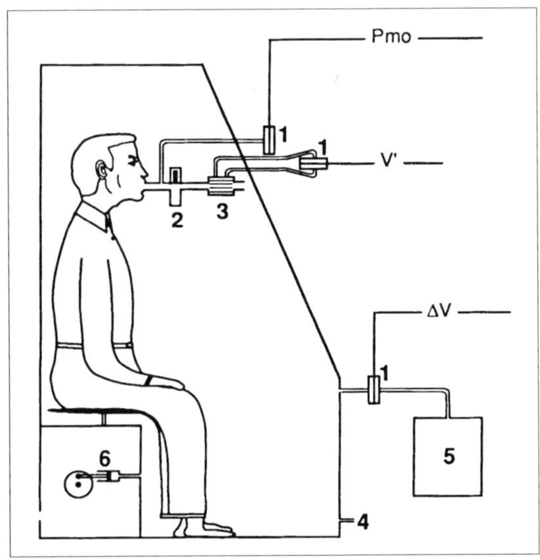

Fig. 1. Constant-volume body plethysmograph. (1) Pressure transducers; (2) flow interruptor; (3) flowmeter; (4) leak; (5) reference chamber; (6) calibration pump; *Pmo*, mouth pressure; $\dot{V}$, airway flow; *ΔV*, plethysmographic volume signal

graph) or to a spirometer (volume-type plethysmograph). These instruments are sometimes referred to as constant pressure plethysmographs, which is improper because some pressure difference is necessary to drive gas through the flowmeter or the spirometer. With flow-type plethysmographs the signal is integrated analogically or digitally to obtain ΔV. All three types have their limitations in terms of the frequency range over which they may accurately measure volume changes. In the pressure-type plethysmograph the relationship between the signal and the actual ΔV decreases when the frequency decreases; this is due both to the leaks and to the fact that the gas compression regime in the chamber switches from being isothermal (Boyle's law) at low frequency to being adiabatic (Poisson's law, 40% "stiffer" gas) when the frequency increases. Common pressure plethysmographs are unsafe below 0.2 Hz, unless they have been calibrated at the frequency of interest. In contrast, flow and volume plethysmographs are reliable at low frequencies only. This is due to gas compression in the chamber related to the above-mentioned pressure changes necessary to drive the gas through the flowmeter or spirometer. The output of these instruments may be corrected by adding to the measured ΔV an estimate of the part lost by compression [11], computed from box pressure changes and from the compliance of the gas in the box (Vbox/1.4 PB for adiabatic compression, with Vbox the volume of gas in the box).

Beside the chamber and its transducer, the set-up includes a breathing circuit comprising, from the mouthpiece outward: a pressure tap connected to a transducer for measuring Pmo (Eq. 6), a flow interruptor (or shutter) to occlude the airway when measuring TGV, and a flowmeter with its differential pressure transducer to measure $\dot{V}$(Fig. 1).

While measuring $\dot{V}$ and Pmo does not pose many difficulties, such is not the case for ΔV which, as mentioned above, is of the order 6 ml in normal adults breathing quietly. In a common 600 l constant volume plethysmograph, the corresponding change in box pressure is about 0.01 hPa, which is barely one order of magnitude above ambient pressure noise in a quiet building. With flow-type plethysmographs, the pressure drop across the flowmeter (usually a large screen set in the wall of the box) is still smaller. It is therefore necessary to use very sensitive and stable pressure transducers with a high signal-to-noise ratio. The influence of the ambient noise may be decreased by connecting the other side of the transducer to a reference chamber having a similar response to ambient noise (Fig. 1). With volume-type plethysmographs, a spirometric system specially adapted to measuring small volume changes should be used. For all types, the structure of the box should be such that its volume changes in response to transmural pressure variations or motion of the subject are minimal. Finally, the dynamic responses of the box (after correction for gas compression in the flow-type and volume-type instruments) and that of the other channels should be well matched up to 2 Hz for measurements during quiet breathing, and up to 5 Hz for measurements during panting (see later).

Thermal component of ΔV

Several methods have been proposed to minimize or eliminate the thermal component of ΔV.

- The *panting method* [3] consists in having the subject rebreathe with a small tidal volume and high frequency (typically 0.3 l at 2 Hz) through a large instrumental dead space. It is believed that, provided the front of gas remains inside the dead space, the thermal and water vapor exchanges are minimal. It has been shown, however, that the thermal factor is still substantial at 2 Hz [5], which leads to some underestimation of Raw. In many subjects, particularly those with airway obstruction, panting is accompanied by a progressive undesirable increase in TGV. On the other hand, panting increases the signal-to-noise ratio and keeps the glottis wide-open [12].
- *Conditioning the inspired gas to BTPS* [13]: for this, the breathing circuit is connected to a gas conditioner maintaining inspired air saturated with water vapor at 37°C. With this method, measurements may be performed during normal breathing. Rebreathing from a closed circuit also decreases the variations of respiratory exchange ratio during the respiratory cycle and minimizes the gas exchange factor [3].
- *Correcting the data*: the thermal component of ΔV is not strictly in phase with volume [4, 5], but contaminates the resistive component in phase with flow. Corrections based on subtracting from ΔV a term proportional to volume [14] are therefore inadequate. On the other hand, most of the thermal artefact may be eliminated using a correction based on the inspired gas mean temperature and on a thermal time constant of 100-200 ms, depending on the equipment [15].

Calibration

Pressure plethysmographs are usually provided with a small reciprocating pump delivering a fixed stroke volume (20-100 ml) at a frequency of 1-3 Hz (Fig. 1). This permits calibrating pressure changes in the box in terms of volume changes. If the calibration is performed when the box is empty, a correction factor must be applied to account for the decrease in Vbox when the subject is inside. Volume plethysmographs are calibrated with a syringe and flow plethysmographs may be calibrated either using rotameters, or more conveniently by the so-called integral method using a syringe [16].

Protocol

Once the subject is seated inside the box and the box is closed, a waiting period of 1-2 min is allowed for reaching thermal equilibrium, as shown by a reasonably stable box pressure or volume signal, or by a box flow signal close to zero. Box calibration is performed while the subject holds his breath. Then, the subject is asked to place the mouthpiece in position and to support each cheek with one hand. The shutter is closed at end-expiration for a period of 2-5 s to record the ΔV/Pmo relationship (Eq. 6) while the subject makes breathing efforts with an amplitude of about 10 hPa and a frequency of 1-2 Hz (1 Hz is preferable in subjects with severe airway obstruction to minimize the difference between Pmo and PA [18]). Subsequently, the shutter is opened and the subject is asked to continue panting or to breathe quietly for a few seconds (depending on the method used to eliminate the thermal component of ΔV) while the $\Delta V/\dot{V}$ relationship (Eq. 5) is recorded. Both the ΔV/Pmo and $\Delta V/\dot{V}$ relationships must be closely inspected and, unless digital drift correction is provided, measurements with excessive drift of ΔV should be rejected. ΔV/Pmo relationships should be linear with minimal phase lag. Glottis closure or occlusion of the mouthpiece with the tongue are frequent causes of faulty manoeuvers. $\Delta V/\dot{V}$ may be non-linear, asymmetrical, and present a substantial degree of looping in severely obstructive patients (Fig. 2a). Three to five satisfactory measurements are usually obtained. Variants of this protocol may be used but it is essential that ΔV/Pmo and $\Delta V/\dot{V}$ are measured at precisely the same lung volume, or that any change in volume between the two measurements is measured and used to correct the value of TGV entered in Eq. 5.

Data Processing

All modern plethysmographic equipment include a computer system to record and analyze the signals. After proper low-pass analog filtering, the signals are sampled and digitized at a frequency of 50-200 Hz by an analog-digital conversion board connected to the computer. The signals are usually visualized so that poorly performed manoeuvers or excessively drifting records may be rejected. A moderate drift may be eliminated by the computer programme [19]. The data analysis consists in computing the slopes of the ΔV/Pmo and $\Delta V/\dot{V}$ relationships. For ΔV/Pmo, this is usually done by linear regression between the two variables. For $\Delta V/\dot{V}$, the problem is complicated by the fact that the relationship, as mentioned above, may be nonlinear, asymmetrical and exhibit some looping. Then, the relationship does not have a unique slope and may be characterized in various ways.

- By computing the slope over a specific range of flows, most frequently ±0.5 l/s (Fig. 2b).
- By relating the difference between the inspiratory and expiratory maxima of ΔV to the difference between the flows at the same instants ("total" Raw or Raw, tot [20]) (Fig. 2a). This approach has been proposed for the case where the expiratory limb of the $\Delta V/\dot{V}$ relationship exhibits a substantial amount of looping, suggesting the occurrence of expiratory flow limitation. Then, it expresses the resistance of the compressed airways and the result is likely to be effort-dependent.
- By computing the effective resistance (Raw,eff) as obtained from the ratio of the area of ΔV/V loop to the area of the $\dot{V}$/V loop (where V is obtained by integrating the flow signal) [21]. This approach may also be useful when $\Delta V/\dot{V}$ is nonlinear or exhibits some looping. Then, Raw,eff is the value of the constant resistance which would give the same amount of mechanical work as that corresponding to the observed $\Delta V/\dot{V}$.

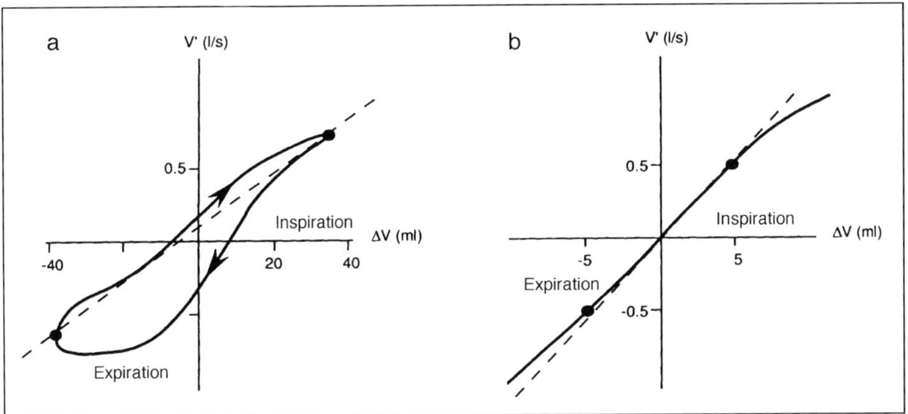

Fig. 2 a,b. Computation of $\Delta V/\dot{V}$ slope for Raw measurements (a) from the extremes of ΔV (b) in the ±0.5 l/s flow range

Whatever the method used to characterize the slopes of the $\Delta V/\dot{V}$ (S1) and $\Delta V/Pmo$ (S_2) relationships, the value of Raw is obtained by combining Eqs. 5 and 6:

$$Raw = -(S_1/S_2) - Req \tag{7}$$

Req may be either measured separately or obtained on the same respiratory cycles as Raw by recording simultaneously Pmo and computing the slope of the $Pmo/\dot{V}$ relationship.

Raw is usually expressed in hPa s/l. Raw has been shown to decrease with increasing lung volume [22], due to the increasing outward stress applied by lung tissue or intrathoracic pressure around the airways. To take this factor into account, one frequently computes specific airway resistance (sRaw) as given by the product of Raw and TGV (units of hPa s). When Req is comparatively low and may be neglected, an approximate value of sRaw may be obtained directly from Eq 5 by multiplying $\Delta V/\dot{V}$ by PB-PH_2O. Then, one may dispense with the occlusions manoeuvers necessary to measure TGV. Beside Raw and sRaw, one may also express the results in terms of their reciprocals, airway conductance (Gaw=1/Raw, units of $l\ s^{-1}\ hPa^{-1}$) and specific airway conductance (sGaw=1/sRaw, units of $hPa^{-1}\ s^{-1}$).

Reference values

Airway resistance exhibits a substantial intra-individual [19] and interindividual variability and is poorly related to age and stature in adults. The mean, standard deviation (SD) and limits of normality (mean plus or minus 1.64 SD) of Raw and sGaw in adult men and women with the panting method, obtained by pooling the data from a number of studies [3, 13, 23-28], are given in Table 1, along with the values observed in a large series of healthy subjects during quiet

Table 1. Airway resistance and specific conductance in normals

Sex	Raw (hPa s/l)			sGaw (hPa^{-1} s^{-1})		
	N	*Mean ± SD*	*Upper Limit*	*N*	*Mean ± SD*	*Lower Limit*
Panting method[a]						
Male	145	1.40±0.48	>2.19	198	0.216±0.080	<0.085
Female	36	1.50±0.48	>2.28	65	0.231±0.078	<0.104
Quiet breathing[b]						
Male	908	1.81±0.61	>2.81	–	–	–
Female	281	1.99±0.59	>2.96	–	–	–

[a] Data pooled from a number of small series [3, 13, 23-28]
[b] Amrein et al. [29]

breathing by Amrein et al. [29]. For both men and women, the upper limit of normality of Raw is about 2.2 hPa s/l with the panting method and 3.0 hPa.s/l when measurements are made during quiet breathing with the inspired gas conditioned to BTPS. The difference probably reflects the influence of panting on laryngeal resistance [12]. In contrast with adults, Raw is significantly correlated to body height (H) in children, and the following relationships have been obtained by Tammeling and Quanjer [30] who compiled data from the literature: Raw=7.0 $H^{-2.5}$ hPa s/l; Gaw=0.143 $H^{2.5}$ l hPa^{-1} s^{-1} s; Gaw=0.25 $H^{-0.2}$ hPa^{-1} s^{-1} (H is expressed in m).

Measurement of total respiratory resistance by forced oscillations

As mentioned above (Eq. 2), total respiratory resistance (Rrs) is the coefficient of proportionality between the resistive component of the pressure applied to the total respiratory system (Prs) and the gas flow in the airways. Prs is the difference between mouth pressure (Pmo) and the pressure applied to the passive structures of the chest wall. The latter is the sum of the pressure at the body surface (Pbs, usually equal to PB) and of the combined stresses applied to these structures by the respiratory muscles (Pmus):

$$\text{Prs} = \text{Pmo} - (\text{Pmus} + \text{Pbs}) \qquad (8)$$

As Pmus cannot be directly measured there are only two possibilities for obtaining Prs. The first is to measure Prs during artificial ventilation in subjects who voluntarily relax their respiratory muscles or are paralysed (Pmus=0). The second is the forced oscillation (FO) method [31] which may be applied during spontaneous breathing. Additional advantages of the method are that it is strictly noninvasive, requires only passive cooperation from the subject, and in contrast with spirometric maneuvers [32], does not modify the bronchomotor tone [33]. For these reasons, it is increasingly used to explore bronchial reactivity, particularly in children [34-37]. In addition, as measurements may be done over a large range of frequencies, it provides information on the frequency dependence of resistance, a characteristic feature of mechanical nonhomogeneity of the lung [38, 39].

Principle

The FO method is based on: 1) the observation that the frequency content of Pmus during breathing is fairly narrow (about 0.2-2 Hz for quiet breathing) [40]; and 2) the possibility to separate the various frequency components of a signal, using Fourier harmonic analysis. The method consists in applying flow or pressure variations to the respiratory system at frequencies outside the range of Pmus, and in extracting and analysing the corresponding frequency components of Prs and $\dot{V}$.

If one applies to the respiratory system with an external generator a sinusoidal flow input having a frequency (f) outside the frequency range of Pmus, and an amplitude ($\dot{V}o$) small enough to ensure linear behaviour:

$$\dot{V}_f = \dot{V}o \cdot \sin(\omega t) \tag{9}$$

with $\omega=2\pi f$, then the resulting component of Prs (Prs_f) is also a sine wave:

$$Prs_f = Po \cdot \sin(\omega t+\varphi) \tag{10}$$

with an amplitude (Po) and a phase with respect to $\dot{V}_f$ (φ) which depends on the resistive, elastic and inertive properties of the system (Fig. 3). The relationship between Prs_f and $\dot{V}_f$ is called the total respiratory impedance at frequency f (Zrs); it is characterized by the amplitude ratio of the variables, also called the modulus of the impedance ($Po/\dot{V}o$ denoted $|Zrs|$), and by the phase angle or argument (φ). Using the simple trigonometric relationship $\sin(a+b)=\sin(a)\cos(b)+\cos(a)\sin(b)$, Prs_f may be written as the sum of two terms, a sine term which is in phase with $\dot{V}_f$, and a cosine or out-of-phase term which is in phase with acceleration:

$$Prs = Po \cdot \cos(\varphi) \cdot \sin(\omega t) + Po \cdot \sin(\varphi) \cdot \cos(\omega t) \tag{11}$$

Identifying Eq. 11 with the simple linear model of the respiratory system (Eq. 2), the first term corresponds to the resistive component of Prs (in-phase with flow):

$$Po \cdot \cos(\varphi) \cdot \sin(\omega t) = Rrs \cdot \dot{V}o \cdot \sin(\omega t) \tag{12}$$

from which:

$$|Zrs| \cdot \cos(\varphi) = Rrs \tag{13}$$

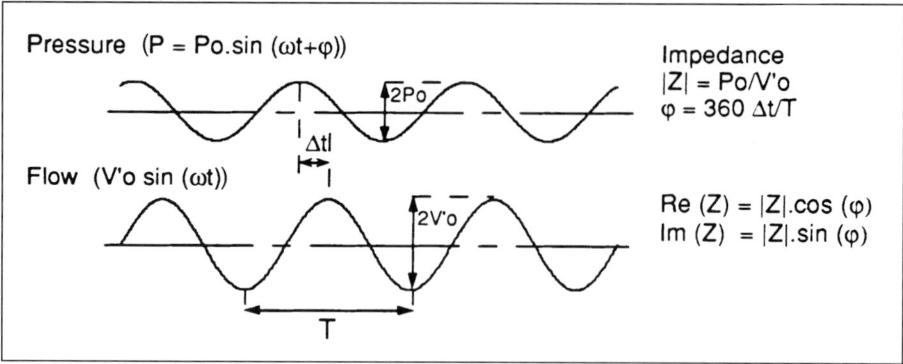

Fig. 3. Relationship between flow and pressure signals when measuring a mechanical impedance by forced oscillations with a sinusoidal input. *Po* and *V'o*, amplitude of pressure and flow signals, respectively; ω, circular frequency ($\omega=2\pi f$ with *f* the oscillation frequency); *T=1/f Δt*, time elapsed between pressure and flow maxima or minima. */Z/* and *φ*, modulus and phase of impedance, respectively; *Re(Z)* and *Im(Z)*, real and imaginary parts of impedance, respectively

Then, Rrs may easily be computed from the amplitude ratio and phase angle of pressure and flow. |Zrs|•cos (φ) is the real or resistive part of the impedance (Re(Zrs)).

The second term in Eq. 11 corresponds to the sum of the elastic and inertive pressures. The components of V and $\dot{V}$ at frequency f being $V_f = -\dot{V}o \cdot \cos(\omega t)/\omega$' and $\ddot{V}_f = \dot{V}o \cdot \omega \cdot \cos(\omega t)$, one may easily show that:

$$|Zrs| \cdot \sin(\varphi) = Irs \cdot \omega - Ers/\omega \tag{14}$$

from which Irs and Ers may be computed provided measurements are made at two or more oscillation frequencies. |Zrs|•sin(φ) is the imaginary part of the impedance (Im(Zrs)), also called reactance (Xrs).

Respiratory impedance may be characterized either by |Zrs| and φ, or, more commonly, by Re(Zrs) and Im(Zrs). The first set may be derived from the second by:

$$|Zrs| = [Re(Zrs)^2 + Im(Zrs)^2]^{1/2} \tag{15}$$

$$\varphi = \tan^{-1} [Im\,(Zrs)/Re\,(Zrs)] \tag{16}$$

Pressure oscillations may be applied at the airway opening or around the chest wall. Also, one may measure airway flow or chest flow. There are, therefore, several ways to perform forced oscillation measurements [41]; the resulting impedances are different, due to alveolar gas compression. Eq. 2 and the derived Eqs. 13 and 14 are not an acceptable model of the respiratory system at high frequencies, when pressure is applied at one end of the system and flow is measured at the other end (transfer Zrs: its real part becomes negative at about 35 Hz in humans). In what follows, I will only consider the measurement of Rrs by applying pressure oscillations at the airway opening, and measuring flow at the same place (input impedance), which is by far the most usual approach. Also, I will keep to pressure oscillations at frequencies in the range between the highest harmonics of spontaneous breathing (>3 Hz) and 40 Hz. The validity of Eq. 2 also deteriorates at higher frequencies, due to acoustic resonance in the airways [42].

Equipment

A typical FO set-up, as described by Grimby et al. [43], is shown in Figure 4. It includes a pressure or flow generator connected to the subject's airway by a flowmeter. Airway pressure is sampled at a tap next to the mouthpiece. The subject breathes through a side tube branched between the flowmeter and the generator; the length and diameter of the tube are such that it has low impedance at breathing frequencies (low resistance) and, to minimize the loss of FO signal, high impedance at the oscillation frequencies (high inertance). To avoid rebreathing, the circuit may be rinsed by a bias flow from a high impedance source. Commonly, the generator is made of a powerful loud-speaker (50-100 W) enclosed in a box and supplied with the excitation signal through a power amplifier, but small reciprocating pumps have also been used [31]. Nowadays, the set-up is always completed by a computer equipped with digital-analog and analog-digital conversion boards, which are used to generate the excitation signal and to sample, digitize and analyse the pressure and flow signals.

FO measurements require much higher dynamic performances from the pressure and flow transducers than measurements during spontaneous breathing. Ideally, the pressure and flow should be measured with minimal amplitude (±2%) and phase (±2°) distortion up to the highest excitation frequency, or their

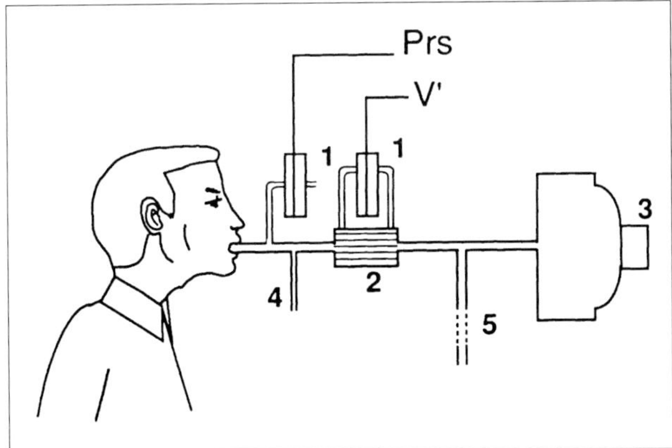

Fig. 4. Typical set-up to measure total respiratory impedance. (1) pressure transducer; (2) flowmeter; (3) pressure generator (loud speaker); (4) high impedance bias flow line to minimize rebreathing; (5) side tube for spontaneous breathing

amplitude and phase responses should be measured and corrected for. The response of pressure transducers depends heavily upon the length and diameters of the connecting tubes and must be reassessed if they are modified [44]. Among resistive flowmeters, the screen-type has a good frequency response provided the pressure taps are placed extremely close to the screen, but the Fleisch capillary type is equivalent to a resistance-inertance (R-I) system with a I/R ratio of about 2.1 ms, and requires correction above a few Hz [45]. Another problem with flowmeters is the so-called common mode rejection ratio (CMRR) [46]. The difference to be measured across the resistive element by a differential pressure transducer is typically one order of magnitude lower than the pressure oscillations applied to the subject. Measuring accurately a small difference between two large signals requires a transducer with high dynamic symmetry. The latter is assessed by applying the same signal to both sides of the transducer simultaneously and taking the ratio between the amplitude of the observed signal (A1, ideally zero) and that of the applied pressure (A2):CMRR=20 log A2/A1 (dB). The CMRR required for accurate measurements depends on the relative impedances of the flowmeter and of the subject. For common flowmeters, it should be at least 60 dB for measurements in moderately obstructive patients. As the best CMRR achievable with available differential transducers is about 70 dB, it is technically difficult to make measurements in highly obstructive patients. An easy way to check if the CMRR is adequate in practice is to see if the data remain the same (except for the sign) when connecting the proximal side of the transducer to the distal pressure tap of the flowmeter and vice versa. It is also profitable to test frequently the equipment on a known and steady mechanical analog of the respiratory system. Calibration methods have been described to assess the response of the equipment and to correct the data [47]. At large frequencies, the classic pressure and flow measurements may be replaced by the measurement of the pressures at both ends of a long rigid tube [48]. A number of recommendations concerning the technical characteristics of FO set-ups have been issued by a working group of the EEC (European Economic Community) [49].

Various types of excitation signals may be used. The simplest is a sine wave, which provides a value of Rrs at a single frequency (generally between 5 and 20 Hz). It is sufficient for a number of porposes, and allows following the changes of Rrs during breathing with a time resolution equal to the reciprocal of the frequency [50]. When measurements at several frequencies are needed, either to study the frequency dependence of Rrs, or to compute Ers and Irs, one may either repeat the measurements with different sine waves, or use a signal containing either an infinity of random frequency components (white noise [51]) or a predetermined set of frequencies (pseudorandom noise (PRN) [52]). In cases where the respiratory system is strongly non-linear, it is better to use noninteger-multiple frequency components to avoid "cross-talk" between frequencies [53]. To promote linear behaviour, the peak-to-peak amplitude of the applied pressure input is usually limited to 2 hPa. An example of recording is shown in Figure 5.

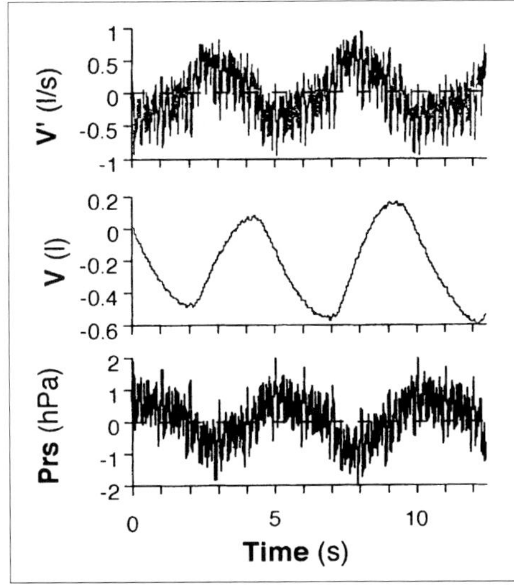

Fig. 5. Recording during forced oscillation measurements. Input signal is the sum of 10 sine waves with noninteger-multiple frequencies ranging from 4 to 29 Hz. *V'*, flow; *V*, volume; *Prs*, pressure applied to the respiratory system

Upper airway artefact

Beside the adequacy of the equipment, the most serious problem when measuring Rrs by the forced oscillation method, particularly in patients, is the shunt impedance of upper airway walls [54]. Indeed, the walls of the mouth cavity, pharynx, and upper trachea constitute an elastic pathway in parallel with the respiratory system, such that part of the flow passing through the flowmeter does not enter the chest. According to the association of impedances in parallel (Ohm's law):

$$Zrs^{\circ} = Zrs \cdot Zuaw/(Zrs + Zuaw) \quad (17)$$

where Zrs° is the measured impedance and Zuaw is the lumped impedance of upper airway wall. The difference between Zrs° and Zrs is larger when Zrs is high and Zuaw is low. Typically, the upper airway walls have a resistance around 20 hPa s/l at 4 Hz, decreasing to about 10 hPa s/l at 20-30 Hz, and a reactance increasing from -50 hPa s/l at 4 Hz to almost 0 at 30 Hz [55]. The resulting error may be quite substantial in obstructive patients, even if they support their cheeks with the palms to increase Zuaw: the upper airway shunt is responsible for a frequency-dependent underestimation of Rrs and a shift to the right of the reactance curve [54]. Two approaches may be used to decrease the artefact.

- Measure Zuaw and correct the data for it [51]. Zuaw may be obtained by measuring the input impedance at the mouth when the subject performs a Valsalva manoeuver to close tightly the glottis (Zrs tending to infinity). Then, except for the compressibility of the small amount of gas in the upper airway, what is measured is the impedance of airway walls. The problem with this approach is that it requires much cooperation from the subject.
- Apply the pressure input around the head ("head generator" method) instead of at the mouth (Fig. 6) [56]. In so doing, except for the small pressure drop

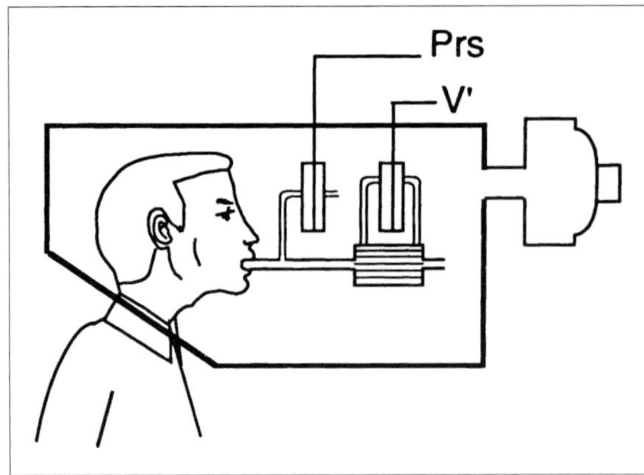

Fig. 6. Measurement of respiratory input impedance with head generator to decrease the upper airway shunt. The pressure input is applied around the head so as to minimize transmural pressure across upper airway walls

across the flowmeter and along the upper airways themselves, the same pressure is applied inside and outside the upper airway walls, which minimizes their motion. The head generator improves the sensitivity of FO measurements of Rrs during bronchomotor challenges in children [36].

Protocol

The measurements are usually performed in sitting subjects wearing a noseclip and, unless a head generator is used, supporting firmly their cheeks and mouth floor without compressing the pharynx. Neck flexion and hyperextension should be avoided. The sampling period usually covers a few respiratory cycles (typically 15-30 s) and, if possible, the measurements are repeated 3-4 times to assess the variability and reject outlying data.

Data analysis

The pressure and flow signal are first analogically low-pass filtered to eliminate all the frequency components (noise) above the frequencies of interest. Then, they are sampled and digitized at a rate which is usually 8-16 points per oscillation cycle for a sinusoidal input, and a little above twice the highest frequency of interest for multifrequency signals. The digitized signals are high-pass filtered to eliminate the low-frequency breathing components. For a sinusoidal input, the Fourier coefficients of Prs (Ap, Bp) and $\dot{V}$(Av, Bv) are computed at the frequency of interest by:

$$A = \sum_{i=1}^{k \cdot n} X_i \cdot \cos(2 \cdot \pi \cdot i/n) \quad (18)$$

$$B = \sum_{i=1}^{k \cdot n} Xi \cdot \sin(2 \cdot \pi \cdot i/n) \quad (19)$$

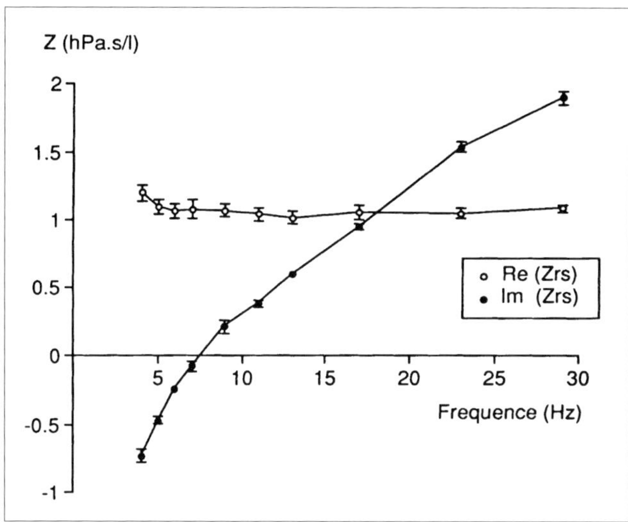

Fig. 7. Impedance data obtained in a healthy subject with an input pressure signal containing 10 noninteger-multiple frequencies applied at the mouth (Fig. 5). Data corrected for upper airway shunt; mean values and standard deviations of 7 consecutive measurements

where k is the number of oscillation cycles over which the analysis is made, n is the number of points sampled per cycle, and X stands for either Prs or $\dot{V}$. For multifrequency signals, this is achieved at all frequencies of interest using a classic algorithm, the fast discrete Fourier transform [57]. In both instances, the Fourier coefficients are combined to obtain Re(Zrs) and Im(Zrs) at each frequency component:

$$\text{Re (Zrs)} = (\text{Ap} \cdot \text{Av}+\text{Bp} \cdot \text{Bv})/(\text{Av}^2+\text{Bv}^2) \quad (20)$$

$$\text{Im (Zrs)} = (\text{Bv} \cdot \text{Ap}-\text{Bp} \cdot \text{Av})/(\text{Av}^2+\text{Bv}^2) \quad (21)$$

Variants of these equations may also be used [58]. Finally, when necessary, the data are corrected for the frequency response of the equipment and for the impedance of upper airway walls, if available. Beside Re(Zrs) and Im(Zrs), it is usual to compute a coherence function [51] which expresses how tight is the relationship between pressure and flow, and may be used as a criterion to reject noisy data. These computations are performed on-line in a matter of seconds or less, and the data are immediately displayed for inspection. An example of impedance data from 4 to 29 Hz in a healthy subject is shown in Figure 7.

Interpretation of Rrs measurements

Abnormalities of tissue resistance in the usual frequency range (4-40 Hz) of FO measurements have not been described. Threfore, an increased Rrs points to airway obstruction. Studying the frequency dependence of Rrs may provide some additional information. In normal subjects Rrs varies little over that frequency range. Assuming that the measurements are technically correct and that the upper airway artefact has been properly eliminated, a negative frequency dependence of Rrs suggests a systematic change in the distribution of the flow oscillation in the lung with increasing frequency. This may occur either because the lung is mechanically nonhomogeneous [38], or because, due to severe peripheral airway obstruction, an increasing part of the flow is shunted by the compliant walls of the intra-thoracic airways [39]. There are observations in favour of the second mechanism in chronic obstructive pulmonary disease (COPD) patients [51, 59]. One may consider three types of abnormalities: 1) an increased Rrs without negative frequency dependence suggests central airways obstruction; 2) an increased Rrs at the lowest frequencies only, with a negative frequency dependence, suggests peripheral airway obstruction; and 3) an increased Rrs at all frequencies, but predominating at lower frequencies, suggests a combination of central and peripheral airway obstruction.

Indices and reference values

When multifrequency inputs are used, Rrs is usually averaged over some frequency range. It is sometimes expressed in terms of its reciprocal, total respiratory conductance (Grs), but specific values (Rrs•TGV) are rarely computed because TGV is not available. The frequency dependence of Rrs may be expressed by the slope of the Rrs-f curve over some frequency range (units of hPa•s^2/l). Then, the intercept of the slope at f=0, termed zero-frequency Rrs (Ro), is usually reported. Alternatively, the Rrs-f curve is caracterized by the coefficients of a mechanistic model [60]. Prediction equations for Rrs derived from observations in healthy adults and children are given in Table 2. Rrs was found to vary significantly with body height in adults and with the square of body height during growth in children.

Table 2. Prediction equations of total respiratory resistance (hPa s/l)

Subjects	Sex	N	Equation	SD	Reference
Adults					
	male	407[a]	2.50	0.60	[52]
		126[a]	8.73 - 0.034 H	0.64	[61]
		110[b]	7.64 - 0.030 H	0.61	[62]
	female	100[a]	3.05	0.60	[61]
		105[b]	6.98 - 0.024 H	0.83	[62]
Children					
	male	58[c]	$6.79\ 10^4\ H^{-1.93}$	–	[63]
	female	63[c]	$2.22\ 10^5\ H^{-2.17}$	–	[63]
	both	138[d]	$9.3\ 10^{-4}\ H^2 - 0.342\ H + 34.9$	–	[64]

SD, residual standard deviation; *H*, height in cm
[a] Mean Rrs from 4 to 24 Hz, pressure applied at the mouth
[b] At 10 Hz, pressure applied around the head
[c] At 3-10 Hz, pressure applied at the mouth
[d] Mean Rrs from 6 to 10 Hz

Plethysmography or forced oscillations?

Of the two techniques described in this chapter, which should be recommended? Each has its merits and drawbacks.

Equipment

The FO method is cheaper but a body plethysmograph may also be used for other purposes.

Technical difficulty

Both are technically rather demanding. Basically, the signal-to-noise ratio of plethysmographic measurements is low and a well-designed body box is necessary to measure Raw in normal humans (smaller signal than in patients) with an acceptable accuracy. With FO, the signal-to-noise ratio is good, but the best differential pressure transducers used in the best conditions are barely good enough for measuring the high impedances of certain patients. Note that plethysmographic measurements are technically more difficult in normals, and FO measurements are more difficult in patients.

Physiological artefacts

The thermal factor is a substantial cause of error in plethysmography, particularly in normals where the error is relatively large. With FO, an artefactual negative frequency dependence of Rrs may be created by the upper airway shunt, particularly in obstructive patients. Again, plethysmography is easier in patients and FO is easier in normals. Both artefacts may be avoided, but it takes some additional equipment and trouble.

Practicality

FO is easier for the subject and somewhat faster. Data analysis was difficult in the past, particularly for FO, but no longer presents a problem nowadays with digital data processing.

Information

Plethysmography is more specific but provides a value of Raw at a single frequency; measurements may be repeated at intervals of a few seconds to study fast changes in airway patency. FO is less specific, but provides additional information which may help locating the problem; it has potentially a much higher time resolution.

And why not both together?

Estimating alveolar pressure changes by plethysmography during forced oscillation measurements has been recently proposed to partition Zrs into its airway and tissue components [65]. The thermal artefact of plethysmography was eliminated by breathing BTPS gas, and the upper airway artefact of FO by correcting the data for Zuaw. The method makes its possible to study the frequency dependence of both airways and tissue resistances and reactances. It appears to be reliable in healthy subjects, but has not yet been evaluated in patients.

References

1. Mead J, Milic-Emili J (1964) Theory and methodology in respiratory mechanics with glossary of symbols. In: Fenn WO, Rahn H (eds) Respiration. Handbook of Physiology. Vol I. American Physiological Society, Washington DC, pp 363-376
2. Fredberg JJ, Keefe DH, Glass GM, Castile RG, Frantz ID (1984) Alveolar pressure nonhomogeneity during small-amplitude high-frequency oscillation. J Appl Physiol 57:788-800
3. DuBois AB, Botelho SY, Comroe JH (1956) A new method for measuring airway resistance in man using a body plethysmograph: values in normal subjects and in patients with respiratory disease. J Clin Invest 35:327-335
4. Peslin R, Jardin P, Hannhart B (1976) Modeling of the relationship between volume variations at the mouth and chest. J Appl Physiol 41:659-667
5. Peslin R, Duvivier C, Vassiliou M, Gallina C (1995) Thermal artifacts in plethysmographic airway resistance measurements. J Appl Physiol 79:1958-1965
6. Jaeger MJ, Bouhuys A (1969) Loop formation in pressure vs. flow diagrams obtained by body plethysmography. In: DuBois AB, Van de Woestijne KP (eds) Progress in respiration research. Vol 4. Karger, Basel, pp 116-130
7. DuBois AB, Botelho SY, Bedell GN, Marshall R, Comroe JH (1956) A rapid plethysmographic method for measuring thoracic gas volume: a comparison with a nitrogen washout method for measuring functional residual capacity in normal subjects. J Clin Invest 35:322-326
8. Comroe JH, Botelho SY, DuBois AB (1959) Design of a body plethysmograph for studying cardiopulmonary physiology. J Appl Physiol 14:439-444
9. Mead J (1960) Volume displacement plethysmograph for respiratory measurements in humans subjects. J Appl Physiol 15:736-740
10. Peslin R (1984) Body plethysmography. In: Techniques in the Life Sciences. Resp Physiol 4(14):1-26
11. Clément J, Van de Woestijne KP (1969) Pressure correction in volume and flow-displacement body plethysmography. J Appl Physiol 27:895-897
12. Stanescu DC, Pattijn J, Clément J, van de Woestijne KP (1972) Glottis opening and airway resistance. J Appl Physiol 32:460-466
13. Jaeger MJ, Otis AB (1964) Measurement of airway resistance with a volume displacement body plethysmograph. J Appl Physiol 19:813-820
14. Smidt U, Muysers K, Buchheim R (1969) Electronic compensation of differences in temperature and water vapor between inspired and expired air and other signal handling in body plethysmography. In: DuBois AB, Van de Woestijne KP (eds) Progress in respiration research. Vol 4. Karger, Basel, pp 39-49
15. Peslin R, Duvivier C, Malvestio P, Benis AB (1996) Correction of thermal artifacts in plethysmographic airway resistance measurements. J Appl Physiol 80:2198-2203
16. Varène P, Vieillefond H, Saumon G, Lafosse JE (1974) Etalonnage des pneumotachographes par méthode intégrale. Bull Physiopath Resp 10:349-360
17. Peslin R (1983) Lung mechanics II: resistance measurements. Bull Europ Physiopath Resp 19(Suppl 5):33-38

18. Stanescu DC, Rodenstein D, Caubergh M, Van de Woestijne KP (1982) Failure of body plethysmography in bronchial asthma. J Appl Physiol 52:939-948
19. Peslin R, Gallina C, Rotger M (1987) Methodological factors in the variability of lung volume and specific airway resistance measured by body plethysmography. Bull Eur Physiopathol Respir 23:323-327
20. Ulmer WT, Reichel G, Nolte D (1970) Die Lungenfunktion. Thieme Verlag, Stuttgart, pp 134-146
21. Matthys H, Orth U (1975) Comparative measurements of airway resistance. Respiration 32:121-134
22. Butler J, Caro CG, Alcala R, DuBois AB (1960) Physiological factors affecting airway resistance in normal subjects and in patients with obstructive respiratory disease. J Clin Invest 39:584-591
23. Briscoe WA, DuBois AB (1858) The relationship between airway resistance, airway conductance and lung volume in subjects of different age and body size. J Clin Invest 37:1279-1285
24. Nadel JA, Comroe JH (1961) Acute effects of inhalation of cigarette smoke on airway conductance. J Appl Physiol 16:713-716
25. Schmidt AM, Cohn JE (1961) Modified body plethysmograph for study of cardiopulmonary physiology. J Appl Physiol 16:935-938
26. Cohn JE, Donoso HD (1963) Mechanical properties of lung in normal men over 60 years old. J Clin Invest 42:1406-1410
27. Pelzer AM, Thompson ML (1966) Effect of age, sex, stature and smoking habits on human airway conductance. J Appl Physiol 21:469-476
28. Mitchell M, Watanabe S, Renzetti AD (1967) Evaluation of airway conductance in normal subjects and patients with chronic obstructive pulmonary disease. Am Rev Respir Dis 96:685-691
29. Amrein R, Keller R, Joos H, Herzog H (1970) Valeurs théoriques nouvelles de l'exploration de la fonction ventilatoire du poumon. Bull Physiopath Resp 6:317-349
30. Tammeling GJ, Quanjer PH (1980) Contours of breathing. Boehringer, Ingelheim, pp 202-205
31. DuBois AB, Brody AW, Lewis DH, Burgess BF (1956) Oscillation mechanics of lung and chest in man. J Appl Physiol 8:587-594
32. Gayrard P, Orehek LJ, Grimaud C, Charpin J (1975) Bronchoconstrictor effects of a deep inspiration in patients with asthma. Am Rev Respir Dis 111:433-439
33. Peslin R, Saunier C, Gallina C, Duvivier C (1994) Small-amplitude pressure oscillations do not modify respiratory mechanics in rabbits. J Appl Physiol 76:1011-1013
34. Solymar L, Aronsson PH, Engstrom I, Bake B, Bjure J (1984) Forced oscillation technique and maximum expiratory flows in bronchial provocation tests in children. Eur J Respir Dis 65:486-495
35. Duiverman EJ, Neijens HJ, Van der Snee-van Smaalen M, Kerrebibn KF (1986) Comparison of forced oscillometry and forced expirations for measuring dose-related responses to inhaled methacholine in asthmatic children. Bull Europ Physiopath Respir 22:433-436
36. Marchal F, Mazurek H, Habib M, Duvivier C, Derelle J, Peslin R (1994) Input respiratory impedance to estimate airway hyperreactivity in children: standard method versus head generator. Eur Respir J 7:601-607
37. Bouaziz N, Beyaert C, Gauthier R, Monin P, Peslin R, Marchal F (1996) Respiratory system reactance as an indicator of the intrathoracic airway response to methacholine in children. Pediatr Pulmonol 22:7-13
38. Otis AB, McKerrow CB, Bartlett RA, Mead J, McIlroy MB, Selverstone NJ, Radford EP

(1956) Mechanical factors in distribution of pulmonary ventilation. J Appl Physiol 8:427-443
39. Mead J (1969) Contribution of compliance of airways to frequency-dependent behavior in the lungs. J Appl Physiol 26:670-673
40. McCall CB, Hyatt RE, Noble FW, Fry DL (1957) Harmonic content of certain respiratory flow phenomena in normal individuals. J Appl Physiol 10:215-218
41. Peslin R, Fredberg JJ (1986) Oscillation mechanics of the respiratory system. In: Macklem PT, Mead J (eds) The respiratory system. Mechanics of breathing. Handbook of Physiology. Vol III. American Physiological Society, Bethesda, pp 145-178
42. Dorkin HL, Lutchen KR, Jackson AC (1988) Human respiratory input impedance from 4 to 200 Hz: physiological and modeling considerations. J Appl Physiol 64:823-831
43. Grimby G, Takishima T, Graham W, Macklem P, Mead J (1968) Frequency dependence of flow resistance in patients with obstructive lung disease. J Clin Invest 47:1455-1465
44. Farré R, Peslin R, Navajas D, Gallina C, Suki B (1989) Analysis of the dynamic characteristics of pressure transducers for studying respiratory mechanics at high frequencies. Med Biol Eng Comput 27:531-537
45. Peslin R, Morinet-Lambert J, Duvivier C (1972) Etude de la réponse en fréquence de pneumotachographes. Bull Physiopath Respir 8:1363-1376
46. Peslin R, Jardin P, Duvivier C, Begin P (1984) In-phase rejection requirements for measuring respiratory input impedance. J Appl Physiol 56:804-809
47. Farré R, Navajas D, Peslin R, Rotger M, Duvivier C (1989) A correction procedure for the asymmetry of differential pressure transducers in respiratory impedance measurements. IEEE Trans BME 36:1137-1140
48. Cauberghs M, Van de Woestijne KP (1983) Mechanical properties of the upper airway. J Appl Physiol 55:335-342
49. Van de Woestijne KP, Desager KN, Duiverman EJ, Marchal F (1994) Recommendations for measurement of respiratory input impedance by means of the forced oscillation method. Eur Respir Rev 4:235-237
50. Peslin R, Ying Y, Gallina C, Duvivier C (1992) Within-breath variations of forced oscillation resistance in healthy subjects. Eur Respir J 5:86-93
51. Michaelson ED, Grassman ED, Peters WR (1975) Pulmonary mechanics by spectral analysis of forced random noise. J Clin Invest 56:1210-1230
52. Landser FJ, Clément J, Van de Woestijne KP (1982) Normal values of total respiratory resistance and reactance determined by forced oscillations. Influence of smoking. Chest 81:586-591
53. Daroczy B, Fabula A, Hantos Z (1991) Use of noninteger-multiple pseudorandom excitation to minimize nonlinear effects on impedance estimation. Eur Respir Rev 1:183-187
54. Peslin R, Duvivier C, Gallina C, Cervantes P (1985) Upper airway artefact in respiratory impedance measurements. Am Rev Respir Dis 132:712-714
55. Peslin R, Duvivier C, Jardin P (1984) Upper airway walls impedance measured with head plethysmograph. J Appl Physiol 57:596-600
56. Peslin R, Duvivier C, Didelon J, Gallina C (1985) Respiratory impedance measured with head generator to minimize upper airway shunt. J Appl Physiol 59:1790-1795
57. Harris FJ (1978) On the use of windows for harmonic analysis with the discrete Fourier transform. IEEE Trans BME 66:51-83
58. Navajas D, Farré R, Rotger M, Peslin R (1988) A new estimator to minimize the error due to breathing in the measurement of respiratory impedance. IEEE Trans BME 35:1001-1005
59. Ying Y, Peslin R, Duvivier C, Gallina C, Felicio da Silva J (1990) Respiratory input and

transfer mechanical impedances in patients with chronic obstructive pulmonary disease. Eur Respir J 3:1186-1192

60. Lorino AM, Zerah F, Mariette C, Harf A, Lorino H (1997) Respiratory resistive impedance in obstructive patients: linear regression analysis vs viscoelastic modelling. Eur Respir J 10:150-155
61. Pasker HG, Mertens I, Clément J, Van de Woestijne KP (1994) Normal values of total respiratory input resistance and reactance for adult men and women. Eur Respir Rev 4:134-137
62. Peslin R, Teculescu D, Locuty J, Gallina C, Duvivier C (1994) Normal values of total respiratory input impedance with the head generator technique. Eur Respir Rev 4:138-142
63. Hantos Z, Daroczy D, Gyurkovits K (1985) Total respiratory impedance in healthy children. Pediatr Pulmonol 1:91-98
64. Hordvik NL, Konig P, Morris DA, Kreutz C, Pimmel RL (1985) Normal values for forced oscillatory respiratory resistance in children. Pediatr Pulmonol 1:145-148
65. Peslin R, Duvivier C (1998) Partitioning of airway and respiratory tissue mechanical impedances by body plethysmography. J Appl Physiol 84:553-561

Chapter 5

Oscillatory mechanics: principles and clinical applications

U. LUCANGELO

The forced oscillation technique (FOT) was first used in 1956 by Du Bois et al. [1] to measure the impedance of the respiratory system (Z_{rs}). They resorted to an especially designed piston pump which generated a sinusoidal pressure wave at the mouth of the subject during a short period of voluntary apnoea. The respiratory system reacted to this stimulation with a sinusoidal isofrequency airflow wave. The characteristics of the wave depended solely on the mechanical properties of the respiratory system, i.e. on its impedance, impedance being defined as the ratio between externally imposed pressure oscillation and induced airflow variation. The authors also stimulated the respiratory system with a sequence of variable frequency waves in order to show that Z_{rs} was frequency-dependent. This obviously required repeated periods of apnoea, and therefore the procedure was particularly slow and ill-fitted for clinical application. Moreover, the analysis of results was particularly difficult because of the complex mathematical calculations involved, and this further limited the diffusion of FOT. Today, calculation problems are solved by computers, which can also be used as sinusoidal wave generators, in which case, the respiratory system is stimulated by a single complex signal comprising different sinusoidal waves at varying frequencies.

Pressure and flow signals are subsequently analysed, frequency by frequency, by a mathematical procedure known as Fourier analysis. Calculations can be performed automatically by a computer which applies the Fast Fourier Transform (FFT), i.e. Fourier analysis adapted to this specific application. Thus, today the value of Z_{rs} can be obtained for each frequency almost in real time while the subject is being stimulated by a single complex signal. This greater ease of use has led to renewed interest in FOT as a clinical monitoring system of the respiratory function.

The object of this chapter is to highlight the elementary principles underlying FOT and to list its most current clinical applications.

A basic knowledge of the physical principles of FOT is essential both for a correct clinical interpretation of data and to avoid methodological mistakes during the use of this technique. For this reason, alternating quantities and their laws are going to be outlined first, and then the elementary AC electric circuitry that is best suited for the understanding of the physical-clinical results of FOT will be discussed.

Physical bases of FOT

Definitions on alternating quantities

An alternating function is defined as any function of time which meets both the condition of periodicity and that of having an average null value for every period.

To meet the first condition, the function must take the full range of its possible values within a given time T, and then repeat exactly the same pattern throughout every following interval, the duration of which must be T. The time T is the period of the function and is measured in seconds.

To meet the second condition, the entire sequence of negative and positive values taken by the function in every period must be distributed over time in such a way as to have an average value of zero. This means that an alternating function must change sign at least once in every period.

In accordance with the foregoing definitions, an alternating quantity is defined as any physical quantity which varies with time following a periodic alternation. This means that the algebraic change of sign corresponds physically to a change in the sense of the function.

Two further elements characterise alternating quantities: period and form. The period of an alternating quantity is defined as the constant time span between the instant at which the said quantity has a given value and the first subsequent instant at which it takes that same value again, after having taken the full range of positive and negative values it may take. The period T is measured in seconds; its inverse is the number of periods per second, i.e. frequency f in hertz (Hz), hence:

$$f = \frac{1}{T} \qquad (1)$$

The form of an alternating quantity is defined by the rule according to which the quantity varies within a period. The most frequent alternating form is the sinusoid, i.e. alternating current and voltage, as well as soundwaves; the forced oscillation technique is based on the latter.

Sinusoidal alternating quantities

Sinusoidal quantities are represented by a harmonic function of the sine type:

$$y = Y_M \sin \omega t \qquad (2)$$

where Y_M is the amplitude or maximum value taken by the function, w angular velocity and t time.

The variable ω represents the angular velocity of a body which rotates around an axis, i.e. the ratio between its angular displacement and time (t). It is measured in degrees (°), revolutions, or radians (rad). A radian is the central angle of a circle determined by an arc which is of the same length as the circle's radius. Since the circumference (crf) is equal to the length of the radius (r) multiplied by 2π:

$$crf = 2\pi \bullet r \tag{3}$$

the angular displacement corresponding to one revolution is 2π radians.

Therefore, 1 revolution=360°=2π radians; hence 1 radian=360°/2π=57.3°.

If a body describes an angle of δ radians in t seconds, its angular velocity ω, expressed in radians per second, is equal to the ratio between the angle (in radians) and the time t needed for this displacement:

$$\omega(^{rad}/_{sec}) = \frac{\delta}{t} \tag{4}$$

These details are necessary in order to clarify the fact that angular velocity is also a function of frequency (f), since if 1 rps=2π rad/s, then ω (rad/s)=2π rps=2π f, where f is frequency in rps (revolutions per second).

Thus, the subsequent instantaneous values y of function (1) vary proportionally to the sine of a uniformly increasing angle, such as the angle described by a segment which rotates around an axis at constant angular velocity ω.

In Figure 1, the magnitude and sign of these values are represented by the projections of the rotating segment Y_M=OM on the axis of ordinates. While the rotating segment describes the first quadrant, from 0° to 90°, from the reference

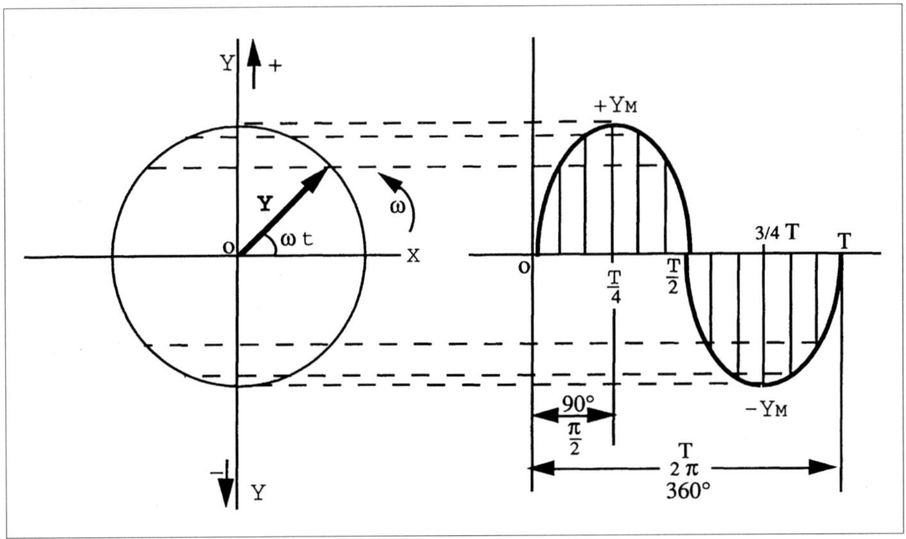

Fig. 1. Segment OM rotates around the origin at constant angular velocity: its projection y on the Cartesian axis of ordinates varies in accordance with a sinusoidal law

axis OX, its projection on the y-axis increases from zero to the entire value of the radius OA; the sine of the angle α described by the segment varies from zero to one and thus function y takes the full range of values from zero to the maximum value Y_M.

On the other hand, in the second quadrant (from 90° to 180°), the projection of the rotating segment decreases from OA to zero: the sine of the angle α varies from one to zero and function y decreases proportionally from Y_M to zero. In the subsequent half revolution (from 180° to 360°), the same sequences are repeated, but signs change, and so on in all subsequent revolutions.

The curve represented by function y as defined above is a sinusoidal curve of amplitude Y_M which can be easily drawn as shown in Figure 2.

The period T of function y (Fig. 2) is equal to the time needed by the rotating segment to describe a complete revolution: if ω is angular velocity in radians per second, therefore:

$$T = \frac{2\pi}{\omega} \tag{5}$$

The axis of abscissas of the sinusoidal curve can thus be graduated in seconds, in radians and in degrees. A period T is equal to 2π radians or 360°; half a period, to π radians or 180°, and so on.

Frequency (f) is equal to the number of periods per second, hence:

$$f = \frac{1}{T} = \frac{\omega}{2\pi} \tag{6}$$

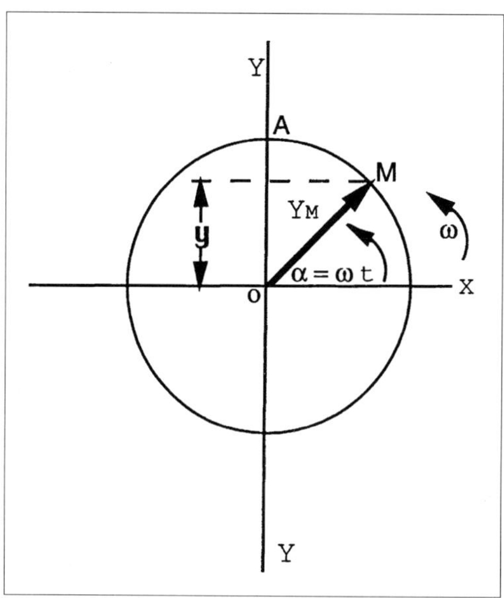

Fig. 2. Construction of a sinusoidal curve with a rotating segment

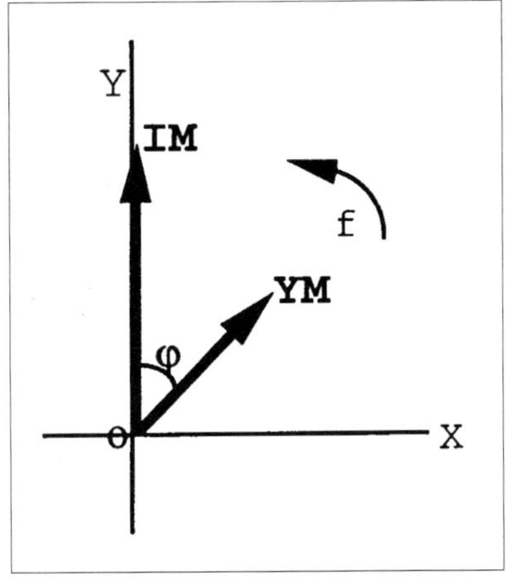

Fig. 3. Vectorial representation of sinusoidal quantities

All the values taken sequentially by the quantity in time are represented (in the set scale) by the projections of the rotating segment on the Cartesian y-axis – obviously, the segment must rotate around an axis at a given angular velocity.

$$\omega = \frac{2\pi}{T} - 2\,\pi f \qquad (7)$$

The maximum value Y_M or amplitude is reached in every period; all the other values of y are instantaneous values at a given instant t. The constant parameter $\omega = 2\,\pi f$ is also called pulsatance.

Sinusoidal quantities can also have a vectorial representation, as shown in Figure 3. A rotating vector is drawn with its own direction, intensity and sense, within a Cartesian coordinate system. The length of the vector corresponds to the maximum amplitude of the sinusoidal quantity Y_M and the vector itself is assumed to rotate around the origin of the Cartesian axes at a number of revolutions per second equal to frequency. Its orientation in space indicates phase in respect of a reference (normally, the x-axis). The angle φ between two vectors represents their phase difference [2, 3].

Outlines of elementary alternating current circuitry

The elements which comprise elementary electric circuits are resistance (R), inductance (L) and the capacitor (C). As will be the shown in the next paragraph, each of these is a biological analogue of the linear, single-compartment model of the respiratory system. The equivalent electric circuit which best describes it is called R-L-C, since it consists of a resistance, an inductance and a capacitor connected in series. The theoretical understanding of the working of the following electric circuits can therefore prove instrumental in interpreting the behaviour of the respiratory system with FOT.

The behaviour of the electric components R, C and L varies depending on whether direct current or alternating current is used [3]. In the former case, the value of the current (I) flowing through the resistance R is equal to the potential difference across the resistance, divided by the resistance R itself, in accordance with Ohm's law.

$$I = \frac{V}{R} \tag{8}$$

The capacitor C behaves as an open circuit since current may not flow through it, while inductance L behaves as a short circuit since it offers virtually no resistance to the current which flows through it.

The situation changes entirely when alternating current is used, i.e. when the components R, C and L are fed a current which varies with time in accordance with the function $i=I_M \sin \omega t$.

In an alternating current circuit comprising only a resistance, voltage (v) and current (i) reach both zero and maximum value at the same time (Fig. 4). In this case voltage and current are said to be in phase. This can be demonstrated by measuring voltage (Vr) across the resistance, which, in accordance with Ohm's law, is $Vr=R \cdot i$. If current is defined by the function $i=I_M \sin \omega t$, then $Vr= R \cdot I_M \sin \omega t$; hence, Vr varies with time in accordance with the same sinusoidal rule which applies to current.

Let us now consider the circuit in Figure 5, which comprises a resistance R and an inductance L, which are fed alternating current. Voltage V, measured across the circuit, is the sum of two voltage drops: a resistive one, $Vr=R \cdot i$, and an inductive one, $V_L=L\frac{di}{dt}$, hence $v=Ri+L\frac{di}{dt}$.

The current circulating in the coil and in the resistance is equal; yet, the voltage of the latter is in phase with current, while the voltage across the coil is

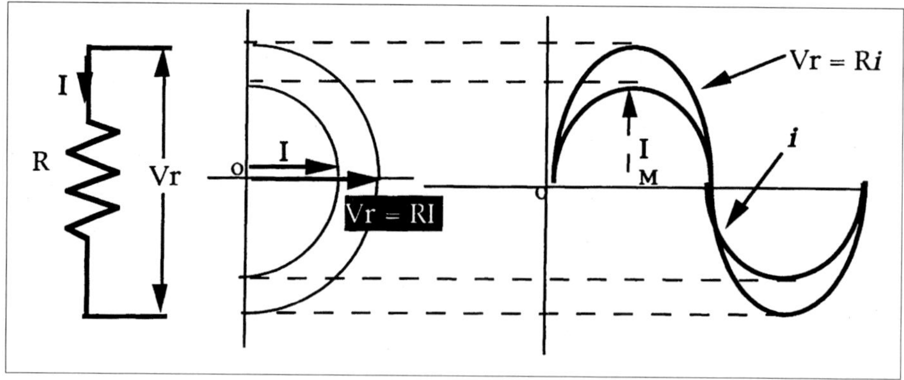

Fig. 4. Electric circuit: vectorial and graphic representation of a purely reactive circuit. The voltage and current waves are represented by the quantities $Vr=R \cdot i$ and $i=I_M \sin \omega t$, respectively, which are in phase

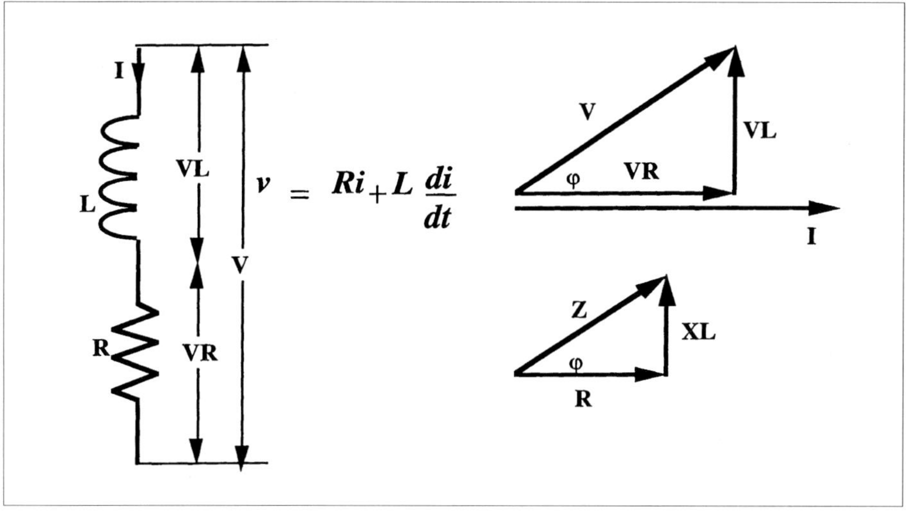

Fig. 5. Ohmic-inductive (R-L) circuit, with corresponding diagrams

out of phase by 90°; thus, there is a phase difference of 90° between the voltage drops across the coil and the resistance, respectively, as shown by the vectors in Figure 5.

To determine voltage V across the circuit, the two voltages must be added vectorially because of the aforementioned phase difference. The drop Vr across the resistance is in phase with the vector current at 0°. The drop Vx across the inductance is in advance by 90° with respect to current. A right triangle (called triangle of voltages) of base Vr, height Vx and hypotenuse V is thus obtained. The value of V can therefore be easily calculated by applying the Pythagorean theorem:

$$V = \sqrt{Vr^2 + Vx^2} \tag{9}$$

It is therefore clear that the electric behaviour of an inductance varies enormously, depending on the type of current it is fed. If it is alternating current, the coil's turns offer opposition to the flow of current, and thus generate an effect of self-inductance, which in turn depends on inductance (number of turns), on pulsatance ω and therefore on frequency f.

The quantity defined by the product ωL is called inductive reactance (X_L). It is also called "apparent resistance" since it causes a potential drop equal to that which is needed to counter the effects of self-inductance.

Reactance X_L is measured in ohm; fundamentally, it corresponds to the reactive inertial effect which offers opposition to current variations in the circuit. Reactance is also essentially different from ohmic resistance, which gives rise to dissipation of energy (which is converted into heat) in accordance with the

Joule effect. Hence, the higher inductance L and frequency f, the greater the reactive effect, in accordance with the formula

$$X_L = \omega L = 2\pi f L \tag{10}$$

where f is frequency in hertz and L inductance expressed in Henry (H).

Ohm's law may however be applied also to reactance X_L, even if the latter represents an "apparent resistance".

It is therefore possible to state that the voltage across resistance R is equal to $V_r = R \cdot i$ and, by analogy, the voltage across reactance X_L is equal to $V_x = X_L \cdot i$. By substituting the appropriate values in (9), the following expression is obtained:

$$V = I \sqrt{R^2 + X_L^2} \tag{11}$$

and by dividing the whole expression by I, the ratio between alternating voltage and current, i.e. the impedance (Z) of the R-L circuit is obtained:

$$\frac{V}{I} = Z = \sqrt{R^2 + X_L^2} \tag{12}$$

This relation shows that, by virtue of the combined effect of resistance R and reactance X_L, the opposition offered by the circuit to the flow of current is a "total apparent resistance", normally called impedance Z. The vectorial representation of Z is a right triangle (the impedance triangle) with base R, height X_L and hypotenuse Z, and with the same phase angle φ that there is between the voltages.

Like an inductance, a capacitor which is fed alternating current will also behave as a reactance X, which is called capacitive reactance (X_c) and is frequency-dependent, in accordance with the following formula, in which capacitance (C) is expressed in Farad (F):

$$X_c = \frac{1}{\omega C} = \frac{1}{2\pi f C} \tag{13}$$

This means that a capacitor C, when inserted in an alternating current electric circuit, does not function as a break (open circuit): on the contrary, electric current keeps flowing through the circuit while the capacitor is charged and discharged.

The mutual relations between the components of an R-C circuit are essentially the same as those of an R-L circuit, except that there is a diametrically opposite phase angle (-90°) between capacitive reactance X_c and the corresponding voltage V_c on the one hand, and current and the voltage drop across the resistance on the other, as shown in Figure 6.

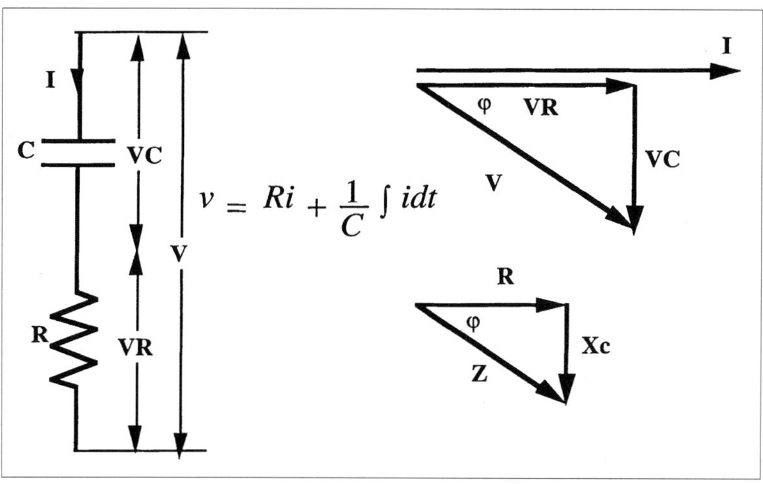

Fig. 6. Ohmic-capacitive (R-C) circuit, with corresponding diagrams

As in the case of an R-L circuit, voltage V measured across an R-C circuit is the sum of two voltage drops $v=Ri+\frac{1}{C}\int idt$: a resistive one $Vr=R\cdot i$, and a capacitive one $Vc=\frac{1}{C}\int idt$, which is however in delay (phase angle of -90°) in respect of the former. The corresponding triangle of voltages has the voltage drop VR as base, the voltage drop VC as height and V as hypotenuse. Therefore, the Pythagorean theorem may be applied:

$$V = \sqrt{V_R^2 + V_C^2} \tag{14}$$

hence $V=I\sqrt{R^2 + X_C^2}$ (15); the corresponding value of the impedance of the ohmic capacitive system will be

$$Z \sqrt{R^2 + X_C^2} = \sqrt{R^2 + \frac{1}{\omega C}} \tag{16}$$

When the three fundamental components are connected in series in a single R-L-C circuit, the voltage drops and impedance can be calculated by a combination of the previous methods.

The voltage V measured across the circuit in Figure 7 is the sum of three voltage drops: a resistive one $Vr=R\bullet i$, an inductive one $V_L=L\frac{di}{dt}$ and a capacitive one $Vc=\frac{1}{C}\int idt$, hence $v=Ri+L\frac{di}{dt}+\frac{1}{C}\int idt$.

The resistive voltage drop is in phase with the current, while the two other voltage drops are in opposition between them. The phase angle of the inductive voltage drop V_L is 90° with respect to current, while that of the capacitive voltage drop V_C is the opposite (-90°). V_L and V_C can thus be represented as two diametrically opposite vectors; the resultant voltage V_X is the algebraic sum of the two drops.

If capacitive reactance X_C is greater than inductive reactance X_L, then V_C is greater than V_L, and V_X (the resultant of their algebraic sum) must be oriented in accordance with the sense of V_L, as can be seen in the voltage diagram in Fig. 7.

The Pythagorean theorem may be applied to this triangle of voltages as well, hence

$$V = \sqrt{Vr^2 + Vx^2} = \sqrt{Vr^2 + (V_L - V_C)^2} \tag{17}$$

and therefore

$$V = I \sqrt{R^2 + (V_L - V_C)^2} \tag{18}$$

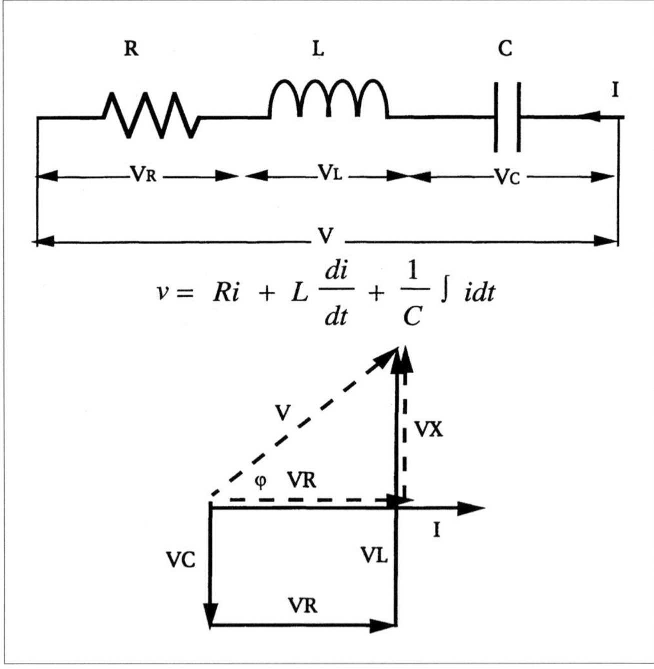

Fig. 7. Inductive circuit (R-L-C circuit with X_L>X_C), with the corresponding vectorial diagram of voltages

The resultant effect of the two reactances X_L and X_C is therefore equal to that of an equivalent reactance X, equal to their difference, i.e.:

$$X = X_L - X_C = \omega L - \frac{1}{\omega C} \tag{19}$$

and the impedance Z of the circuit is therefore

$$Z = \sqrt{R^2 + X^2} = \sqrt{R^2 + (X_L - X_C)^2} \tag{20}$$

In conclusion, reactances are added when connected in series, but the sum of a capacitive reactance X_C and an inductive reactance X_L is actually a difference, since they are opposite in sign. There is therefore a compensation between these two reactances, which means that the overall reactance of the circuit may be actually smaller than either of the two individual reactances. Hence, the greater of these two opposite reactances will prevail on the smaller, and will thus give an inductive or capacitive nature, respectively, to the whole circuit.

If X_L is greater than X_C, the resultant reactance $X=X_L-X_C$ is positive and the circuit is inductive, as in Fig. 7, while if X_C is greater than X_L, the resultant reactance $X=X_L-X_C$ is negative and the circuit is capacitive.

Resonance

Resonance may be exhibited by the abovementioned circuit when $X_L=X_C$ and therefore the resultant reactance $X=X_L-X_C=0$.

Under these conditions, the whole circuit behaves as a purely resistive circuit because of the mutual compensation between the opposite effects of inductance and capacitance.

The resonance of the circuit is determined by the equality $\omega L = \frac{1}{\omega C}$ whence $\omega^2 LC = 1$.

Resonance is thus a function of the respective values of inductance L, capacitance C and frequency.

For every couple of values L and C, there exists always one single resonance frequency fr determined by the relation

$$wr = 2\pi fr = \frac{1}{\sqrt{LC}} \text{ (21), whence } fr = \frac{1}{2\pi\sqrt{LC}} \tag{22}$$

Equivalence between the mechanical and electrical model of the respiratory system

Respiratory Mechanics defines the behaviour of the lung and chest when subjected to changes in pressure (Prs), flow ($\dot{V}$) and volume (V) induced by the respiratory muscles and by the mechanical ventilatory support which cyclically act on the system.

The simplest model of the respiratory system, which is still currently used, is a series combination of a tube and a balloon, i.e. a resistance (R) and an elastance (E): a rough representation of the anatomy of an alveolus with its bronchial duct.

This model, that will be called mechanical model, can be applied both during spontaneous ventilation and during constant flow passive ventilation. The following mathematical equation, known as motion equation, describes its behaviour:

$$Prs = Ers \bullet V + Rrs \bullet \dot{V} + Irs \bullet \ddot{V} \qquad (23)$$

where Prs is the pressure applied to the respiratory system, V volume, $\dot{V}$ airflow and $\ddot{V}$ its acceleration.

Prs and $\dot{V}$ may be measured directly at the patient's mouth, respectively with a pressure transducer and with a pneumotachograph. Airflow acceleration and volume are derived mathematically from the recording of the airflow wave, since $\dot{V}$ is the first derivative and $\ddot{V}$ the second derivative of volume V.

The respective values of the three unknown quantities Ers, Rrs and Irs can therefore be obtained by fitting Eq. (23) to the sampled values of Prs, V, $\dot{V}$ and $\ddot{V}$ [4, 5].

The term Ers•V corresponds to the pressure which must be applied in order to balance elastic forces, and depends on both the volume insufflated in excess of resting volume (Vo) and on the elastance of the respiratory system (Ers). The term Rrs•$\dot{V}$, on the other hand, corresponds to the pressure which must be applied to balance frictional forces, and is due chiefly to the resistance offered to flow. Lastly, the product Irs•$\ddot{V}$ corresponds to the pressure loss which is needed to win the system's inertia. This effect is called inertance of the respiratory system (Irs) and depends on acceleration $\ddot{V}$.

Therefore, Prs corresponds to the sum of the resistive, elastic and inertial pressure drops of the respiratory system; in this there is an analogy to what has been described above for voltage V across the R-C-L circuit. This parallelism between the mechanical and the electrical model is not fortuitous, on the contrary: these two systems are – to a certain extent – equivalent, as the following differential equations demonstrate.

The following expression can be obtained by rewriting Eq. 23 with a different notation:

$$Prs = Ers \bullet V + Rrs \frac{dV}{dt} + Irs \frac{d^2V}{dt^2} \quad (24)$$

Let us now consider the equation $v = Ri + L\frac{di}{dt} + \frac{1}{C}\int idt$, which quantifies voltage across an R-C-L electric circuit; Eq. 25 and 26 are obtained from it, respectively, by calculating its first derivative and then by rearranging its terms:

$$\frac{dV}{dt} = R\frac{di}{dt} + L\frac{d^2i}{dt^2} + \frac{1}{C}i \quad (25)$$

$$\frac{dV}{dt} = \frac{1}{C}i + R\frac{di}{dt} + L\frac{d^2i}{dt^2} \quad (26)$$

A comparison between the terms of (24) and those of (26)

$$Prs = Ers \bullet V + Rrs \frac{dV}{dt} + Irs \frac{d^2V}{dt^2} \quad (24)$$

$$\frac{dV}{dt} = \frac{1}{C} R \frac{di}{dt} + L\frac{d^2i}{dt^2} \quad (26)$$

shows that there is an analogy between the mechanical and electric quantities, and this analogy can be used to convert the "anatomical" model which describes the respiratory system into an equivalent electrical model.

The electrical model can thus be used as a "simulator" of the respiratory system, just by substituting a resistance R for Rrs, a capacitor C for Crs (which is

Table 1. Analogous quantities in mechanical and electrical systems

Mechanical			**Electrical**		
Quantity	*Symbol*	*Units*	*Quantity*	*Symbol*	*Units*
Volume	V	liter	Change	Q	coulomb
Flow	$\dot{V}$	1/sec	Current	I	ampere
Pressure	Prs	hPa	Voltage	V	volt
Resistance	Rrs	hpa/1/s	Resistance	R	ohm
Compliance	Crs	1/hPa	Capacitance	C	farad
Inertance	Irs	hpa/1/s^2	Inductance	L	henry
Reactance	Xrs	hpa/1/s	Reactance	X	ohm

equivalent to the inverse of Ers), and an inductance L for Irs. Obviously, the conditions of equivalence between the two systems must be met (Tab. 1). If this is the case, then it is possible to derive an electrical equivalent from a highly complex mechanical model; the equivalent is indeed as complex, but it can be studied easily through the application of the laws of electrical engineering.

Forced oscillation techniques and linearity of the system

Eq. 23 analytically describes a linear single-compartment system; therefore, if the model is applicable, this means that the respiratory system follows a linear behaviour too. It follows that Rrs, which correlates pressure with flow, is constant and therefore, in particular, flow-independent; and that elastance Ers, which correlates pressure with volume, is constant and therefore volume-independent. Actually, the pressure-volume curves of the respiratory system show that elastic properties are not linear. The linear part of the pressure-volume curve is close to functional residual capacity (FRC), so that Ers is constant and independent of volume only for small volume changes which are close to FRC, and therefore within the tidal volume (Vt) range. Likewise, the pressure-flow relation too is linear within the same Vt range [6, 7].

FOT can therefore be used if and only if the linearity conditions of the system are met and if the sinusoidal stimulation applied to the system does not alter its balance [9, 10]. For this reason the amplitude between the two peaks of the pressure wave does not exceed 2 hPa, as shown in Figure 8. When the respiratory sys-

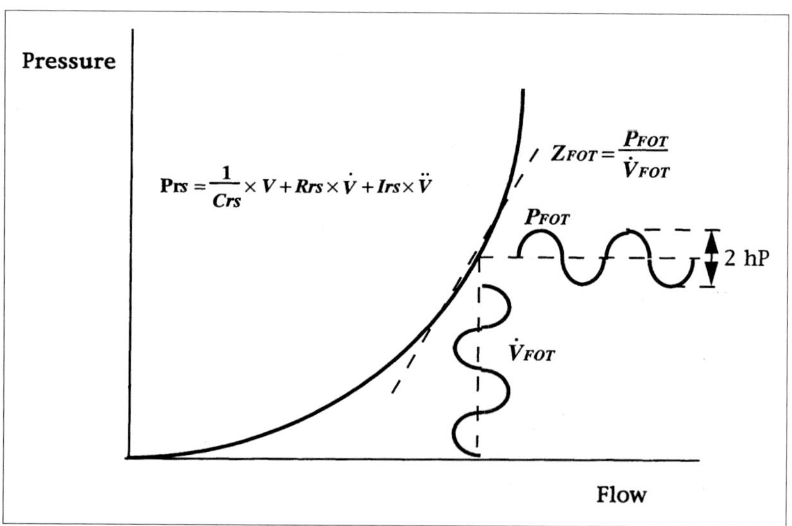

Fig. 8. Pressure-flow relation of the respiratory system. FOT can be applied only within the system's range of linearity. If the input waveform's amplitude is such that it can remain within this range, then the output waveform will exhibit no distortion

tem is linear, oscillation can be superimposed on spontaneous breathing and it is possible to calculate impedance values separately for each frequency.

Moreover, if the frequency of the sinusoidal wave does not exceed 2 Hz (120 breaths/minute), a simplified motion equation can be applied, since the effect of gas and lung tissue inertia is negligible. Eq. 23 is reduced to

$$Prs = Ers \cdot V + Rrs \cdot \dot{V} \quad (24)$$

Functional principles of FOT

The sinusoidal pressure wave generated by FOT (PFOT) excites the respiratory system and thereby induces a volume (VFOT) and a flow ($\dot{V}$FOT), which will have the same frequency as PFOT although they will be out of phase in time.

The relation between the sinusoidal pressure wave and the airflow wave it induces is called impedance of the respiratory system (Zrs). There is a clear equivalence with the electrical model, since pressure is analogous to voltage and flow to electric current, and therefore their relation represents an electric impedance.

The impedance of the respiratory system

$$Z_{rs} = \sqrt{R_{rs}^2 + X_{rs}^2}$$

comprises an Rrs, which is also called effective resistance (Ref) since it is frequency-independent, and a reactance

$$Xrs = \omega Irs - \frac{1}{\omega Crs}$$

which represents Crs and Irs.

The component which may be ascribed to compliance (Crs) is a function of the volume variation of the system, and is inversely correlated with the frequency of the induced oscillation. On the other hand, the component which may be ascribed to inertia is a function of acceleration, which is directly proportional to frequency.

Therefore, for frequencies <2 Hz, $Xrs = -\frac{1}{\omega Crs}$ and reflects only the elastic load of the respiratory system, the effect of inertance being negligible. In accordance with this definition, the Xrs of an elastic load is negative, which means that flow leads pressure.

For frequencies >2 Hz, the Irs component may not be neglected and it affects Xrs, which becomes positive. In this case flow lags pressure and accounts for most of the inertial load.

When the frequency of the induced oscillation has changed, the components of Xrs are affected to the contrary since they are opposite in sign. As in the R-L-C circuit, there is a frequency at which reactances have the same absolute value and neutralize each other. At this resonance frequency (fo), the impedance of the lungs and chest can be entirely ascribed to the resistive component.

Equipment

FOT can be applied under both spontaneous and mechanical ventilation. In both cases, pressure and flow transducers must be used and connected to a mouthpiece, or to an endotracheal tube, as suitable. Oscillation can be applied directly at the mouth to obtain Zrs, or at the chest surface to obtain respiratory transfer impedance (Ztr) [10].

Figure 9 describes the connections between the various components used to study an intubated patient subjected to mechanical ventilation by FOT.

The oscillatory wave is currently produced by a loudspeaker connected to the patient by suitable circuits. Pressure oscillation is produced by the movement of the loudspeaker enclosed in a container which acts as a resonance chamber. The loudspeaker, being a device that converts electric current variations into sound vibrations, must meet specific requirements and must therefore be chosen accurately.

Currently available loudspeakers are magnetostatic, i.e. they comprise a permanent magnet that generates a constant magnetic field; the field encompasses a coil, which is fed variable intensity electric current. Each turn of the coil, when it is fed current and is simultaneously under the influence of the external magnetic field, is subjected to a force which is proportional to the intensity of current itself. The coil therefore oscillates in accordance with current variations

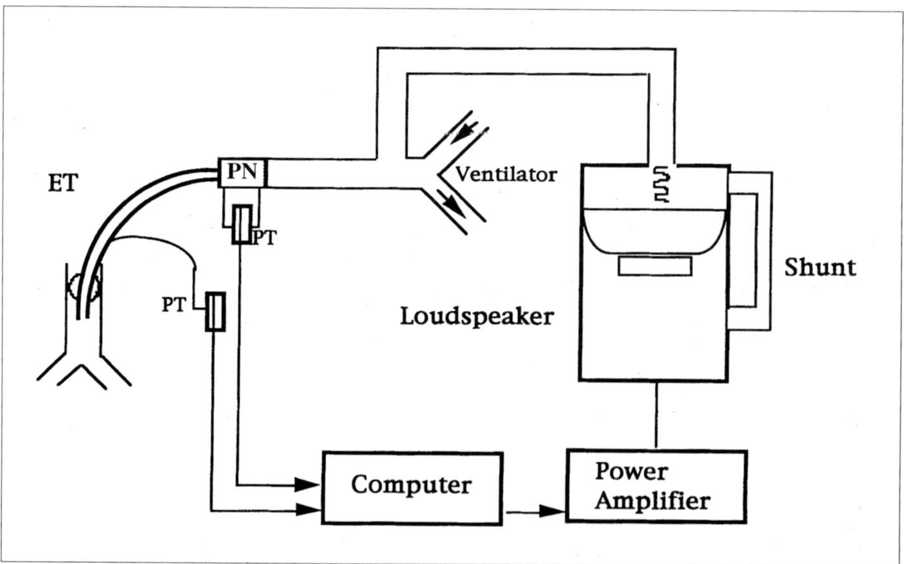

Fig. 9. Experimental set-up. *Pn*, pneumotachograph, *Pt*, differential pressure transducer, *ET*, endotracheal tube

and triggers a vibration in a connected membrane, which then compresses and rarefies adjacent air and generates sound propagation in the environment. Since the force which affects the membrane is proportional to the current which flows through the coil, the frequency of the membrane's and of the current's vibrations must be identical – in this case the loudspeaker is said to be distortion-free. In principle, a good loudspeaker should introduce absolutely no distortion in the entire range of sound frequencies; in fact, a loudspeaker reproduces high sound frequencies better if its vibrating membrane is small, and low frequencies if it is large. This is due to the fact that a large membrane can move more slowly, as is suitable for low frequencies, and by impacting a considerable volume of air it can produce the required sound intensity. On the other hand, a small membrane can move more rapidly, as is suitable for high frequencies, but not for low ones, since the volume of air impact is so small that it cannot produce the required sound intensity.

For this reason, loudspeakers are classified into various categories, in accordance with their intrinsic characteristics and therefore with their ability to reproduce a certain frequency range with high fidelity. The frequencies used in FOT are comprised in a low range: from 5 to 30 Hz. For this reason, the loudspeakers resorted to are woofers or, better still, subwoofers.

The impedance of the respiratory system and its clinical applications

Clinically speaking, the vast majority of data on the respiratory system is not drawn from "total" Zrs, but rather from the separate analysis of Rrs and Xrs within a variable frequency range (2÷0 Hz). It is thus possible to ascertain whether the relevant quantities change in accordance with the status (health vs. lung pathology) of the subject being studied.

Figure 10 illustrates the behaviour of Rrs and of the reactance of the respiratory system as a function of frequency variations in a healthy subject. As can be seen, Rrs remains almost constantly around the value of 2.5 hPa/l/s throughout the frequency range, while reactance Xrs exhibits a marked frequency-dependence below the value of about 8 Hz. The resonance frequency of the system corresponds to the exact frequency value for which Xrs is equal to zero and Zrs is associated only to the resistive load of the system.

The normal values of Rrs are around 2÷3hPa/l/s [12-15] and the resonance frequency is around 9 Hz [15] with an interindividual variation ranging between 7 and 13 Hz [16].

Làndsér et al. [17] have shown that the value of Rrs correlates with the weight, height and age of the subject, and that in women it is 15% higher than in men [18].

In children, Rrs values tend to decrease with puberty and to reach normal adult values around the age of 18 [19, 20].

Some authors have suggested that, under baseline conditions, both the frequency-dependence of Rrs, and the resonance frequency of the respiratory system can be used as sensitive monitors of an early obstruction of the airways [21, 22].

On the other hand, if there is an overt obstructive disease, Rrs undergoes at least a two- or threefold increase in respect of normal values, and loses its characteristic frequency-independence: it reaches its maximum value at low frequencies, and then undergoes a considerable decrease when frequency rises. This pattern has been explained with the inhomogeneity of lung compartments [11].

Xrs varies as well: it becomes increasingly negative at low frequencies and causes an upward shift in the resonance frequency of the system, which is reached around 31 Hz [15, 23, 24].

Rrs follows the same pattern in patients suffering from chronic obstructive pulmonary disease (COPD) and asthma. These patients often require bronchodilation, which can be non-invasively monitored by FOT during spontaneous ventilation [25, 26].

If an oesophageal tube is used during forced oscillation to assess pleural pressure, the impedance of the respiratory system Zrs can be analysed into a lung-dependent (Z_L) and a chest wall-dependent (Z_{CW}) component. Under spontaneous ventilation, it is thus possible to measure the mechanical proper-

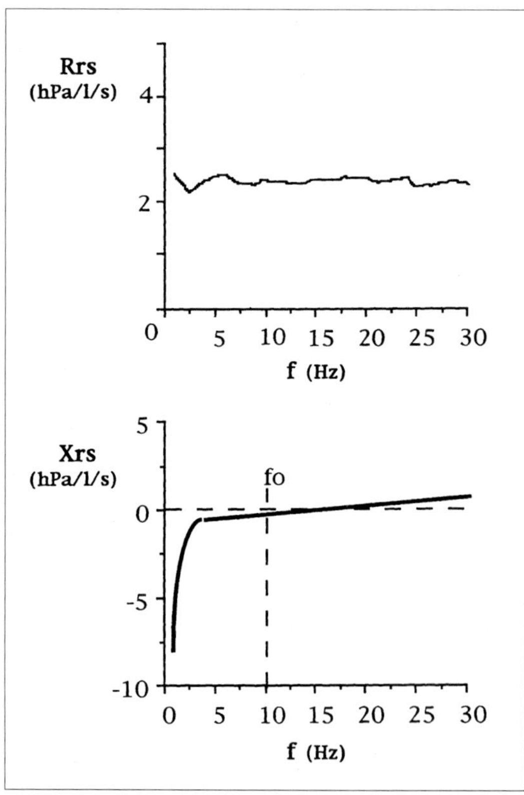

Fig. 10. Behaviour of Rrs and Xrs as a function of frequency in a healthy subject. The frequency value corresponding to zero Xrs is the resonance frequency of the system (fo)

ties of the lung separately from those of the chest wall. Therefore, Rrs will be equal to the sum of lung resistance (RL) and chest wall resistance (RCW), and likewise Xrs will be equal to the sum of XL and XCW.

Nagels et al. [13] studied 15 healthy subjects and 7 COPD patients in the sitting position during quiet breathing at three different volumes. The results obtained in healthy subjects suggested that the variations in Rrs and Xrs with frequency and volume should be correlated chiefly with variations in RL and XL, since RCW and XCW varied only slightly. The same behaviour was exhibited in COPD patients, except that Rrs values were increased while Xrs had fallen.

The mean value of the resonance frequency was 3 Hz for the lung and 7 Hz for the whole respiratory system in healthy subjects, while in COPD patients it reached 19 Hz for the lung and was above 20 Hz for the respiratory system.

In conclusion, this study has demonstrated that about 75% of Rrs, 25% of Crs and pratically the entire Irs-related component may be attributed to the lung component.

FOT has been used also in restrictive diseases of the lungs and chest wall. Some studies have been focused on patients with fibrosing alveolitis [23] and with kyphoscoliosis and ankylosing spondylitis [27]. These have shown modest increases in Rrs and reduced values of reactance Xrs with an increase in the resonance frequency.

Owing to its non-invasiveness and to the limited degree of cooperation required from the patient, FOT is widely used both in pediatrics and in pneumology. It can also be applied in intensive care, both to patients suffering from altered states of consciousness, who require non-invasive monitoring of respiratory mechanics, and to intubated and mechanically ventilated patients. In the latter, the presence of the endotracheal tube offers a non-linear resistance to PFOT, and this causes artefacts in the measurements [28].

Various solutions have been proposed for this problem: the first consists in measuring pressure directly in the trachea by introducing a thin catheter through the endotracheal tube. The second, put forward by Navajas et al. [29], is based on the utilisation of a special endotracheal tube: it comprises a catheter, embedded in the wall of the cannula, which was especially developed for the measurement of pressure at the distal end of the tube. With these procedures, it is now possible to study respiratory mechanics with FOT both under general anaesthesia and in intensive care.

The simplest way to measure Zrs directly in curarized patients undergoing anaesthesia is to replace the ventilator with a loudspeaker, which acts as a sinusoidal pressure generator, for 32 seconds. Navajas et al. [30] applied this procedure to assess the response of the respiratory system within the frequency range 0.25-32 Hz. Their results have highlighted a strong negative frequency-dependence of Rrs between 0.25 and 2 Hz. At higher frequencies, Rrs showed a modest negative frequency-dependence. The high values of Rrs found at the spontaneous breathing frequency were attributed to chest wall viscoelasticity.

In 1994, the same author [31] proposed an alternative way of measuring Zrs during mechanical ventilation without disconnecting the ventilator from the patient: the acoustic generator of sinusoidal waves was connected directly to the expiratory outlet of a Siemens 900-C ventilator.

Thus, the loudspeaker was protected from the high insufflation pressures produced by the ventilator: during the inspiratory phase the expiratory valve remained closed; during the expiratory phase, it was the inspiratory valve that closed, while the expiratory valve was open and allowed the transmission of the oscillatory wave. With this method, the study of chest and lung mechanics during expiration is now possible both in curarized patients and in those under assisted ventilation.

Lastly, Peslin et al. [32] have proposed a technically brilliant way to explore the whole respiratory cycle during mechanical ventilation, while preventing the loudspeaker's membrane from being damaged by the high pressure produced during the ventilator's inspiratory phase. To this end, the authors have enclosed the loudspeaker in a container fitted with a pneumatic shunt, as shown in Figure 9. Thus, the pressure wave hits the front and the back of the membrane simultaneously, so that no pressure gradient is created across it.

Conclusions

Today, technological developments and technical simplifications allow us to predict that FOT will be used by an increasing number of doctors, not only in intensive care, pneumology, pediatrics and neonatology, but also in fields like medical epidemiology or occupational medicine, which require non-invasive methods of mass screening.

References

1. Du Bois AB, Brody AW, Lewis DH, Burgess BF Jr (1956) Oscillation mechanics of lungs and chest in man. J Appl Physiol 8:587-594
2. Crawford FS Jr (1968) Wave. Mc Graw Hill, New York
3. Livieri L, Ravelli E (1962) Elettrotecnica. CEDAM, Milano
4. Hantos Z, Daroczy B, Klebniczki J, (1982) Parameter estimation of transpulmonary mechanics by a nonlinear model. J Appl Physiol 52:955-963
5. Bates JHT, Shardonofsky F, Steward DE (1989) The low-frequency dependence of respiratory system resistance and elastance in normal dogs. Respir Physiol 78:369-382
6. Iemsripong K, Hyatt RE, Offord KP (1976) Total respiratory resistance by forced oscillation in normal subjects. Mayo Clin Proc 51:553-556
7. Horowitz JG, Siegel SD, Primiano FP, Chester EH (1983) Computation of respiratory impedance from forced sinusoidal oscillations during breathing. Computers and biomedical research 16:499-521
8. Desager KN, Buhr W, Willemen M, Van Bever HP, De Backer W, Vermeire PA, Làndsér FJ (1991) Assessment of the linearity of the respiratory system in infants using the forced oscillation technique. Eur Respir Rev 1(3):191
9. Van de Woestijne KP (1991) Recommendations and future plans. Eur Respir Rev 1(3):236-237
10. Lutchen KR, Sulluvan A, Arbogast FT, Celli BR, Jackson AC (1998) Use of transfer

impedance measurements for clinical assessement of lung mechanics. Am Respir Crit Care Med 157:435-446
11. Michaeleson ED, Grassman ED, Peters WR (1975) Pulmonary mechanics by spectral analysis of forced rando noise. J Ciln Invest 56:1210-1230
12. Hayes DA, Pimmel RL, Fillton JM, Bromberg PA (1979) Detection of respiratory mechanical disfunction by forced random noise impedance parameters. Am Rev Respir Dis 120:1095-1100
13. Nagels J, Landsér FJ, Van der Linden L, Clément J, Van de Woestijne KP (1980) Mechanical properties of lungs and chest wall during spontaneous breathing. J Appl Physiol 49(3):408-416
14. Navajas D, Farrè R, Mar Rotger M, Milic-Emili J, Sanchis J (1988) Effect of body posture on respiratory impedance. J Appl Phisiol 64(1):194-199
15. Wouters EFM, Làndsér FJ, Polko AH, Visser BF (1988) Physiologic analysis of extended-spectrum oscillometry. Respiration 54:263-270
16. Peslin R, Fredberg JJ (1986) Oscillation mechanics of the respiratory system. In: Fishman AP (ed) Handbook of physiology. The respiratory system. Vol III. Am Physiol Soc, Bethesda
17. Landsér FJ, Clement J, Van de Woestijne KP (1981) Normal values of total respiratory resistance and reactance determined by forced oscillation. Chest 81:586-591
18. Fisher AB, DuBois AB, Hyde RW (1968) Evaluation of forced oscillation technique for the determination of resistance to breathing. J Clin Invest 47:2045-2057
19. Clément J, Dumoulin B, Gubbelman R, Hendriks S, Van de Woestijne KP (1987) Reference values of total respiratory resistance and reactance between 4 and 26 Hz in children and adolescents aged 4-20 years. Bull Eur Physiopathol Respir 23:441-448
20. Desager KN, Buhr W, Willemen M, Van Bever HP, De Backer W, Vermeire PA, Làndsèr FJ (1991) Measurement of total repiratory impedance in infants by the forced oscillation technique. J Appl Physiol 71(2):770-776
21. Grimby G, Takishima T, Graham W, Macklem P, Mead J (1968) Frequency dependence of flow resistance in patients with obstructive lung disease. Clin Inv 47:1455-1465
22. Hayes DA, Pimmel RL, Fullton JM, Bromberg PA (1979) Detection of respiratory mechanical dysfunction by forced random noise impedance parameter. Am Rev Respir Dis 120:1095-1100
23. Van Noord JA, Clément J, Chauberghs M, Mertens I, Van de Woestijne KP, Demedts M, (1989) Total respiratory resistance and reactance in patients with diffuse interstitial lung disease. Eur Respir J 2:846-852
24 Pasker HG, Schepers R, Clément J, Van de Woestijne KP (1996) Total respiratory impedance measured by means of the forced oscillation technique in subject with and without respiratory complaints. Eur Respir J 9:131-139
25. Hayden MJ, Petak F, Hantos Z, Hall G, Sly PD (1998) Using low-frequency oscillation to detect bronchodilator responsiveness in infants. Am J Respir Crit Care Med 157: 574-579
26. Takishima T, Hida W, Sasaki H, Suzuki S, Sasaki T (19981) Direct - writing recorder of the dose - response curves of the airway to methacholine. Chest 80: 600-606
27. Van Noor JA, Cauberghs M, Van de Woestine KP, Demedts M (1991) Total respiratory resistance and reactance in ankylosing spondylitis and kyphoscoliosis. Eur Respir J 4:945-951
28. Michelis A, Làndsér FJ, Caubergs M, Van de Woestijne KP (1988) Measurement of total respiratory impedance via the endotracheal tube; a model study. Clin Resp Physiol 22:615-620

29. Navajas D, Farré R, Rotger M, Canet J (1988) Recording pressure at the distal end of the endotracheal tube to measure respiratory impedance. Eur Respir J 2:178-184
30. Navajas D, Farré R, Canet J, Rotger M, Sanchis J (1990) Respiratory input impedance in anesthetized paralyzed patients. J Appl Physiol 69(4):1372-1379
31. Navajas D, Farré R, Rotger M, Torres A (1994) Monitoring respiratory impedance by forced oscillation in mechanically-ventilated patients. Eur Respir Rev 4:216-218
32. Peslin R, Da Silva JF, Duvivier C, Chabot F (1993) Respiratory mechanics studied by forced oscillations during artificial ventilation. Eur Respir J 6:772-784

Chapter 6

Resistance measurement in ventilator-dependent patients

A. Rossi

Movement of any flow ($\dot{V}$) through a pipe requires a driving pressure to overcome frictional resistance. The magnitude of flow depends on the difference in pressures (ΔP) across the pipe and the resistance (R) offered by the pipe itself [1]:

$$\dot{V} = \Delta P / R \quad (1)$$

Flow resistance is proportional to the length (l) of the pipe and varies inversely with the fourth and fifth power of the radius (r) for laminar and turbulent flow, respectively, as described by the Poiselle's law:

$$R = \eta \cdot l \cdot 8 / \pi r^4 \quad (2)$$

where η represents the viscosity of the gas and $8/\pi$ is a constant.

It is generally accepted that, in normal subjects, airway resistance is linear during quiet breathing and can be expressed as a single number, according to Eq. 1 in general, about 2-4 cm H_2Osl^{-1}. However, airway resistance (Raw) is only 1 component of total respiratory system's resistance (Rrs), which also includes tissue resistance of the lung (RTL), thus giving total pulmonary resistance (RL), and chest wall resistance (RW) (discussed below) [2]. The resistive characteristics of the respiratory system were first described by Rohrer with the equation:

$$Pres = K_1\dot{V} + K_2\dot{V}^2 \quad (3)$$

where K_1 and K_2 are constants. Another equation has also been used:

$$Pres = a\,\dot{V}^b \quad (3a)$$

where Pres is the resistive pressure drop, a is the value of Pres at $\dot{V}$ of 1 l/s and b is a dimensionless index describing the shape of the pressure-flow relationship-concavity and convexity to the $\dot{V}$ axis are represented by $b<1$ and $b>1$, respectively. When both components of Eq. 3 are divided by $\dot{V}$ (see also Eq. 1), the result is:

$$R = K_1 + K_2\dot{V} \quad (4)$$

This is a first degree equation, where K_1 represents the value of resistance extrapolated to zero and K_2 represents the slope of the increase in R with increasing flow ($\dot{V}$) Eq. 4 is the basis for one of the tenets of respiratory mechanics, namely that, at a given lung volume resistance should increase with increasing flow. Another basic tenet is that at a given flow, resistance should decrease with increasing lung volume because of a decrease in airway resistance due to bronchial dilatation. Assuming that the flow-dependent pressure losses within the thorax are also reduced because the linear velocity of thoracic tissues decreases with increasing lung volume, total respiratory system resistance (Rrs) should decrease with increasing volume, thus Eq. 4 becomes:

$$Rrs = Rt + K_1 + K_2\dot{V} \quad (5)$$

where Rt represents thoracic tissue resistance. Equation 5 assumes that the thoracic tissues exhibit ohmic (Newtonian) behaviour. However, a recent series of studies on respiratory mechanics have shown that this is not the case. In fact, Rt measured during constant flow inflation from relaxed functional residual capacity (FRC) is not constant but increases with the duration of inspiration (Ti) and decreases progressively with increasing flow at fixed lung volume. As a consequence, Rrs initially decreases with increasing flow as a result of the stress relaxation until at high flow the term K_2 becomes predominant.

Endotracheal tubes

In ventilator-dependent patients, a significant component of the total flow resistance is provided by endotracheal tubes, which have highly curvilinear flow-resistive properties [3]. In normal subjects, flow is laminar during tidal ventilation and becomes turbulent only with increasing ventilatory demands. As a result, Eq. 1 has been commonly used when assessing normal breathing. By contrast, in intubated patients, Eqs. 3 and 3a have been used to describe their pressure-flow characteristics. The flow resistance offered by the endotracheal tubes increases markedly with increasing flow and varies with the size of the tube.

Flow resistance is increased in all patients with acute respiratory failure (ARF) due to airway diseases, such as asthma or an exacerbation of COPD. Abnormal flow resistance has been also found in some patients with acute respiratory distress syndrome (ARDS) and pulmonary oedema, particularly in the early stages [4]. Various explanations have been offered for this finding including: 1) inflammatory fluid and cellular debris in the bronchial lumen; 2) reflex bronchoconstriction; 3) decreased FRC; and 4) reduction in the number of ventilating airways. Some authors have reported essentially normal values of airway resistance in ARDS patients, although total respiratory system resistance may be increased. Bronchodilator-induced smooth muscle relaxation decreases flow resistance in ventilator-dependent patients with ARDS [5]. This suggests that increased tone of bronchial smooth muscle also plays a role. Total flow resistance includes the resistance of the endotracheal tube, which can be greater in vivo than in vitro due to secretions in the lumen, or kinking and compression of the tube. In this context, the resistance of ventilator devices and valves should also be taken into account.

Time constant

A factor influencing the dynamics of breathing, the intrapulmonary distribution of inspired gas, and the rate of lung emptying is the time constant (τ), which is normally computed from the following formula:

$$\tau = C \cdot R \text{ or } \tau = R/E \tag{6}$$

If the respiratory system is characterised by a single compliance (C) and single resistance (R), as in the case of the rigid pipe-compliant balloon model, it is also defined by a single τ-in normal subjects this is about 0.2 s (C=0.1 l/cm H_2O and R=2 cm H_2Osl^{-1}). About 64% of a volume will be exhaled during a time interval equal to 1 τ; therefore, an expiratory time >4 τ (i.e., >0.8 s in normals) is necessary for complete expiration. Clearly, as dictated by Eq. 6, a low compliance and normal resistance will be associated with a short τ, thus favouring rapid expiration, whereas a high compliance and high resistance will effect a longer τ and will require a longer expiratory time to decompress the lungs. In addition, the viscoelastic properties of the respiratory tissues also affect lung emptying. In ventilator-dependent patients, the situation becomes complicated by several events.

- Due to the high flow-dependent resistance of endotracheal tubes and the additional resistance of ventilator tubings, valves, and devices, the resistive properties of the patient-endotracheal tube-ventilator circuit ensemble cannot be described by a single resistance. The endotracheal tubes negate a single τ.
- The lungs of patients with ARF present an inhomogeneous distribution of pathologic changes with considerable regional differences in the mechanical properties of the lungs [5], and lung mechanics cannot be described by a single τ.
- Expiratory flow limitation plays a greater role than ohmic resistance in retarding expiratory flow, particularly in patients with acute-on-chronic ventilatory failure, and thus, factors other than the value of τ govern the time course of expiration.

In summary, the endotracheal tubes, together with other factors such as lung inhomogeneity and expiratory flow limitation, exclude application of a single τ in ventilator-dependent patients.

Intrinsic PEEP

In mechanically ventilated patients, alveolar pressure can remain positive if the time available to breathe out is shorter than the time required for lung volume to return to V_r. this can be the consequence of: 1) reduced lung elastic recoil; 2) increased flow resistance; 3) expiratory flow limitation; 4) excessive tidal volume; and 5) short T_E, (due for istance to high breathing frequency or shorter duty cycle). Under these circumstances, expiration is not completed before the onset of the next mechanical lung inflation and the end-expiratory lung volume (EELV) will stabilize above relaxed FRC or Vr [6, 7]. The end-expiratory elastic recoil (Pel,rs) due to incomplete expiration has been termed auto PEEP, inadverted PEEP, endogenous PEEP, internal PEEP, and intrinsic PEEP. Basically, in mechanically-ventilated patients, factors causing the elevation of EELV and intrinsic PEEP (PEEPi) and determining its magnitude are:

- abnormal patient respiratory mechanics, i.e., high resistance and compliance, and expiratory flow limitation;
- added flow resistance, i.e., endotracheal tube and ventilator circuits and valves;
- ventilatory pattern, with large V_T, high frequency, short T_E (due to the ventilator setting, a patient's own ventilatory pattern and demand, or both), and the end-inspiratory pause.

In other words, all mechanisms that either decreasing expiratory flow or shortening T_E promote PEEPi, in ventilator dependent patients. Recently it has been shown that another factor promoting PEEPi is the brief end-inspiratory pause (<0.5s), which is often set to improve gas exchange. An end-inspiratory pause not only increases inspiratory time, and hence decreases T_E at any given frequency, but also decreases the driving pressure available to produce expiratory flow, due to the decrease in Pel,rs as a result of stress relaxation [8].

PEEPi has important implications for all ventilator-dependent patients. Among other adverse effect, PEEPi can depress cardiac output, and it poses an inspiratory threshold load for inspiration. The latter consequence is relevant only with assisted modes, wherease the former has to be taken into account regardless of the ventilator mode. From a monitoring standpoint, PEEPi can be suspected, though not quantified, from the shape of the expired flow-time or flow-volume relationship: if flow does not become nil toward the end of expiration and at the onset of inspiration flow increases abruptly from expiratory to inspiratory there may be PEEPi unless expiratory muscle activity is present. Dynamic hyperinflaction is almost systematically associated with PEEPi.

Dynamic pulmonary hyperinflation (DPH)

During controlled ventilation, and often during assisted ventilation, the presence of PEEPi implies dynamic pulmonary hyperinflation, i.e., an increase in end-expiratory lung volume (EELV) above Vr, the difference between EELV and Vr being defined as ΔFRC. The measurement of ΔFRC has been used by William and Tuxen in asthmatic patients to quantify the degree of pulmonary hyperinflation; they termed this quality V_{EI}, i.e. V_T plus ΔFRC. These authors recommended monitoring V_{EI} in patients with acute asthma to prevent excessive alveolar overdistension and barotrauma. They have shown that keeping V_{EI}<20 ml/Kg can improve survival in asthma. This manoeuvre is simple and suitable for bedside monitoring in relaxed patients. However, with extreme airway obstruction even 30 s may not be sufficient to reach Vr, particularly in presence of patient's inspiratory efforts or because of the need to reinstitute ventilation to prevent deterioration in arterial blood gases.

References

1. Brandi G (1981) Fisica medica. Piccin, Padova
2. Milic-Emili J (1990) Flow resistance in anesthesia. Acta Anaesthesiol Scand 34:42-45
3. Wrigth PE, Marini JJ, Bernard GR (1989) In vitro versus in vivo comparison of endotracheal tube airflow syndrome. Am Rev Respir Dis 139:1169-1174
4. Broseghini C, Brandolese R, Poggi R et al (1988) Respiratory resistance and intrinsic positive end-expiratory pressure (PEEP) in patients with the adult respiratory distress syndrome (ARDS). Eur Respir J 1:726-731
5. Pesenti A, Pelosi P, Rossi N et al (1997) Respiratory mechanics and bronchodilator responsiveness in patients with the adult respiratory distress syndrome. Intensive Care Med 23:58-64
6. Rossi A, Polese G, Brandi G, Conti G (1995) The intrinsic positive end expiratory pressure (PEEPi): physiology, implications, measurement and treatment. Intensive Care Med 21:522-36
7. Rossi A, Ganassini A, Polese G, Grassi V (1997) Pulmonary hyperinflation and ventilator-dependent patients. Eur Respir J 10:1663-1674
8. Georgopoulos D, Mistrouska I, Markopoulou, Patakas D, Anthoninsen NR (1995) Effects of breathing pattern on mechanically ventilated patients with chronic obstructive pulmonary disease and dynamic hyperinflation. Intensive Care Med 21:880-6

Chapter 7

Mechanical models of the respiratory system: linear models

W.A. Zin, R.F.M. Gomes

The respiratory system, as well as its pulmonary and chest wall components, is comprised of a multitude of elements.

The undisputed necessity to interpret the meaning of measurable variables such as volume, airflow, and pressure under both physiological and pathological conditions has imposed the need for relatively simple models able to describe as accurately as possible the mechanical behaviour of the system. The components of such models and their associated parameters should have reasonable physiological counterparts, naturally.

One-compartment model

The simplest model of the respiratory system, which is still the most commonly used, incorporates two lumped elements: one resistance (associated with the pipe) and one elastance (balloon), as depicted in Figure 1a. The equation of motion of the respiratory system describes its behaviour:

$$P(t) = R\dot{V}(t) + EV(t) \tag{1}$$

where P is the driving pressure, R is the resistance of the pipe to airflow ($\dot{V}$), E is the balloon elastance, V represents the change in volume of the balloon above its relaxed configuration, and *t* is time. This single-compartment linear model assumes that R and E are independent of $\dot{V}$ and V, respectively, and that inertial forces are negligible. The latter postulate is probably acceptable within the physiological breathing frequencies up to 2 Hz [1].

The electrical analogue of the linear one-compartment model (Fig. 1b) associates an ohmic resistance to a capacitance of magnitude 1/E, which are subjected to the same flow.

From the mechanical point of view (Fig. 1c), the deformation (i.e. volume V) results from the movement of a Voigt body (one dashpot and a spring arranged in parallel constitute a Voigt body).

The values for R and E can be determined during continuous breathing by fitting Eq. 1 to P, $\dot{V}$, and V using multiple linear regression [2, 3] or the electrical subtraction method [4]. Alternatively, R and E can be obtained during relaxed expiration [5].

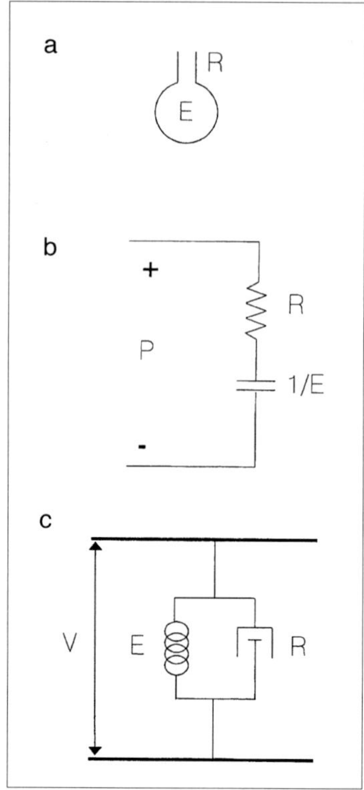

Fig. 1a-c. Linear one-compartment model. (a) Anatomic representation; (b) electrical representation; (c) rheological representation by a Voigt body

Although attractive, the linear single-compartment model cannot explain certain mechanical phenomena presented by the respiratory system, such as: 1) the slow decay in pressure observed after an end-inspiratory occlusion [6-8]; 2) the double-exponential profile of expiration sometimes found in animals and human beings [9, 10]; 3) the frequency dependence of resistance and elastance in the range of 0-2 Hz [3, 11-14]; and 4) the quasi-static pressure-volume hysteresis in isolated lungs. Therefore, in order to better describe the respiratory system mechanical behaviour more complex models are required.

Two-compartment models

Linear two-compartment models increase the mechanical degrees of freedom of the system, and explain frequency dependence of respiratory parameters, stress adaptation, and the two-exponential decay of expired volume under relaxed conditions. They are divided into two main types: gas redistribution and rheologic models.

Gas redistribution models

These models describe mechanical properties of the respiratory system based on inhomogeneities of gas distribution within the lungs. In this context, they can be divided into two sub-types: parallel and series redistribution.

The *parallel gas redistribution model* [15] consists of two alveolar compartments with elastances E_1 and E_2 served by paralled airways with fixed resistances R_1 and R_2 (Fig. 2a). Additionally, a resistance common to the two compartments can be added to the model to represent central airways resistance [16]. Electrically, the model is made up of two serially arranged RC elements organized in parallel (Fig. 2b). Mechanically (Fig. 2c), the model serially associates two Voigt bodies characterized by their respective springs (E_1 and E_2) and dashpots (R_1 and R_2). The total deformation (i.e. volume V) is the sum of each of their respective deformations. This model associates stress adaptation to parallel Pendelluft, which consists of alveolar pressure equilibrium during airflow interruption, and depends on the difference between the two peripheral time constants (τ=R/E), and on volume history.

In the *serial gas redistribution model* [17], homogeneous lungs (represented by an alveolar compartment with elastance E_2 and distal airways with resistance R_2) are served by central airways with an elastance E_1 and a resistance R_1 (Fig. 3a). The electrical analogue of this model (Fig. 3b) is comprised of a resistance R_1 in series with R_2 and E_2, which, in turn, are in parallel with a capacitance 1/E. This capacitance behaves as a buffer between alveolar and driving

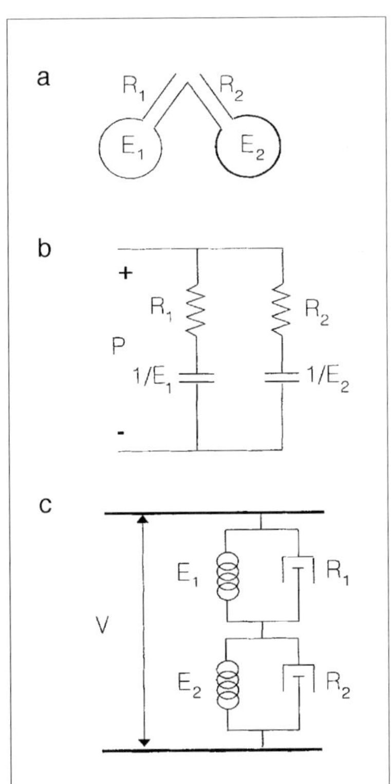

Fig. 2a-c. Linear parallel two-compartment gas redistribution model. (a) Anatomic representation; (b) electrical representation; (c) rheological representation by two Voigt bodies (R_1, E_1 and R_2, E_2)

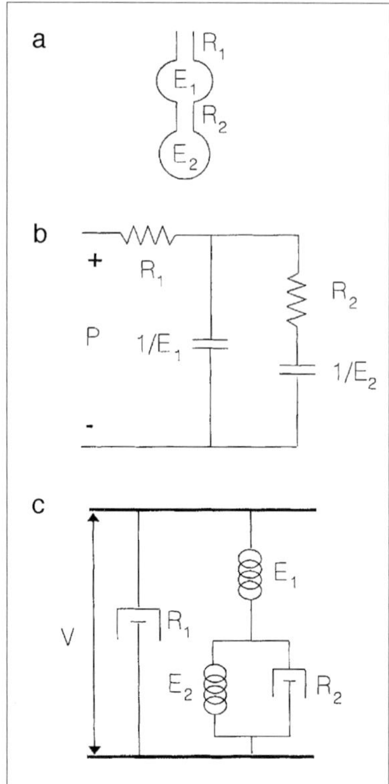

Fig. 3a-c. Linear serial two-compartment gas redistribution model. (a) Anatomic representation; (b) electrical representation; (c) rheological representation by a dashpot (R_1) associated in parallel with a spring (E_1) serially coupled a Voigt body (R_2, E_2)

pressures. Hence, a given fraction of the inspired volume remains in the central airways, depending on central and peripheral time constants (τ_1 and τ_2, respectively), thus decreasing the volume available for gas exchange. The mechanical representation of the model (Fig. 3c) is obtained by substituting mechanical elements in series for electrical ones in parallel (and those in parallel for electrical ones in series), since mechanical bodies in parallel undergo the same deformation rate and are submitted to an identical pressure when arranged in series. This kind of model is particularly useful in the interpretation of pathological conditions, such as chronic obstructive pulmonary disease (COPD). When elastic and resistive data of normal individuals are considered, the serial gas distribution model cannot explain frequency dependence of resistance and elastance in the normal range of breathing frequencies. However, when the peripheral resistance R_2 increases, the model confers a time dependence to R and E compatible with the real behaviour of COPD lungs. Finally, there are alternative anatomical interpretations for E_1, such that it would be associated with either an alveolar gas compliance or a lung region with negligible resistance [18, 19]. However, the original association of E_1 with centrial airway elastance still prevails [18, 20].

As also displayed by the parallel two-compartment model, there is gas redistribution between the compartments after flow interruption. In fact, the behaviour of both models may be identical, depending on the values chosen for the four parameters, since they are described by the same differential equation [21]:

$$P(t) + a\dot{P}(t) = bV(t) + c\dot{V}(t) + d\,\ddot{V}(t) \qquad (2)$$

where $\dot{P}(t)$ is the first time derivative of $\dot{P}(t)$, and $\ddot{V}(t)$ corresponds to second time derivative of V (t).

Rheological models

The rheological models do not assume the existence of an uneven distribution of ventilation. Supporting this notion, no inhomogeneity of gas distribution could be detected under normal conditions [22, 23]. In fact, the rheological models extend the one-compartment model by incorporating a viscoelastic [24, 25] or plastoelastic [26, 27] element in parallel with the Voigt body depicted in Figure 1c.

In the viscoelastic model of the respiratory system (Fig. 4) [24, 25, 28] stress adaptation originates from lung, chest wall tissues, or surfactant viscoelastic properties (R_2 and E_2, Fig. 4c). A Kelvin body, which is made up of a Maxwell body (R_2, E_2) in parallel with E_1, represents the viscoelasticity in Figure 4a. The

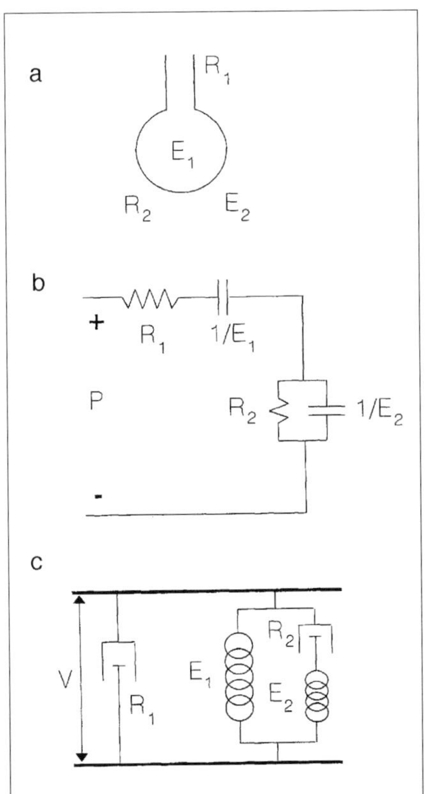

Fig. 4a-c. Linear viscoelastic two-compartment model. (a) Anatomic representation; (b) electrical representation; (c) rheological representation by a dashpot (R_1) associated in parallel with a spring (E_1) coupled in parallel with a Maxwell body (R_2, E_2)

Maxwell body associated in parallel with a Voigt body (R_1, E_1) constitutes the mechanical viscoelastic model of the lung. E_1 represents static elastance, and, according to recent experiments involving alveolar capsules, R_1 corresponds to airway resistance in normal animals [22, 23]. The deformation of the Maxwell body is the sum of the deformations of its resistive and elastic elements, and its slow time constant ($\tau_2=R_2/E_2$) might be responsible for the tissue stress adaptation phenomenon. The electrical analogue of the viscoelastic model is depicted in Figure 4b. Finally, this model is also governed by a differential equation like Eq. 2.

The plastoelastic model differs from the viscoelastic one by the substitution of a dry friction (Coulomb) element for the viscous element (R_2) in the Maxwell body, thus forming the Prandtl body [29]. The Coulomb element will only start moving after a pressure threshold has been reached. Henceforth, energy is continuously dissipated independently of the rate of displacement. This model could account for the quasi-static pressure volume hysteresis in isolated lungs. However, the plastoelastic model is rarely used in vivo under small volume excursions, where its parameter values have sometimes been found difficult to be interpreted mechanically [30, 31].

Multi-compartment models

An attempt to more accurately describe a set of experimental data can be performed by means of multi-compartment models.

Hence, a varying number of Voigt, Kelvin, or Maxwell bodies could be added in parallel to the aforementioned models. In this line, a model has been proposed in which P(t) decreses linearly as a function of the logarithm of the time subsequent to a step change in volume (V), according to the equation [26, 32, 33]:

$$P(t)/V = A - B \cdot \ln t \tag{3}$$

Naturally, the existence of a multitude of time constants is implicit in this particular model. Nevertheless, the multi-compartment models yield a great deal of parameters, whose direct assigment to mechanical elements is unwarranted.

Choosing the appropriate model

The choice of the model will depend upon the intended physiological or pathophysiological goal. In other words, the most adequate model is that whose elements closely reproduce the actual system under study [21, 34]. Thence, it is virtually impossible to use a "perfect" model. However, the use of simple models that satisfactorily represent the general mechanical behaviour of the respiratory system and its lung and chest wall components is of paramount importance to the respirologist.

The models are to be chosen according to the scientific questioning, techniques and methods to be used and, of course, the experimental condition. Furthermore, the easy gathering of the parameters of a given model should never thwart the quest for the most appropriate physiological interpretation of the data.

References

1. Sharp JT, Henry JP, Sweany SK, Meadows WR, Pietras RJ (1964) Total respiratory inertance and its gas and tissue components in normal and obese men. J Appl Physiol 43:503-509
2. Hantos Z, Daróczy B, Klebniczki J, Dombos K, Nagy S (1982) Parameter estimation of transpulmonary mechanics by a nonlinear inertive model. J Appl Physiol 52:955-963
3. Bates JHT, Shardonofsky F, Stewart DE (1989) The low-frequency dependence of respiratory system resistance and elastance in normal dogs. Respir Physiol 78:369-382
4. Mead J, Whittenberger JL (1953) Physical properties of human lungs measured during spontaneous respiration. J Appl Physiol 5:779-796
5. Zin WA, Pengelly LD, Milic-Emili J (1982) Single-breath method for measurement of respiratory mechanics in anesthetized animals. J Appl Physiol 52:1266-1271
6. Hughes R, May AJ, Widdicombe JG (1959) Stress relaxation in rabbits' lungs. J Physiol 146:85-97
7. Don HF, Robson JG (1965) The mechanics of the respiratory system during anesthesia. Anesthesiol 26:168-178
8. Bates JHT, Rossi A, Milic-Emili J (1985) Analysis of the behaviour of the respiratory system with constant inspiratory flow. J Appl Physiol 58:1840-1848
9. Bates JHT, Decramer M, Chartrand D, Zin WA, Böddener A, Milic-Emili J (1985) The volume-time profile during relaxed expiration in the normal dog. J Appl Physiol 59:732-737
10. Chelucci GL, Brunet F, Dall'Alva-Santucci J, Dhainaut JF, Paccaly D, Armaganidis A, Milic-Emili J, Lockhart A (1991) A single-compartment model cannot describe passive expiration in intubated, paralysed humans. Eur Respir J 4:458-464
11. Barnas GM, Yoshino K, Loring SH, Mead J (1987) Impedance and relative displacements of relaxed chest wall up to 4 Hz. J Appl Physiol 62:71-81
12. Brusasco V, Warner DO, Beck KC, Rodarte JR, Rehder K (1989) Partitioning of pulmonary resistance in dogs: effects of tidal volume and frequency. J Appl Physiol 66:1190-1197
13. Hantos Z, Daróczy B, Suki B, Galgoczy G, Csendes T (1986) Forced oscillatory impedance of the respiratory system at low frequencies. J Appl Physiol 60:123-132
14. Hantos Z, Daróczy B, Suki B, Nagy S (1987) Low-frequency respiratory mechanical impedance in the rat. J Appl Physiol 63:36-43
15. Otis AB, McKerrow CB, Bartlett RA, Mead J, McIlroy MB, Selverstone NJ, Radford EP (1956) Mechanical factors in the distribution of pulmonary ventilation. J Appl Physiol 8:427-444
16. Bates JHT, Baconnier P, Milic-Emili J (1988) A theoretical analysis of interrupter technique for measuring respiratory mechanics. J Appl Physiol 64:2204-2214
17. Mead J (1969) Contribution of compliance of airways to frequency-dependence behavior of lungs. J Appl Physiol 26:670-673
18. Eyles JG, Pimmel RL (1981) Estimating respiratory mechanical parameters in parallel compartment models. IEEE Trans Biomed Eng 28:313-317
19. Peslin R (1986) Methods for measuring total respiratory impedance by forced oscillations. Bull Eur Physiopathol Respir 22:621-631

20. Michaelson ED, Grassman ED, Peters WR (1975) Pulmonary mechanics by spectral analysis of forced random noise. J Clin Invest 56:1210-1230
21. Lorino AM, Lorino H, Harf A (1994) A synthesis of the Otis, Mead, and Mount mechanical respiratory models. Respir Physiol 97:123-133
22. Bates JHT, Ludwig MS, Sly PD, Brown K, Martin JG, Fredberg JJ (1988) Interrupter resistance elucidated by alveolar pressure measurements in open-chest normal dogs. J Appl Physiol 65:408-414
23. Saldiva PHN, Zin WA, Santos RLB, Eidelman DH, Milic- Emili J (1992) Alveolar pressure measurement in open-chest rats. J Appl Physiol 72:302-306
24. Mount LE (1955) The ventilation flow-resistance and compliance of rat lungs. J Physiol 127:157-167
25. Bates JHT, Brown KA, Kochi T (1989) Respiratory mechanics in the normal dog determined by expiratory flow interruption. J Appl Physiol 67:2276-2285
26. Hildebrandt J (1970) Pressure-volume data of cat lung interpreted by plastoelastic, linear viscoelastic model. J Appl Physiol 28:365-372
27. Fredberg JJ, Stamenovic D (1989) On the imperfect elasticity of lung tissue. J Appl Physiol 67:2408-2419
28. Sharp JT, Johnson FN, Goldberg NB, van Lith P (1967) Hysteresis and stress adaptation in the human respiratory system. J Appl Physiol 23:487-497
29. Similowski T, Bates JHT (1991) Two-compartment modelling of respiratory system mechanics at low frequencies: gas redistribution or tissue rheology? Eur Respir J 4:353- 358
30. Navajas D, Farré R, Cannet J, Roger M, Sanchis J (1990) Respiratory inputs impedance in anesthetised paralyzed patients. J Appl Physiol 69:1372-1379
31. Shardonofsky F, Sato J, Bates JHT (1990) Quasi-static pressure-volume hysteresis in the canine respiratory system in vivo. J Appl Physiol 68:2230-2236
32. Hildebrandt J (1969) Dynamic properties of air-filled excised cat lung determined by liquid plethysmography. J Appl Physiol 27:246-250
33. Hildebrandt J (1969) Comparison of mathematical models for cat lung and viscoelastic balloon derived by Laplace transform methods from pressure-volume data. Bull Math Biophys 31:651-667
34. Rotger M, Peslin R, Navajas D, Farré R (1995) Lung and respiratory impedance at low frequency during mechanical ventilation in rabbits. J Appl Physiol 78:2153-2160

Chapter 8

Mechanical models of the respiratory system: non-linear and inhomogeneous models

Z. Hantos

Non-linearities and structural complexity are characteristic determinants of the respiratory mechanical system. Although they are inherent properties in both health and disease, it is generally assumed that their effects are predominantly manifested in pathological conditions. The linear and one-compartment models, which are of key importance for an understanding of the fundamentals of mechanical behaviour, may be of restricted validity in pulmonary diseases associated with flow limitation, loss of elastic recoil, peripheral bronchoconstriction and certain other mechanical disorders.

Non-linearity and inhomogeneity are distinct phenomena, even if they often act in an interwoven way and are sometimes subject to conceptual confusion. When speaking about non-linearity, one usually refers to a system whose response (an output quantity) is not proportional to the excitation at its input, as for example in the nasal passages, where the pressure-flow relationship is typically curvilinear. Inhomogeneity in turn is connected to a complex structure in which elements belonging in the same class (i.e. the peripheral airways of comparable morphological generations) possess significantly different parameters, and exhibit locally non-uniform behaviour, resulting in a characteristic change in the global function of the system. Non-linearity and inhomogeneity have different modelling methodologies and, apart from recent efforts, the complexity of each phenomenon has not encouraged combined studies.

The conventional approach

According to the classical concept of respiratory mechanics, the transpulmonary pressure (Ptp) contains three additive components: the elastic, viscous and inertive pressure terms. In the lumped linear model widely used to elucidate the basic mechanical phenomena, each term contains a coefficient of proportionality: the elastance (E) describes the dependence of the elastic pressure component on volume (V) above the resting (end-expiratory) level (P_0), the Newtonian resistance (R) is the coefficient between volume flow ($\dot{V}$) and resistive pressure drop, and the inertance (I) is the proportionality factor between volume acceleration ($\ddot{V}$)and the inertive pressure component:

$$\mathrm{Ptp} = P_0 + E\,V + R\,\dot{V} + I\,\ddot{V} \qquad (1)$$

The parameters of this model, generally with neglect of the inertive term, have been commonly estimated by multiple linear regression since this technique was first proposed by Wald et al. [1]. Mead and Milic-Emili [2] suggested a more general form that allows the specification of non-linear elastic, viscous and inertive relationships:

$$Ptp = f_1(V) + f_2(\dot{V}) + f_3(\ddot{V}) \quad (2)$$

where f_1, f_2 and f_3 denote functions of volume (V), volume flow ($\dot{V}$) and volume acceleration ($\ddot{V}$), respectively. With the assumption of curvilinear pressure-volume and pressure-flow relationships described by third-order polynomials, and a linear relationship between pressure and acceleration, this model has been shown to give an excellent fit to transpulmonary pressure data in mechanically ventilated dogs [3]. The dynamic characteristics (f_1, f_2 and f_3) estimated by non-linear regression represent biomechanically realistic pressure-volume, pressure-flow and pressure-acceleration relationships. The major limitation of this polynomial model was the formal lack of plausible cross-relationships, i.e. the inability to account for the dependence of the viscous pressure drop on the actual lung volume via the altered bronchial diameters [4], or the elastic pressure term on the rate of deformation (i.e. $\dot{V}$) [5, 6]. In general, recent advances in tissue mechanics have brought into question the appropriateness of this time-domain approach. In particular, the non-Newtonian nature of tissue resistance and the characteristic frequency dependences of both resistance and elastance render this model descriptive rather than mechanistic. However, even if serious problems do arise in the interpretation of the parameters, the facts that this method is based on signals recorded during spontaneous breathing or mechanical ventilation and that it is easy to implement computationally make linear and non-linear regression techniques useful tools for assessment of the overall mechanical status of the respiratory system.

Non-linearities and the frequency-domain approach

The analysis of linear systems is supported by well-elaborated and robust methodologies. They offer powerful tools for the collection and interpretation of experimental data; one such is the estimation of the frequency response. By driving a mechanical system with signals of wide frequency spectrum and recording its response, one can acquire large amounts of information for identification of the components of the system. The forced oscillation technique has been applied in respiratory mechanics research for decades [7], and recent investigations of low-frequency mechanical impedance have also been based on this method [8-10]. However, to avoid any violation of linearity, the externally applied driving signal must be kept well below the tidal excursions; if this is not the case, non-linearities result in harmonic distortion and cross-talk that corrupt the impedance spectra [11-13].

The latter fact has challenging implications as concerns mechanical ventilation. If a driving signal of tidal amplitude is composed of frequency components that are not integer multiples of each other, the harmonics produced by non-linearities in the mechanical response will not coincide with the components of the input signal; additionally, higher-order distortions (cross-talk) can be cancelled if neither sums nor differences of the existing components are allowed in the input frequency spectrum. If these specially devised ventilator waveforms are used, adequate tidal ventilation can be maintained, while they simultaneously serve as a forced oscillatory signal identifying the linear subsystem of the fundamentally non-linear respiratory mechanical system [13-16]. Furthermore, the primary data from these measurements reflecting both the amplitude and frequency dependences of respiratory mechanics are adequate material for sophisticated complex models encompassing parts of linear viscoelasticity, airway and tissue non-linearities via the non-linear block-structured modelling approach [17].

Characteristic non-linear phenomena in the respiratory system

Non-linearities in the airways

During quiet breathing, the airflow in the lower airways is laminar and, apart from the bifurcation regions, the velocity profile is parabolic. This flow condition corresponds to the minimum energy loss due to the internal friction of the gas. In the upper airways, however, the abrupt changes in cross-sectional area, especially at the level of the vocal cords, lead to more complex flow patterns even during normal breathing. This means that excessive dissipations dependent on the gas density add to the work of laminar flow, which is a function of the gas viscosity. Higher flow rates and marked geometric irregularities in the upper airways (such as the narrow nasal pathways, and orifice effects at the distal end of cuffed endotracheal tubes or in face masks) make these additional dissipations increasingly important. The first approach combining the pressure losses due to unidirectional laminar and turbulent flows was suggested in 1915 by Rohrer [18]:

$$P_{aw} = K_1 \dot{V} + K_2 \dot{V}^2 \tag{3}$$

where P is the pressure drop across the airways, $\dot{V}$ is the airflow, and the coefficients K_1 and K_2 are linear functions of gas viscosity and density, respectively. For bidirectional (alternating) flows, the appropriate form of this equation is

$$P_{aw} = K_1 \dot{V} + K_2 \dot{V} |\dot{V}|, \tag{4}$$

a graphical representation of which is given in Figure 1a. Subsequent studies have shown that the above equations contain terms that correspond to flows of very low Reynolds' numbers (pressure linearly dependent on flow) and the fully developed orifice flow characteristic of extremely high Reynolds' numbers (the quadratic term), and that in irregular conduits and at intermediate flows the pressure-flow relationship is more complicated [19]. However, Rohrer's model has remained a plausible and easily identifiable model of the rheology of the airways.

Although the irregular geometry of the upper airways causes deviations from the linear pressure-flow relationship, as long as the geometry is fixed, the airway resistance remains a basically unique function of flow. This is no longer the case in several respiratory mechanical disorders characterized by significant transbronchial pressure changes (generally due to a high overall airway resistance), increased airway compliance, decreased parenchymal support and their combinations. The cyclic change in transbronchial pressure related to the more easily measurable lung volume introduces considerable fluctuations in the airway geometry in these pathological conditions. Formally, one can say that P_{aw} becomes a function of both flow and volume, i.e. $P_{aw}=f(V, \dot{V})$. Models implementing this function have been developed to explain the flow limitation occurring in forced expiratory manoeuvres [20]; however, the impact of changing airway geometry on airway resistance is clearly apparent in the expiratory looping of plethysmographic P_{aw}-$\dot{V}$ diagrams recorded during normal breathing (Fig. 1b). Measurement techniques that faithfully reveal the pressure-flow characteristics of the airways may therefore furnish useful information about the structural background of the non-linearities. On the other hand, however, instead of a set of coefficients which describe curvilinear relationships and are difficult to handle, it is sometimes desirable to obtain linear, energetically equivalent quantities to characterize the overall dissipation in the airways [21, 22].

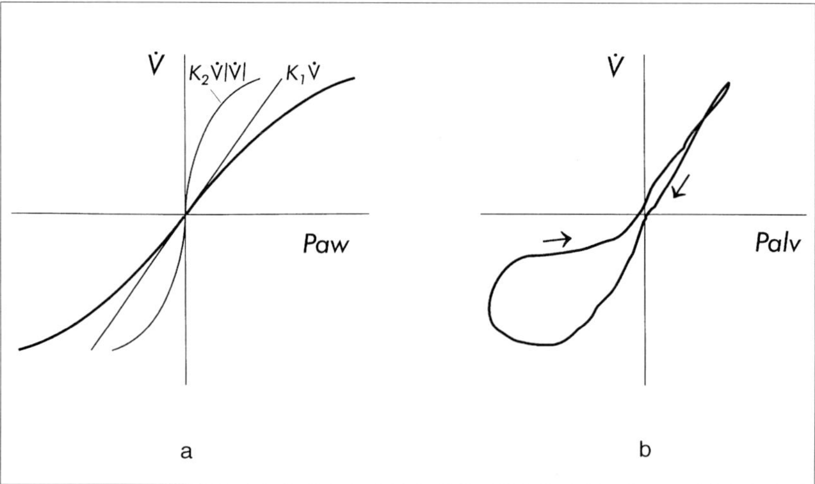

Fig. 1a,b. Airway non-linearities. (a) decomposition of the S-shaped relationship between airway pressure (Paw) and flow ($\dot{V}$) into linear and quadratic terms according to Rohrer [18]; (b) schematic change in airway resistance during the respiratory cycle, manifested in expiratory looping in the plethysmographic relationship between alveolar pressure (Palv) and $\dot{V}$

Tissue non-linearity

The non-linear behaviour of the respiratory tissues has always been regarded as a complex phenomenon: in comparison with airway non-linearities, it is conceptually far more problematic and is subject to much contradiction in the literature. If the (quasi-) static P-v diagram of the lungs is considered, the flattening of the curve at high lung volumes suggests that higher tidal volumes invoke progressively higher elastic forces. Such non-linear stress-strain behaviour has recently been modelled with a network of distributed-parameter pairs of elastin and collagen fibres [23]. Whereas the involvement of stretch-limiting tissue elements may indeed become the dominant factor at extreme volume excursions, the normal range of tidal volumes is characterized by a negative dependence of tissue elastance and resistance on the volume amplitude.

This striking inverse relationship was first analysed by Hildebrandt [5, 6], who measured the mechanical response of excised cat lungs by applying different tidal volumes with both stepwise inputs and sinusoidal oscillations over a wide range of low frequencies. Hildebrandt's study led to two important results, but unfortunately these have often been confused. The first advance was the frequency-domain formulation of a *linear viscoleastic* model derived from an empirical time-domain process of stress relaxation. This model involves a distribution of time constants and can therefore be regarded as a generalized Kelvin or Maxwell body or a multitude of viscoelastic elements [24], and it has been shown to describe accurately the oscillatory mechanics of the lung parenchyma over several decades of frequency [5, 6, 8-10]. The second finding was the systematic decrease in elastance and tissue viscance with increasing amplitude of deformation; this observation was proved to be consistent with the behaviour of an array of *plastoelastic* elements (Prandtl bodies, Fig. 2) connected to one of linear viscoelastic elements (spring-dashpot combinations). The Prandtl bodies contain units of dry friction, the threshold forces of which follow a distribution, similarly as do the elastic units. The system would be relatively rigid at small amplitudes of deformations, where in a significant number of plastoelastic elements, the threshold forces are not overcome, and maximally compliant at large deformations where all friction elements slip (Fig. 3). The morphological correspondence of these mechanical model components is not clear. In the lungs, as pointed out by Fredberg and Stamenovic, [25], plastic properties can be involved in several substructures where dissipative and elastic processes are coupled: cross-bridges of the contractile elements, the surface-active monolayer, the fibre networks and the alveolar wall.

The degree to which the non-linear phenomena contribute to the overall dissipative and elastic properties of the lungs may not seem very important. In Hildebrandt's study, a four-fold increase in tidal volume (VT) resulted in an approximately 24% fall in elastance at a high mean lung volume, and in a far lower change at a lower volume level [6]. Smaller changes (from 9% to 20%) were observed in the tissue parameters derived from input impedance in open-chest cats [10] and from the transpulmonary impedance of intact dogs [26], over a four-fold and six-fold volume range, respectively. Even a large increase of

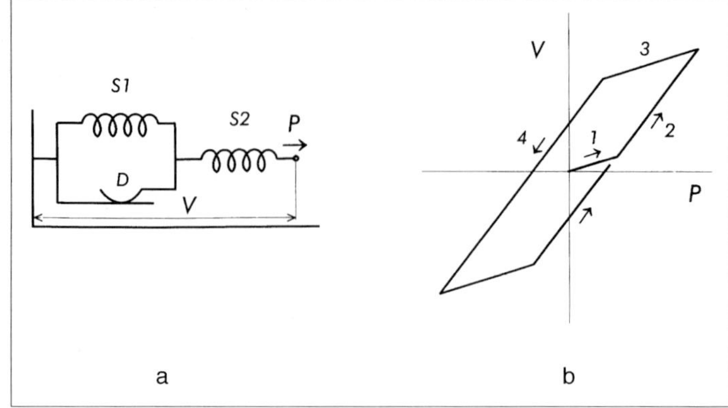

Fig. 2a,b. (a) A Prandtl body, the plastoelastic unit of Hildebrandt's model of tissue non-linearity, consisting of ideal elastic (spring) elements (S1 and S2) and a dry friction (slip) element (D). The force-length relationship of the plastoelastic unit is expressed in terms of pressure (P) and volume (V). (b) During the initial deformation from the resting state (phase 1) only S2 expands; when a threshold pressure (yield point) is reached, D becomes detached and exerts a constant pressure, and both springs expand (phase 2); the reverse deformation starts with S1 fixed again (phase 3) until the lower yield point of D is reached and both springs are compressed (phase 4)

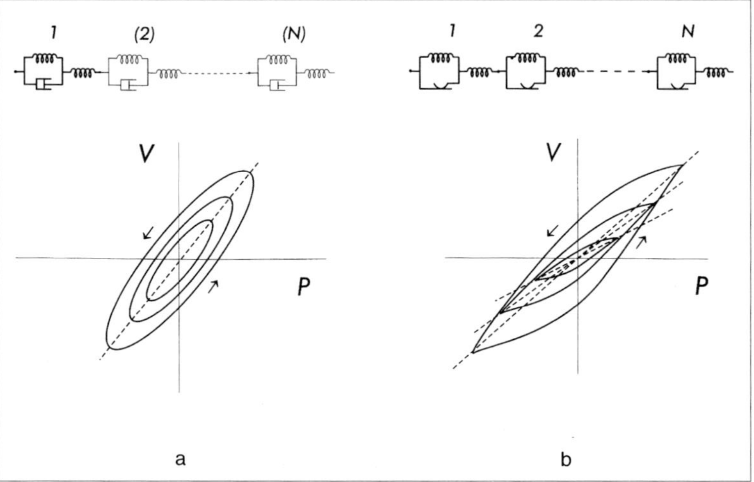

Fig. 3a,b. Arrays of linear viscoelastic (a) and plastoelastic units (b) according to Hildebrandt [6]. Both the slope and hysteresis of the pressure (P)-volume (V) loop of the linear model are independent of the pressure amplitude, for either one unit or the whole array of N units (the frequency dependences of the slope and hysteresis become different if not one unit but an array of different-parameter units is considered). The multitude of plastoelastic units with a distribution of yield points makes the P-V diagram of the plastoelastic array smooth (Fig. 2b). With increasing P, the number of units of exceeded yield points grows, involving more and more springs that expand and thereby making the array more compliant: the mean compliance of the system (the slopes of the dashed lines) increases with the amplitude of the cycling pressure oscillated volume from 15 to 460 ml in thoracotomized dogs led to a moderate decrease of 20%-22% in elastance [27]. The importance of parenchymal non-linearity becomes appreciable beyond the largely theoretical impact if the properties of healthy and injured lungs are compared. Lutchen et al. [16] observed a mild increase (from 19% to 27%) in the amplitude dependence of tissue elastance in a three-fold VT range on infusion of histamine in dogs, but in oleic acid lung injury the VT dependence may become several times stronger than in the control state [28, 29]. These studies suggest that, in addition to the conventional measures of pulmonary mechanics, such as airway and tissue resistances and lung elastance, the altered tissue non-linearity might play an important role in characterizing several other pathological conditions of the lungs.

It is important to note that this kind of tissue non-linearity is stronger in the chest wall than in the lungs. Marked negative dependences of chest wall resistance and elastance were observed in studies with the same measurement technique which revealed negligible non-linearities for the pulmonary tissue [10, 26, 30, 31]. For the total respiratory system, an intermediate degree of amplitude dependence is expected. Any impact of this particular non-linearity would be highly speculative; it is tempting nevertheless to assume that this non-linear behaviour extrapolated to very small deformations may result in a marked increase in tissue rigidity, thereby offering protection against disturbances of non-respiratory origin and increasing the stability of the end-expiratory position.

Recent modelling studies have confirmed that plastoelasticity is a plausible but not unique phenomenon accounting for the negative amplitude dependence of tissue elastance and resistance, and that various models of non-linear viscoelasticity can simulate this tissue property [17, 25, 32-36].

Airway closure and reopening

I address very briefly a characteristic non-linear phenomenon in the lung, the closure and reopening of airways. Although it has long been recognized that these processes are an integral part of the pulmonary P-V relationship [37], the vast majority of experimental and modelling work in this area has focussed on the issue of airway stability at the level of individual airways. An interesting global modelling approach was described by Suki et al. [38], who used a symmetrical airway tree terminating in uniform alveoli to model the reopening of the collapsed lungs. Each airway segment was assigned a threshold opening pressure taken from a wide distribution; airway opening occurred during inflation of the lung when the internal pressure in the particular airway exceeded its threshold value. Simulations demonstrated that the opening of an airway facilitated the opening of a daughter branch and thereby triggered an avalanche process of opening along the whole subtree of the airways. This process was reflected by discrete changes in overall airway resistance, closely resembling the statistical properties of actually measured resistance data in isolated lungs [38, 39]. The impact of this finding is that the stochastic nature of the airway reopening can be utilized in the ventilation strategy by introducing biological variability in the respirator parameters [40].

Models of mechanical inhomogeneity

The failure of the one-compartment model containing one parameter for each of the elastic, viscous and inertive pressure drops (Eq. 1) becomes apparent once the fundamental frequency of breathing or mechanical ventilation is altered significantly. Although recent studies on low-frequency respiratory impedance and tissue mechanics have invalidated most of the assumptions concerning the mechanisms of frequency dependences of resistance and elastance, the model of two parallel compartments put forward by Otis et al. [41] may be considered the archetype of linear inhomogeneous respiratory mechanical models intended to explain the behaviour of the non-uniformly diseased lungs. (I note that, within a narrow frequency range, similar behaviour is exhibited by a one-compartment model suggested by Mead [42], which includes airway wall compliance as a shunt pathway and which is therefore often given the conceptually wrong notation "serial inhomogeneity", as opposed to the parallel inhomogeneity embodied in the Otis model.)

Whereas the Otis model was simple enough for its predictions to be developed mathematically, more complex models of inhomogeneity had to wait until sophisticated computation tools became available. In the meantime, direct measurements of local alveolar pressures shed light on the importance and nature of the regional heterogeneity of lung mechanics [43, 44]. To explain the essentials of the latter, Fredberg et al. suggested a two-generation model in which the single central airway is shared by numerous regional units in parallel, each consisting of the peripheral airway and a local tissue compartment whose parameter values are taken from distributions [43]. This model, illustrated in Fig. 4,

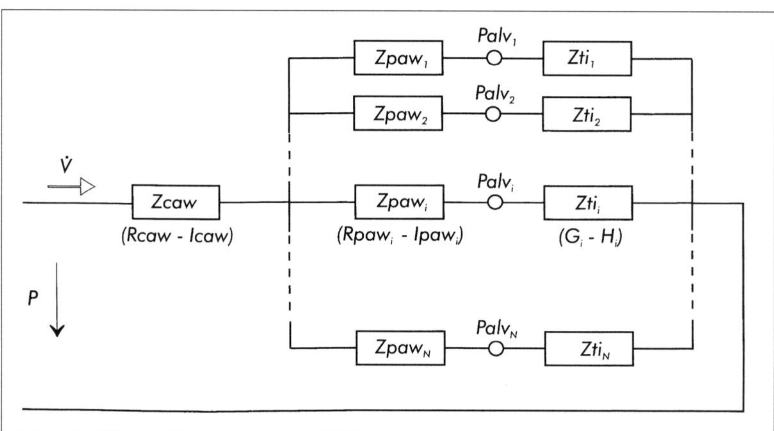

Fig. 4. Distributed-periphery model of the lung proposed by Fredberg et al. [43] and adopted for a simulation study by Hantos et al. [9]. The airways are modelled with a central airway impedance (Zcaw) and N peripheral airways ($Zpaw_i$) in parallel, each consisting of resistances (R) and inertances (I). The tissue units (Zti_i) are constant-phase impedances [9] characterized by tissue damping (G) and elastance (H). The parameter values of $Zpaw_i$ and Zti_i can be given independent distributions to simulate a great variety of inhomogeneity patterns in alveolar pressure ($Palv_i$). The input impedance of the model is the relationship between the transpulmonary pressure (P) and central airflow ($\dot{V}$)

was implemented by assuming resistive and inertive parameters for the airway compartments, while the tissue units were characterized by the coefficients for damping (i.e. tissue viscance) and elastance of the constant-phase tissue model [9]. The simulation studies with this model (an example is presented in Fig. 5) resulted in good qualitative agreement between the modelled and actually measured regional transfer impedances (the relationships between local alveolar pressure and central airflow) for the impedances obtained in the control

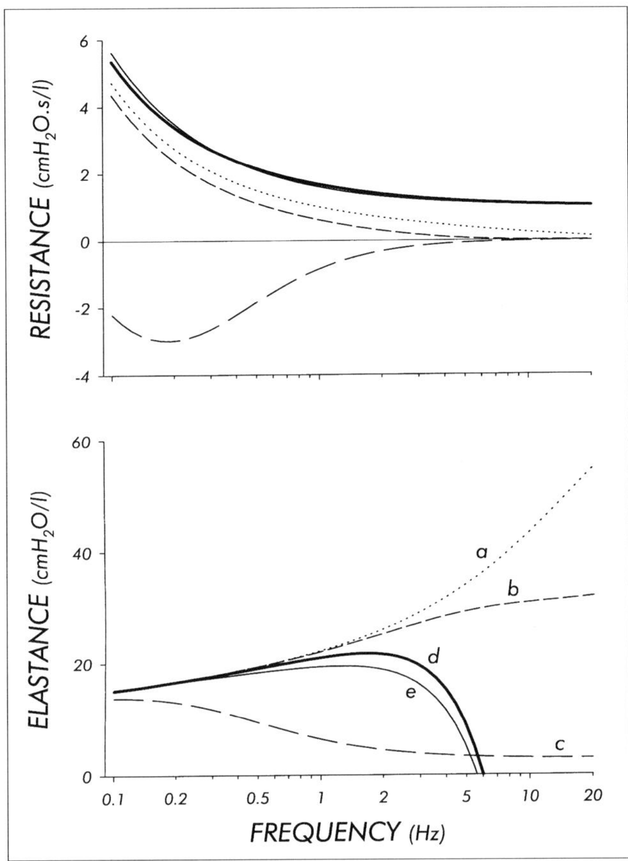

Fig. 5. Results of simulation with the distributed-periphery model shown in Fig. 4, in terms of resistance (top) and elastance (bottom) as functions of frequency. The overall resistance of the peripheral airways was set at 4 Rcaw, and the peripheral constriction was made inhomogeneous by distributing the $Rpaw_i$ values over a 20-fold range. The tissue parameters were perturbated within ±25% of the mean values. Lines a, b and c indicate the transfer tissue impedances (i.e. the relationships between the local $Palv_i$ values and $\dot{V}$) for the minimum, average and maximum $Rpaw_i$ pathway, respectively. In spite of the marked inhomogeneity of the local quantities, the input resistance and elastance computed from the relationship between P and $\dot{V}$ (line d) were well fitted by a lumped-periphery four-parameter model (line e)

state and during histamine-induced constrictions. Another important observation in this study was that, in both the experimental and simulated data, the input impedances were consistent with a four-parameter model containing an airway impedance and a constant-phase tissue unit, even if the regional transfer impedances exhibited markedly different patterns of frequency dependence. This observation leads to the conclusion that even an extremely inhomogeneous lung structure can produce virtually homogeneous behaviour, as seen globally from the input.

Studies using experimental and modelling methods to address peripheral inhomogeneity have refreshed the old concept of "pendelluft". The pattern of interregional flows accompanying the mainstream airflow between the alveoli and the airway opening is a function of the degree of mechanical inhomogeneity and as such is a phenomenon associated with a frequency dependence. Simulations based on the distributed-periphery model [9] predicted that the interregional flows intensifed by the enhanced heterogeneity of the peripheral airways would lead to dissipations inconsistent with a Newtonian resistance, but closely resembling the negative frequency dependence of tissue resistance. In other words, the inhomogeneous constriction of peripheral airways produces a virtual component of tissue damping (as identified in the input impedance of the lungs), which is superimposed on any genuine mechanical change in the tissues evoked by the same constrictor stimulus. Experimental studies applying resident gases of different viscosities before and after pulmonary constriction have confirmed the presence of this virtual component in the constricted lung, demonstrating at the same time that the interregional flows are not detectable during control conditions [45, 46].

Although the studies involving the one-generation distributed-periphery model discussed above [9, 43] were able to demonstrate the basic processes of inhomogeneity, the predictive value of simulation can be increased if more realistic structures are considered. Recent modelling studies have considered the effects of inhomogeneity by applying irregularly branching airway networks based on morphometric data [47] and assuming stochastic processes that determine the degree of the constrictions in the individual airways [48-50].

References

1. Wald A, Jason D, Murphy TW, Mazzia VDB (1969) A computer system for respiratory parameters. Comput Biomed Res 2:411-429
2. Mead J, Milic-Emili J (1964) Theory and methodology in respiratory mechanics with glossary of symbols. In: Fenn WO, Rahn H (eds) Respiration. Handbook of physiology. Vol I. American Physiological Society, Washington, pp 363-376
3. Hantos Z, Daróczy B, Klebniczki J, Dombos K, Nagy S (1982) Parameter estimation of transpulmonary mechanics by a non-linear inertive model. J Appl Physiol 52:955-963
4. Eissa NT, Ranieri M, Corbeil C, Chasse M, Braidy J, Milic-Emili J (1991) Effect of positive end-expiratory pressure, lung volume, and inspiratory flow on interrupter resistance in patients with adult respiratory distress syndrome. Am Rev Respir Dis 144:538-543

5. Hildebrandt J (1970) Dynamic properties of air-filled excised cat lung determined by liquid plethysmograph. J Appl Physiol 27:246-250
6. Hildebrandt J (1970) Pressure-volume data of cat lung interpreted by a plastoelastic linear viscoelastic model. J Appl Physiol 28:365-372
7. Peslin R, Fredberg JJ (1986) Oscillation mechanics of the respiratory system. In: Macklem PT, Mead J (eds) The respiratory system. Handbook of Physiology. Vol III. Mechanics of breathing. American Physiological Society, Bethesda, pp 145-178
8. Hantos Z, Csendes T, Suki B, Nagy S (1990) Modeling of low-frequency pulmonary impedance in the dog. J Appl Physiol 68:849-860
9. Hantos Z, Daróczy B, Suki B, Nagy S, Fredberg JJ (1992) Input impedance and peripheral inhomogeneity of dog lungs. J Appl Physiol 72:168-178
10. Hantos Z, Adamicza Á, Govaerts E, Daróczy B (1992) Mechanical impedances of lungs and chest wall in the cat. J Appl Physiol 73:427-433
11. Daróczy B, Fabula A, Hantos Z (1991) Use of noninteger-multiple pseudorandom excitation to minimize non-linear effects on impedance estimation. Eur Respir Rev 1:183-187
12. Suki B, Lutchen KR (1992) Pseudorandom signals to estimate apparent transfer and coherence functions of non-linear systems: applications to respiratory mechanics. IEEE Trans Biomed Eng 39:1142-1151
13. Lutchen KR, Yang K, Kaczka DW, Suki B (1993) Optimal ventilator waveform for estimating low-frequency mechanical impedance in healthy and diseased subjects. J Appl Physiol 75:478-488
14. Hantos Z, Peták F, Adamicza Á, Daróczy B, Suki B, Lutchen KR (1994) Optimum ventilator waveform for the estimation of respiratory impedance: an animal study. Eur Respir Rev 4:191-197
15. Lutchen KR, Suki B, Kaczka DW, Zhang Q, Hantos Z, Daróczy B, Peták F (1994) Direct use of mechanical ventilation to measure respiratory mechanics associated with physiological breathing. Eur Respir Rev 4:98-202
16. Lutchen KR, Suki B, Zhang Q, Peták F, Daróczy B, Hantos Z (1994) Airway and tissue mechanics during physiological breathing and bronchoconstriction in dogs. J Appl Physiol 77:373-385
17. Suki B, Zhang Q, Lutchen KR (1995) Relationship between frequency and amplitude dependence in the lung: a non-linear block-structured modeling approach. J Appl Physiol 79:660-671
18. Rohrer F (1915) Der Strömungswiderstand in den menschlichen Atemwegen und der Einfluss der unregelmässigen Verzweigung des Bronchialsystems auf den Atmungsverlauf in verschiedenen Lungenbezirken. Pfluegers Arch 162:255-259
19. Jaeger MJ, Matthys H (1968) The pattern of flow in the human upper airways. Respir Physiol 6:113-127
20. Zin WA (1998) Pathophysiology of flow limitation. In: Gullo A (ed) Proceedings of the 12th postgraduate course in critical care medicine. Springer-Verlag, Berlin Heidelberg New York, pp 75-82
21. Varène P, Jacquemin C (1970) Airways resistance: A new method of computation. In: Bouhuys A (ed) Airway dynamics. Physiology and pharmacology. Charles C Thomas, Springfield, pp 99-108
22. Hantos Z, Galgóczy G, Daróczy B, Dombos K (1978) Computation of equivalent airway resistance. A comparison with routine evaluation of plethysmographic measurements. Respiration 36:64-72
23. Maksym GN, Bates JHT (1997) A distributed non-linear model of lung tissue elasticity. J Appl Physiol 82:32-41

24. Fung YC (1981) Biomechanics. Mechanical properties of living tissues. Springer-Verlag, Berlin Heidelberg New York
25. Fredberg JJ, Stamenović D (1989) On the imperfect elasticity of lung tissue. J Appl Physiol 67:2408-2419
26. Barnas GM, Sprung J (1993) Effect of mean airway pressure and tidal volume on lung and chest wall mechanics in the dog. J Appl Physiol 74:2286-2293
27. Suki B, Hantos Z, Daróczy B, Alkaysi G, Nagy S (1991) Non-linearity and harmonic distortion of dog lungs measured by low-frequency forced oscillations. J Appl Physiol 71:69-75
28. Barnas GM, Sprung J, Kahn R, Delaney PA, Agarwal M (1995) Lung tissue and airway impedances during pulmonary edema in the normal range of breathing. J Appl Physiol 78:1889-1897
29. Barnas GM, Stamenović D, Lutchen KR (1992) Lung and chest wall impedances in the dog in the normal range of breathing. J Appl Physiol 73:1039-1046
30. Barnas GM, Mackenzie CF, Skacel M, Hempleman SC, Wicke KM, Skacel CM, Loring SH (1989) Amplitude dependency of regional chest wall resistance and elastance at normal breathing frequencies. Am Rev Respir Dis 140:25-30
31. Barnas GM, Campbell DN, Mackenzie CF, Mendham JE, Fahy BG, Runcie CJ, Mendham GE (1991) Lung, chest wall, and total respiratory system resistance and elastance in the normal range of breathing. Am Rev Respir Dis 143:240-244
32. Suki B, Bates JHT (1991) A non-linear viscoelastic model of lung tissue mechanics. J Appl Physiol 71:826-833
33. Suki B (1993) Non-linear phenomena in respiratory mechanical measurements. J Appl Physiol 74:2574-2584
34. Navajas D, Maksym GN, Bates JHT (1995) Dynamic viscoelastic nonlinearity of lung parenchymal tissue. J Appl Physiol 79:348-356
35. Peslin R, Saunier C, Duvivier C, Marchand M (1995) Analysis of low-frequency lung impedance in rabbits with non-linear models. J Appl Physiol 79:771-780
36. Stamenović D, Lutchen KR, Barnas GM (1993) Alternative model of respiratory tissue viscoplasticity. J Appl Physiol 75:1062-1069
37. Radford EP Jr (1957) Recent studies of the mechanical properties of mammalian lungs. In: Remington JW (ed) Tissue elasticity. American Physiological Society, Washington DC, pp 177-190
38. Suki B, Barabási A-L, Hantos Z, Peták F, Stanley HE (1994) Avalanches and power-law behaviour in lung inflation. Nature 368:615-618
39. Otis DR Jr, Peták F, Hantos Z, Fredberg JJ, Kamm RD (1996) Airway closure and reopening assessed by the alveolar capsule oscillation technique. J Appl Physiol 80:2077-2084
40. Lefevre GR, Kowalski SE, Girling LG, Thiessen DB, Mutch WAC (1996) Improved arterial oxygenation after oleic acid lung injury in the pig using a computer-controlled mechanical ventilator. Am J Respir Crit Care Med 154:1567-1572
41. Otis AB, McKerrow CB, Bartlett RA, Mead J, McIlroy MB, Selverstone NJ, Radford EP Jr (1956) Mechanical factors in distribution of pulmonary ventilation. J Appl Physiol 8:427-443
42. Mead J (1969) Contribution of compliance of airways to frequency-dependent behavior of lungs. J Appl Physiol 26:670-673
43. Fredberg JJ, Keefe DH, Glass GM, Castile RG, Frantz ID III (1984) Alveolar pressure nonhomogeneity during small-amplitude high-frequency oscillation. J Appl Physiol 57:788-800
44. Fredberg JJ, Ingram RH Jr, Castile RG, Glass GM, Drazen JM (1985) Nonhomogeneity

of lung response to inhaled histamine assessed with alveolar capsules. J Appl Physiol 58:1914-1922
45. Lutchen KR, Hantos Z, Peták F, Adamicza Á, Suki B (1996) Airway inhomogeneities contribute to apparent lung tissue mechanics during constriction. 80:1841-1849
46. Peták F, Hantos Z, Adamicza Á, Asztalos T, Sly PD (1997) Methacholine-induced bronchoconstriction in rats: effects of intravenous vs. aerosol delivery. J Appl Physiol 82:1479-1487
47. Horsfield K, Kemp W, Phillips S (1982) An asymmetrical model of the airways of the dog lung. J Appl Physiol 52:21-26
48. Lutchen KR, Greenstein JL, Suki B (1996) How inhomogeneities and airway walls affect frequency dependence and separation of airway and tissue properties. J Appl Physiol 80:1696-1707
49. Thorpe CW, Bates JHT (1997) Effect of stochastic heterogeneity on lung impedance during acute bronchoconstriction: A model analysis. J Appl Physiol 82:1616-1625
50. Lutchen KR, Gillis H (1997) Relationship between heterogeneous changes in airway morphometry and lung resistance and elastance. J Appl Physiol 83:1192-1201

Chapter 9

Mechanical implications of viscoelasticity

J. MILIC-EMILI, E. D'ANGELO

In 1955, Mount [1] assessed the dynamic work per breath ($W_{dyn,L}$) as given by volume-pressure loops in open-chest rats during sinusoidal variations in lung volume. In order to explain the relatively high values of $W_{dyn,L}$ at the lower frequencies and the progressive decrease in dynamic pulmonary compliance with increasing frequency, he proposed a two-compartment viscoelastic model of the lung which "confers time dependency of the elastic properties." In 1967 Sharp et al. [2], who were unaware of Mount's work, proposed a similar viscoelastic model for both lung and chest wall. Until the late 1980s these models were largely ignored. Since then, however, the viscoelastic properties of the respiratory system have been recognized to play an important role in respiratory dynamics. In this review we describe the implications of viscoelastic mechanisms in terms of a) frequency dependence of pulmonary and chest wall elastance and resistance, b) work of breathing, c) passive lung deflation, and d) forced vital capacity (FVC).

While in normal subjects the frequency dependence of pulmonary elastance (E_L) and resistance (R_L) is probably due entirely to the viscoelastic properties of the lung tissues, in patients with pulmonary disease this phenomenon is due in part to time constant inequality within the lung. The latter was first described in a 1956 paper by Otis et al. [3] which, unlike that of Mount, became immediately popular. In addition to the parallel model of Otis et al., Mead [4] subsequently introduced a series model of time constant inequality of the respiratory system, which could also account for frequency dependence of E_L and R_L in patients with lung disease.

Since the parallel and series time constant inequalities should play an appreciable role only in lung disease, the normal lung was not expected to exhibit frequency dependence of E_L and R_L. Accordingly, until recently the experimental findings on normal subjects, which were in contrast to this notion, tended to be dismissed as artifactual. As a result, until the 1980s the understanding of respiratory dynamics in normal subjects has been hampered.

Viscoelastic model

The lungs of chest wall comprise a large number of elements. This complexity, coupled with the necessity to study respiratory mechanics in physiology and clinics, has generated the need for a relatively simple model that can mimic the mechanical behavior of the respiratory system. Based on the pioneering work of Mount [1] and Sharp et al. [2], Bates et al. [5] proposed the eight-parameter spring-and-dashpot model of the respiratory system, shown in Figure 1.

The viscoelastic model in Figure 1 has been validated in normal anesthetized paralyzed humans [6-8], and the values of the various parameters are given in Table 1. The viscoelastic time constants of the lung ($\tau_{2,L}$) and chest wall ($\tau_{2,w}$) are given by R_{2L}/E_{2L} and $R_{2,w}/E_{2,w}$, respectively; Rint,L corresponds to airway resistance (Raw). At present, the precise structural basis of the viscoelastic elements of the model in Figure 1 is unknown.

Table 1. Average values (±SD) of respiratory parameters in Fig. 1 of 18 normal anesthetized paralyzed humans (from [7], except for Rint,L and Rint,w which are from [8])

	R_2 (cm H_2O sl^{-1})	E_2 (cm H_2O/l^{-1})	t_2 (s)	Est (cm H_2O/l^{-1})	Rint (cm H_2O s l^{-1})
Lung	3.4±1.0	3.2±1.1	1.1±0.4	8.2±1.7	1.1±0.4
Chest wall	2.1±0.6	1.7±0.4	1.3±0.3	6.3±1.1	0.4±0.1

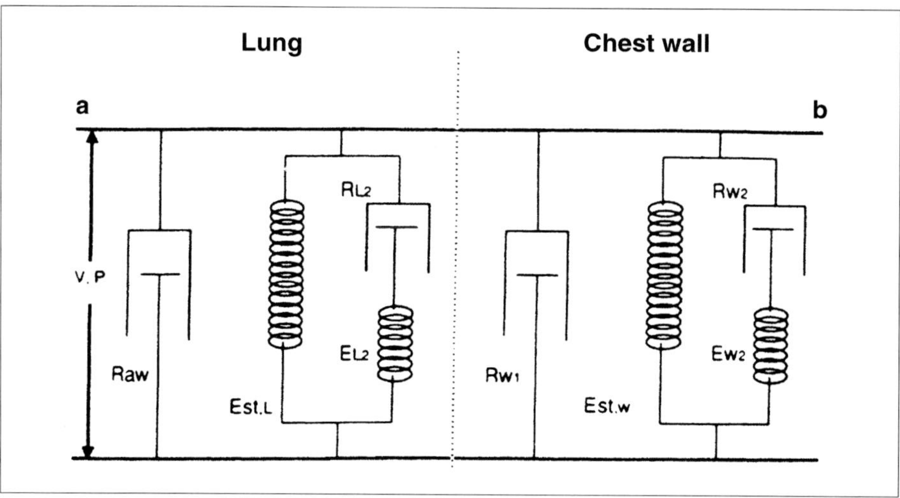

Fig. 1a,b. Scheme of spring-and-dashpot model proposed by Bates at al. [5] for interpretation of respiratory mechanics with airway interruption method in normal subjects. Both lung (a) and chest wall (b) include a resistive component (dashpot; Rint,L and Rint,w respectively) in parallel with a Kelvin body, i.e. (1) an elastic component (spring) accounting for the static elastances of two compartments (Est,L, and Est,w, respectively) and (2) a series spring-and-dashpot element (Maxwell body; R_{L2}, E_{L2} and R_{w2}, E_{w2}, respectively) which imparts viscoelastic behavior to the relevant compartment. The distance between two horizontal bars is analogue of lung volume (V) and tension between these bars is analogue of pressure applied to respiratory system (P)

Time dependence of elastance and resistance

The viscoelastic elements within the pulmonary and chest wall tissues confer time dependence of elastance and resistance to the lung and chest wall. Indeed, at high respiratory frequencies (f) the springs E_2 in Figure 1 will oscillate so fast that there will be insufficient time for their tension to be dissipated through the dashpots R_2. By contrast, at low frequencies, the dashpots R_2 are given time to move and dissipate the elastic energy stored in E_2. In the limit, as frequency tends to zero, the springs E_2 should remain at fixed length (i.e. the resting length at which tension is zero). This implies that the dynamic lung and chest wall elastances (Edyn) should increase with increase with f. At high frequencies, Edyn should approach Est+E_2, while Edyn should reflect Est at f close to zero.

During sinusoidal breathing, the contribution of the viscoelastic properties (ΔE) to Edyn should change with f according to the following function [7]:

$$\Delta E = \omega^2 \tau^2{}_2 E_2 / (1 + \omega^2 \tau^2{}_2) \qquad (1)$$

where ω is angular frequency ($2\pi f$). Figure 2 shows the relation of ΔE_L and ΔE_W to frequency computed according Eq. 1, using the average values of the viscoelastic constants in Table 1. Shown on the right ordinates of Figure 2 is dynamic elastance (Edyn=ΔE+Est), expressed as a fraction of corresponding Est: Edyn,L and Edyn,W increase with frequency, approaching plateau values (Est+E_2) at a frequency of about 0.5 Hz. At these frequencies, Edyn,L is 38%

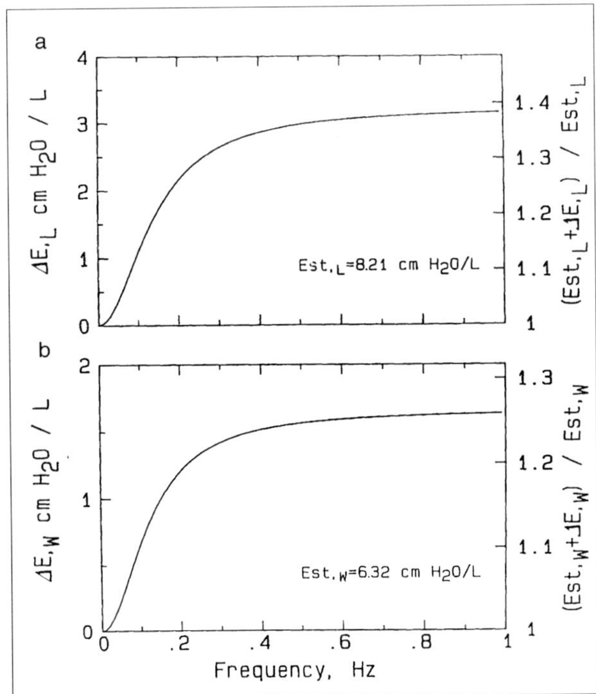

Fig. 2a,b. Relationship of ΔE of lung (a) and chest wall (b) to respiratory frequency computed according Eq. 1 using average values of E_2 and τ_2 in Table 1. Shown on right ordinates is dynamic elastance (Est + ΔE), expressed as a fraction of Es,t. (From [7])

higher than Est,L while the corresponding increase for the chest wall is 26%. In the past, such an increase in lung elastance between 0 and 0.5 Hz would have been considered to be pathological [9].

During sinusoidal breathing, the effective pulmonary and chest wall resistance (ΔR) owing to viscoelastic mechanisms should decrease with frequency according to the following function [7]:

$$\Delta R = R_2/(1 + \omega^2 \tau^2{}_2) \qquad (2)$$

Figure 3 illustrates the relationship of ΔRL and ΔRw to frequency computed according Eq. 2, using the average values of the viscoelastic constants in Table 1. Both ΔRL and ΔRw decrease with increasing frequency, becoming negligible at f >0.5 Hz.

Frequency dependence of pulmonary and chest wall elastance and resistance has also been described in normal subjects using the forced oscillation technique [10, 11], as well as in patients with obstructive lung disease [12]. According to the model in Figure 1 and Eq. 2, RL and Rw at high frequencies should reflect Raw and Rint,w, respectively. Indeed, the values of Rw obtained with the forced oscillation technique in relaxed normal subjects [11] and in normal spontaneously breathing subjects [10] at frequencies between 2 and 9 Hz were close to the values of Rint,w in Table 1.

Time dependence of pulmonary elastance can also be caused by time constant

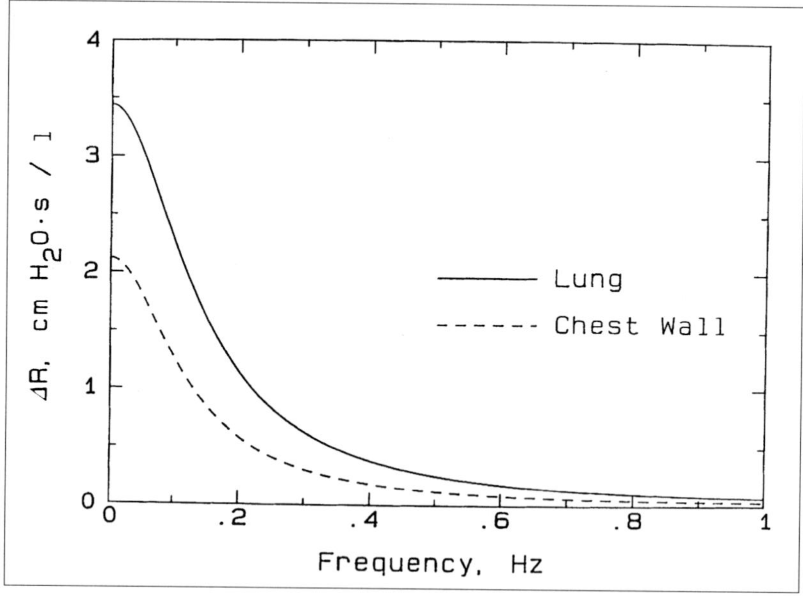

Fig. 3. Relation of effective resistance (ΔR) due to viscoelasticity of lung and chest wall to respiratory frequency computed according Eq. 2 using average values of constants R_2 and τ_2 in Table 1. (From [7])

inequality within the lung [3, 4, 13]. In normal subjects, however, such contributions appear to be negligible. In patients with pulmonary disease, time constant inequality within the lung probably contributes substantially to the observed increase in the magnitude of time dependence of both elastance and resistance [14, 15].

Equations 1 and 2 do not take into account the contributions due to the so-called quasistatic hysteresis. However, during tidal breathing these are negligible in normal lungs [16].

Viscoelastic work

Although at $f<0.2$ Hz the values of ΔR of both lung and chest wall are relatively high (Fig. 3), the corresponding dynamic work of breathing is only a small fraction of the total work of breathing in both normal subjects [6] and patients with pulmonary disease (see Chapter 15). In fact, in terms of the total cost of breathing the dynamic work due to viscoelasticity is negligible, particularly at $f>0.2$ Hz. The same is in general also true for the dynamic work due to time constant inequality.

Expiratory flow

While part of the work done on viscoelastic elements is dissipated as heat, part of the elastic energy stored during inspiration in springs E_2 can be recovered during expiration to overcome expiratory airway resistance. Indeed, at $f>0.5$ Hz, virtually all of the energy stored in springs E_2 during inspiration should be available to drive expiration (see Fig. 2). Thus, during increased ventilation (i.e., muscular exercise) some of the requirements for increased expiratory flow rates are intrinsically met by the increase in $Edyn_{,L}$ and $Edyn_{,w}$ because of the higher frequency of breathing. Since the elastic energy stored in the lung and chest wall is greater with rapid than with slow inspirations, lung deflation should be faster following rapid inflation. Augmentation of the expiratory-driving pressure through a viscoelastic mechanism was originally described by Mortola et al. [17], who found that passive lung deflation was slower if the expiration was preceded by an end-expiratory hold of about 5s. This phenomenon can be readily explained by the fact that during the prolonged end-inspiratory hold the effective elastic recoil pressures of the lung and chest wall decrease progressively owing to the stress relaxation which characterizes viscoelastic behavior [6, 7]. As described below, viscoelastic mechanisms have important effects not only in relaxed expiration but also on forced expiratory maneuvers.

Relaxed expiration

The first mechanical model of the respiratory system [18] consisted of a single compartment of constant elastance (Ers) served by a pathway of constant resistance (Rrs). One the basis of this model, characterized by a single time constant

($\tau rs = Rrs/Ers$). Brody [19] theorized that the time-course of decay in volume (V) during passive expiration should be described by the following single-exponential function:

$$V(t) = V_0 \cdot e^{-t/\tau rs} \tag{3}$$

where t is time and V_0 is initial volume above the relaxation volume of the respiratory system. Until recently, Eq. 3 was the kernel of various methods for measurement of respiratory mechanics [20, 21]. However, Bates et al. [22, 23] showed that in anesthetized paralyzed dogs the time course of volume decay during passive expiration is better described by a double-exponential function:

$$V(t) = A \cdot e^{-t/\tau'} + B \cdot e^{-t/\tau''} \tag{4}$$

This behavior, which was attributed to viscoelastic mechanisms, has also been observed in normal anesthetized paralyzed humans [24] and in patients with adult respiratory distress syndrome (ARDS) [25]. It should be stressed that τ' and τ'' are complex parameter that does not correspond to τrs in Eq. 3 and τ_2 ($=R_2/E_2$), respectively.

Time dependence of FVC maneuver

Pulmonary function is commonly assessed by spirometry whose origin can be traced to the measurement of the slow vital capacity (VC) introduced in 1846 by Hutchinson [26]. It became apparent, however, that VC measurements did not evaluate the predominant ventilatory defect in diseases (i.e., asthma and emphysema) characterized by a decreased ability to exhale air at normal rates. In 1947 Tiffeneau and Pinelli [27] made this possible with the introduction of the measurement of volumes exhaled during the forced vital capacity (FVC) maneuver in a given period of time (i.e. forced vital capacity in 1s, FEV_1). Extensive guidelines have been provided for the measurement procedure of FVC [28, 29]. In these guidelines, however, the inspiratory maneuver preceding the expiratory effort was not standardized. In practice, the FVC maneuver is preceded by maximal inspirations made at different speeds and variable pauses at full inspiration. However, the time course of the inspiration preceding the FVC maneuver has a marked effect on peak expiratory flow (PEF), FEV_1 and the maximal expiratory flow volume (MEFV) curves in both normal subjects [30] and patients with obstructive [31-33] or restrictive lung disease [34], as well as cystic fibrosis [35].

Figure 4 depicts the time course of flow and volume during two FVC maneuvers performed by a patient with chronic obstructive lung disease (COPD): the results on the left were preceded by a rapid maximal inspiration without an end-inspiratory pause (maneuver 1), while the results on the right were obtained after a slow inspiration with an end-inspiratory pause of several seconds (maneuver 2). During maneuver 2 there was a marked reduction in both PEF and FEV_1, but not in FVC. Table 2 provides the average differences in PEF and FEV_1 between maneuvers 1 and

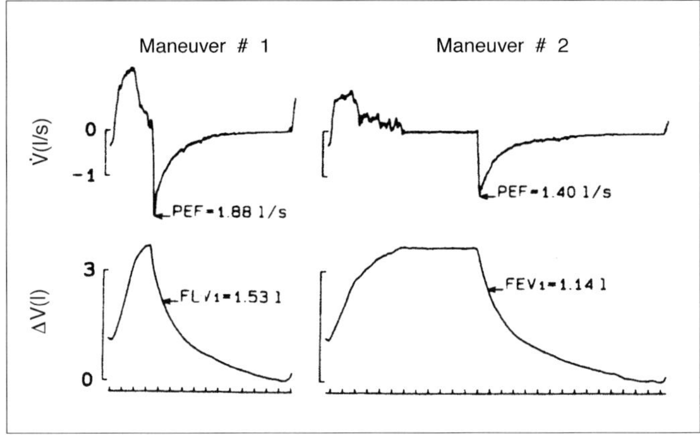

Fig. 4. Tracings showing the time course of changes in flow at the mouth ($\dot{V}$) (*top*) and in lung volume (ΔV) (botton) in a COPD patient during a forced vital capacity (FVC) maneuver preceded by a rapid inspiration without breath hold at end inspiration (*Maneuver 1*) and a slow inspiration with a 5 s breath hold (*Maneuver 2*). With maneuver 2 the peck expiratory flow (PEF) and forced expiratory volume in 1s (FEV_1) were 23% lower than with maneuver 1, while FVC did not change. (Modified from [31])

Table 2. Average differences in peak expiratory flow (PEF) and forced expiratory volume in 1 s (FEV_1) between forced vital capacity maneuvers 1 and 2 in normal subjects and in patients with chronic obstructive pulmonary disease (COPD) or asthma

	N	ΔPEF[b] (l/s)	ΔPEF/PEF (2)[c] (%)	ΔFEV_1[b] (l)	$\Delta FEV_1/FEV_1$ (2)[c] (%)	Reference
Normal	13	1.28	17	0.19	5	[30]
COPD	13	0.71	30	0.24	23	[31]
Asthma	8	1.12	15	0.17	7	[32]

[a] Maneuver 1 was performed after rapid inspiration (usually lasting less than 1.5s) from functional residual capacity and with an end-inspiratory pause of less than 0.3s. For maneuver 2, the corresponding values were 3-5 s and 4-6 s, respectively

[b] Differences are expressed in absolute units

[c] Differences are expressed as percentage changes relative to values obtained with maneuver 2

2 of normal subjects and patients with asthma or COPD. These differences are expressed in both absolute units and as percentage changes relative to values obtained with maneuver 2. Time dependence of PEF and FEV_1 was present in all instances, while FVC did not change significantly. The absolute values of ΔPEF and ΔFEV_1 were higher in normal subjects and asthmatic patients than in patients with COPD; the opposite was true when differences were expressed as a percentage of the corresponding values obtained with maneuver 2. This discrepancy reflects the greater severity of airway obstruction of COPD patients [33].

Time dependence of PEF and FEV_1 has also been found in normal and asthmatic children by Matsumoto et al. [36]. In contrast, Sette et al. [37] found no difference in PEF between maneuvers 1 and 2 in children with asthma. This discrepancy, however, merely reflects the fact that in the asthmatic children PEF was measured with a peak flow meter which was inserted into the mouth after inhalation to total lung capacity (TLC). This necessarily involves an obligatory end-inspiratory pause even with maneuver 1, which may last several seconds depending on the coordination of the children and on the instruction that they have received. As a result of the "spurious" obligatory pause, the difference in PEF between maneuvers 1 and 2 is necessarily reduced or may even be abolished, depending on the duration of the pause. In this regard it should be stressed that routine spirometry involves equipment which is inserted in the mouth either before the maximal inspiration or after inhalation to TLC. In the latter instance, the maneuvers are never if type 1.

Although several factors may contribute to the time dependency of MEFV, this phenomenon should be mainly due to the fact that in maneuver 1 the effective elastic recoil pressure of the lung ($P_{el,L}$) is higher as a result of viscoelastic behavior of lung tissue [30, 33]. Because the magnitude of the maximal flows ($\dot{V}_{max}$) depends on $P_{el,L}$ [38], the maximal flows are necessarily higher with maneuver 1 than 2. In this context, it should be stressed that the higher $P_{el,L}$ obtained with fast inspiration can be completely dissipated during a 5 s breath hold at TLC; hence, to achieve the highest expiratory flows it is necessary to inhale as fast as possible and exhale without pausing at end inspiration [30].

In normal subjects the differences in PEF and FEV_1 between maneuvers 1 and 2 averaged 1.28 l/s and 0.19 l, respectively. In normal non-smoking adults such a change in PEF and FEV_1 would, on average, be expected over an age span of about 30 years [30]. Clearly, in epidemiological studies the inspiratory maneuver before FVC needs to be standardized. The same is valid for patients with COPD and asthma. However, in this case the time dependence of FVC has an important bearing also in the assessment of the response to bronchodilators. According to the American Thoracic Society recommended criteria for response to bronchodilator drugs, a greater than 12% increase in FEV_1 relative to baseline represents a significant response [39]. However, in view of the marked time dependence of FEV_1 (Table 2), correct delineation with these criteria of responders vs. nonresponders to bronchodilator drugs becomes problematic unless the inspiratory pattern before the FVC maneuver is standardized [33]. Similar considerations apply to the measurement of PEF and MEFV curves.

Finally, it should be noted that the viscoelastic behavior of lung tissues might be functionally important to the extent that it would tend to smooth stress distribution within the lungs and thereby minimize local distortions during sudden displacements. Viscoelasticity also plays an important role in animal and human movement [40].

Acknowledgement The authors thank Ms. Angie Bentivegna for secretarial work.

References

1. Mount LE (1955) The ventilation flow-resistance and compliance of rat lungs. J Physiol 127:157-167
2. Sharp JT, Johnson FN, Goldberg NB, Van Lith P (1967) Hysteresis and stress adaptation in the human respiratory system. J Appl Physiol 23:487-497
3. Otis AB, McKerrow CB, Bartlett RA, Mead J, McIlroy MB, Selverstone NJ, Radford EP (1956) Mechanical factors in distribution of pulmonary ventilation. J Appl Physiol 8:427-443
4. Mead J (1969) Contribution of compliance of airways to frequency-dependent behaviour of lungs. J Appl Physiol 26:670-673
5. Bates JHT, Brown K, Kochi T (1987) Identifying a model of respiratory mechanics using the interrupted technique. Proceeding of the 9th American Conference. IEEE Eng Med Biol Soc, pp 1802-1803
6. D'Angelo E, Calderini E, Torri G, Robatto F, Bono D, Milic-Emili J (1989) Respiratory mechanics in anesthetized-paralyzed humans: effects of flow, volume and time. J Appl Physiol 67:2556-2564
7. D'Angelo E, Robatto FM, Calderini E, Tavola M, Bono D, Torri G, Milic-Emili J (1991) Pulmonary and chest wall mechanics in anesthetized paralyzed humans. J Appl Physiol 70:2602-2610
8. D'Angelo E, Prandi E, Tavola M, Calderini E, Milic-Emili J (1994) Chest wall interrupter resistance in anesthetized paralyzed subjects. J Appl Physiol 77:883-887
9. Woolcock AJ, Vincent NJ, Macklem PT (1969) Frequency dependence of compliance as a test for obstruction in small airways. J Clin Invest 48:1097-1106
10. Hantos Z, Daroczy B, Suki B, Galgoczy G, Csendes T (1986) Forced oscillatory impedance of the respiratory system at low frequencies. J Appl Physiol 60:123-132
11. Barnas GM, Yoshino K, Loring SH, Mead J (1987) Impedance and relative displacements of relaxed chest wall up to 4 Hz. J Appl Physiol 62:71-81
12. Grimby G, Takishima T, Graham W, Macklem PT, Mead J (1968) Frequency dependence of flow resistance in patients with obstructive lung disease. J Clin Invest 47:1455-1465
13. Bates JHT, Bacconier P, Milic-Emili J (1988) A theoretical analysis of interrupter technique for measuring respiratory mechanics. J Appl Physiol 64:2204-2214
14. Eissa NT, Ranieri VM, Corbeil C, Chassé M, Robatto FM, Braidy J, Milic-Emili J (1991) Analysis of behavior of the respiratory system in ARDS patients: effects of flow, volume, and time. J Appl Physiol 70:2719-2729
15. Guérin C, Coussa M-L, Eissa NT, Corbeil C, Chassé M, Braidy J, Matar N, Milic-Emili J (1993) Lung and chest wall mechanics in mechanically ventilated COPD patients. J Appl Physiol 74:1570-1580
16. Shardonofsky FR, Sato J, Bates JHT (1990) Quasi-static pressure-volume hysteresis in the canine respiratory system in vivo. J Appl Physiol 68:2230-2236
17. Mortola JP, Magnante D, Saetta M (1985) Expiratory pattern of newborn mammals. J Appl Physiol 58:528-533
18. Otis AB, Fenn WO, Rahn H (1950) The mechanics of breathing in man. J Appl Physiol 2:592-607
19. Brody AW (1954) Mechanical compliance and resistance ofthe lung-thorax calculated from the flow recorded during passive expiration. Am J Physiol 178:189-196
20. McIlroy MB, Tierney DF, Nadel JA (1963) A new method of measurement of compliance and resistance of lungs and thorax. J Appl Physiol 18:424-427
21. Zin WA, Pengelly LD, Milic-Emili J (1982) Single-breath method for measurement of respiratory system mechanics in anesthetized animals. J Appl Physiol 52:1266

22. Bates JHT, Decramer M, Chartrand D, Zin WA, Boddener A, Milic-Emili J (1985) Volume-time profile during relaxed expiration in the normal dog. J Appl Physiol 59:732-737
23. Bates JHT, Decramer M, Chartrand D, Zin WA, Boddener A, Milic-Emili J (1986) Respiratory resistance with histamine challenge by single-breath and forced oscillation methods. J Appl Physiol 61:873-880
24. Chelucci GL, Brunet F, Dall'Ava-Santucci J, Dhainaut JF, Paccaly D, Armaganidis A, Milic-Emili J, Lockhart A (1991) A single-compartment model cannot describe passive expiration in intubated, paralysed humans. Eur Respir J 4:458-464
25. Chelucci GL, Dall'Ava-Santucci J, Dhainaut JF, Chelucci A, Allegra A, Paccaly D, Brunet F, Milic-Emili J, Lockhart A (1993) Modelling of passive expiration in patients with adult respiratory distress syndrome. Eur Respir J 6:785-790
26. Hutchinson J (1846) On capacity of the lungs, and on the respiratory movements, with the view of establishing a precise and easy method of detecting disease by the spirometer. Lancet i:630-632
27. Tiffeneau R, Pinelli AF (1947) Air circulant et air captif dans l'exploration de la fonction ventilatrice pulmonaire. Paris Med 133:624-628
28. American Thoracic Society (1987) Standardization of spirometry. Am Rev Respir Dis 136:1285-1298
29. Quanjer PhH (1983) Lung volumes and forced ventilatory flows. Report of Working Party. Standal-dization of lung function tests. European Coal and Steel Community. Eur Respir J 6:5-40
30. D'Angelo E, Prandi E, Milic-Emili J (1993) Dependence of maximal flow-volume curves on time-course of preceding inspiration. J Appl Physiol 75:1155-1159
31. D'Angelo E, Prandi E, Milic-Emili J (1994) Dependence of maximal flow-volume curves on time-course of preceding inspiration in patients with chronic obstructive lung disease. Am J Respir Crit Care Med 150:1581-1586
32. Wanger JS, Ikle DN, Cherniack RM (1996) The effect of inspiratory maneuvers on expiratory flow rates in health and asthma: Influence of lung elastic recoil. Am J Respir Crit Care Med 153:1302-1308
33. D'Angelo E, Milic-Emili J, Marazzini L (1996) Effects of bronchomotor tone and gas density on time dependence of forced expiratory vital capacity maneuver. Am J Respir Crit Care Med 154:1318-1322
34. Koulouris NG, Rapakoulias P, Rassidakis A, Dimitroulis J, Gaga M, Milic-Emili J, Jordanoglou J (1997) Dependence of forced vital capacity on time course of preceding inspiration in patients with restrictive lung disease. Eur Respir J 10:2366-2370
35. Braggion C, Pradal U, Mastella G, Coates AL, Milic-Emili J (1996) Effect of different inspiratory maneuvers on FEV, in patients with cystic fibrosis. Chest 110:342-647
36. Matsumoto I, Walker S, Sly PD (1996) The influence of breathold on peak expiratory flow in normal and asthmatic children. Eur Respir J 9:1363-1367
37. Sette L, Del Col G, Comis A, Milic-Emili J, Rossi A, Boner AL (1996) Effect of pattern of preceding inspiration on FEV1 in asthmatic children. Eur Respir J 9:1902-1906
38. Mead J, Turner JM, Macklem PT, Little JB (1967) Significance of the relationship between lung elastic recoil and maximum expiratory flow. J Appl Physiol 22:95-106
39. ATS (1997) Standards for the diagnosis and care of patients with chronic obstructive pulmonary disease (COPD) and asthma. Am Rev Respir Dis 136:225-244
40. Alexander R McNeill (1988) Elastic mechanisms in animal movement. Cambridge University Press, Cambridge

Chapter 10

Alveolar micromechanics

P.V. Romero

The mechanical behavior of the air spaces in the periphery of the lung is the result of a delicate balance of forces acting on the tissue scaffold of lung parenchyma. Static and dynamic properties of such a complex system have been an important field of research for many years. Alveolar space micromechanics have important physiological implications in terms of mechanical interdependence, alveolar stability, and the maintenance of a gas exchanging surface in constant contact with air. The mechanical behavior of such system has to allow the expansion of the alveolar surface at physiological rates at a low energy cost, and without interfering with the exchange process. I will describe how the structure and mechanics of the alveolar space are particularly optimized to reach these goals.

Anatomical structure of the alveolar space

The alveolar septum is made of a single capillary network interlaced with fibers (mainly collagen and elastine), which form a continuum embedded in the connective matrix, the thin membrane of epithelial cells forming the external boundary of this scaffold. This irregular surface is to some extent smoothed by an extracellular layer of lining fluid that is rather thin over the capillaries but forms small pools in the intercapillary cavities. Alveolar lining consists of an aqueous layer called the hypophase which is of variable thickness and is present mainly in the pools, and a layer of surfactant which forms a film on the surface of the hypophase. Because of the relevant physical properties of these structures, septal configuration is not exclusively determined by the structural disposition but results from the molding effect of the two main forces that have to be kept in balance: tissue tension and surface tension.

Structural interaction of tissue fibers and surface lining

Many experimental studies agree in the fact that the dimension of the alveolar surface is governed by the equilibrium between surface and tissue forces. Surface tension arises at any gas-liquid interface because the forces between the molecules of the liquid are much stronger than those between the liquid and the gas. As a result, the liquid surface will tend to become as small as possible. A curved surface, such as that of an alveolus, generates a pressure proportional to the curvature and to the surface tension coefficient g. According to Wilson [1], surface pressure (Ps) can be expressed as a function of the surface-to-volume ratio of the alveolar air space $(S/V)_A$ and surface tension (γ) by:

$$Ps = (2/3) \cdot \gamma \cdot (S/V)_A \tag{1}$$

The greater the surface-to-volume ratio, the greater the mean curvature of the surface and the greater the surface pressure at any value of γ. According to the above equation, the most critical effect of surface tension (γ) is that it challenges the stability of airspaces. As a set of connected bubbles, alveoli are intrinsically unstable: since the small ones have a larger curvature than the large ones, they should collapse and empty into the larger units. However, in normal conditions alveoli are highly stable. This is due to two main mechanisms: the interaction between tissue fibers and surface lining, and the intrinsic properties of surfactant itself.

Alveolar walls contain an intricate fiber system. Thus, when an alveolus tends to shrink, the fibers in the wall of the alveoli are stretched and this will prevent the alveolus from collapsing. This stabilizing phenomenon is known as interdependence [2]. Surfactant lines the complete alveolar suface, and even terminal airways. The surface tension coefficient γ of surfactant is variable: it falls as alveolar surface becomes smaller, and rises when alveolar surface expands [3]. Therefore, as alveolar volume decreases, surface tension decreases and tissue fiber tension increases due to interdependence. This force opposed to the alveolar emptying allows the system to remain stable. If surface tension is modified at the level of the liquid-air interface, the alveolar area will be inversely related to the surface tension at any level of alveolar volume, at least in the range of tidal volumes [4]. This is due to the effect of tissue tensions: as surface tension decreases, the stretching effect of tissue tension is magnified and alveolar area increases, provided that alveolar volume does not vary.

Biomechanics of the alveolar lining layer

Structure and composition

The alveolar epithelial cells are covered by a thin liquid film (less than 0.1 μm). At the air-liquid interface of this film, a layer of surface active material, largely phospholipid, aggregates. This alveolar lining layer has been described as an acellular film that forms a continuous lining over the alveolar epithelial cells and spans the pores of Kohn. It was considered to serve as an anti-desiccant to the lungs until, in 1955, Pattle [5] showed that the lung contained surfactant substances capable of stabilizing tiny bubbles, and even to decrease air-water surface tension to near zero values. Two morphological regions of the alveolar lining layer (ALL) have to be distinguished: the hypophase, and the hypophase-air boundary or surfactant lining. The hypophase often appears as a homogeneous matrix by ultrastructural examination. It contains highly ordered tubular myelin osmophilic figures that form a system of packed square tubules. Tubular myelin is a lipoprotein structure of high surface activity that contains dipalmitoyl lecityn, the major component of pulmonary surfactant. Thickness of the hypophase varies, sometimes hardyly visible by electron microscopy in areas where the epithelial cell surface is flat, and sometimes appearing as deep pools where there are folds or crevices in the epithelium or between capillaries. The air-hypophase boundary can be distinguished from the hypophase by its osmophilic property. It is provided by a duplex lining layer composed mainly of desaturated phospholipids.

Biomechanics

The major fraction of the lung's retractive force is normally derived from the interface between air and lung lining layer. Furthermore, the largest portion of the lung's hysteresis and rheological behavior is attributable to this interface. These effects are well known since, in 1929 von Neergard [6] described the pressure-volume characteristics of the liquid-filled and air-filled lungs (Fig. 1): liquid filling eliminates all air interfaces between cell walls and their lumina, so that interfacial tensions are negligible, and only the resistance of tissue forces remain. For many years knowledge about surface tension in situ was derived from studies based on the difference between air-filled and liquid-filled lungs. In 1977 Hoppin and Hildebrandt [7] presented a number of arguments, including those that relate to possible differences between tissue contribution in air-

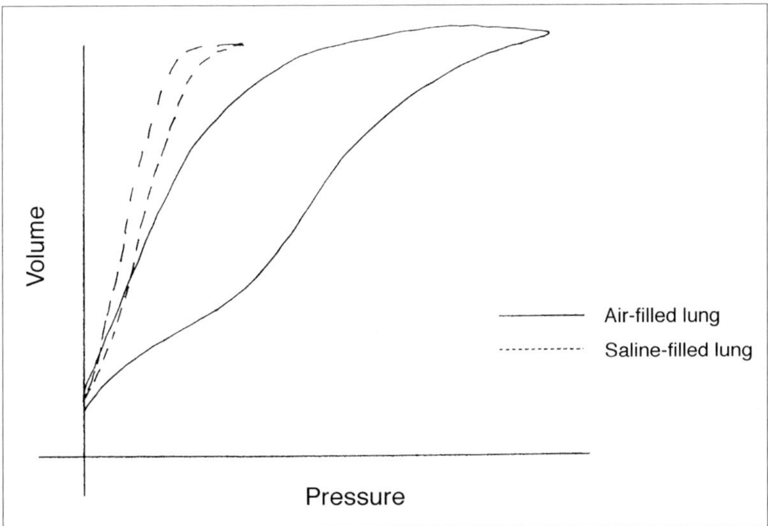

Fig. 1. Volume-pressure diagrams of isolated lungs inflated from minimal lung volume with air or saline. In saline-filled lung the interfacial tension of the lung lining layer is though to be largely eliminated when air is replaced by saline. The saline curve is typically displaced to the left, and has a lower hysteresis than the air-filled curve. A "knee" in the inflation arm of the air-filled loop is characteristically seen

filled and liquid-filled status, which indicated clearly that the use of pressure-volume (PV) diagrams for calculation of γ is unreliable. Between 1976 and 1989 Shürch et al. [8, 9] developed a method of continuously measuring surface tensions in vivo, by monitoring the deformation of test droplets of fluids with different γ deposited on the alveolar surface by means of a micropipette. Surface tension-lung volume and surface tension-recoil pressure relationships have been since then measured in different species. The most important biomechanical features related to surface tension per se can be summarized as follows.

1. The surface tension-lung volume relationship in static conditions is similar for different species, particularly along the deflation limb: surface tension decreases quasilinearly with lung volume from total lung capacity (TLC) to functional residual capacity (FRC) level [4]
2. Static recoil pressure is linearly related to γ, but this relationship differs between species. This difference has been related to the interspecies variability of the alveolar surface to volume ratio and the different participation of lung tissue (tissue component of the recoil pressure, P_t). According to the model proposed by Wilson and Bachofen [10], the component of recoil pressure due to surface tension (P_γ) is directly proportional to $\gamma/V^{1/3}$, where V is the alveolar volume: $P_\gamma = K \cdot \gamma V^{1/3}$
3. There is a prominent hysteresis in the γ-V relationships with values of γ ranging from near zero at low lung volumes during deflation to transiently high tensions near 40 dyn/cm during dynamic inflation. The amplitude of the hysteresis and shapes of γ-V relationships differ between quasistatic and dyamic states and with volume history, and are therefore dependent on the surface film kinetic behavior [11].

Biomechanics of lung tissue

Biomechanical structure of lung tissue

The major constituents of tissue matrix are elastic and collagen fibers, proteoglycans, fibronectin, and the constituents of the basement membranes of endothelium and epithelium. The fiber strands (mainly elastin and collagen) form the scaffold of alveolar walls, and allow the plastic deformation of the lungs during respiration.

Collagen is a basic structural element for soft and hard tissues in animals. It gives mechanical integrity and strength to our bodies. It is present in a variety of structural forms in different tissues and organs. In the lung, collagen represents 15%-20% of dry weight, the major collagen types being I and III. The primary building unit of collagen is the tropocollagen molecule, which is composed of polypeptide chains. In each tropocollagen molecule there are three aminoacid chains coiled into a left-handed helix. The molecule itself consist of a right handed superhelix formed by these three chains. Basically a collection of tropocollagen molecules forms a collagen fibril. Under electron microscopy, the collagen fibrils appear to be cross-striated with a periodicity of 640Å. This cross-banded staining pattern is a consequence of the parallel arrangement of molecules in the fibril: molecules on adjacent axes are staggered by approximately one-quarter the length of an individual molecule. Bundles of fibrils form fibers. Collagen fibers have great tensile strength due to an extensive system of cross-links between α-chains. The collagen fibers in lung tissue at deflation are loosely arranged and are wavy, so they do not become tight until the parenchyma is distended.

Elastin is a protein found in vertebrates. It is present as thin strands in areolar connective tissue. It forms quite a large proportion of the material in the walls or arteries, and in lung tissue. The function of elastin in lung parenchyma is to provide elasticity to the tissue, especially at lower stress levels. Elastic fibers are composed of an amorphous elastin component and a highly structured microfibrilar component. The microfibrils are found at the periphery of the fiber, but in larger fibers they also occur as fine bundles in the interior of the amorphous core. It is believed that the amorphous core represents the actual elastin, and thus has the elastic properties typical of elastic fibers, namely a relatively high extensibility and a low tensile strength when compared with collagen fibers. In fact, elastin is the most linearly elastic biosolid material known: its loading curve is almost a straight line. Loading and unloading do lead, however, to two different stress-strain curves (hysteresis), showing the existence of an energy dissipation mechanism in the material.

Biomechanics

The first information about lung tissue mechanical properties was derived from the liquid pressure-volume diagram (Fig. 1), established by von Neergard [4]: liquid filling eliminates all air interfaces between cell walls and their lumina, so that interfacial tensions are negligible and only the resistance of tissue forces remain. The early model of Setnikar and Meschia [12] explained the liquid PV diagram as representing the resistance of elastin to stretch over most of the volume range, while collagen, which is poorly extensible, would establish resistance to stretch at the highest lung volumes. Since then, many studies have analyzed the stress-strain relationships of small pieces of lung parenchyma, assumed to be a model for the tissue network of the alveolar wall. Although reservations have to be acknowledged, the comparison of the tissue stress-strain behavior with PV diagrams from liquid-lung was fairly good, and the hypothesis first proposed by Setnikar and Meschia (SM) was straightened. Karlinsky et al. in 1976 [13] found that in liquid-filled excised lungs destruction of elastin by the enzyme elastase raised the compliance in the low and middle volume ranges but affected neither volume nor compliance at high transpulmonary pressures. Destruction of collagen by collagenase increased compliance at high lung volumes but left the behavior at low lung volumes the same. Similar results have been observed by Moretto et al. [14] in alveolar wall preparations. These results agreed with the SM model. Morphologic studies have shown that in relaxed state the elastic fibers form a network of more or less straight fibers, whereas the collagen fibers appear to be wavy. Elastin and collagen were considered to be structured as complete and independent networks. According to the SM model the system will function as follows: if the tissue is stretched, the elastic fibers elongate until the collagen fibers are straight. Then, the low extensibility of collagen would prevent further stretching of the tissue. This model would predict a biphasic length-tension relationship with an abrupt decrease in compliance near maximum lung volumes. However, the stress-strain loop of lung tissue is smoothly curved over its entire range (Fig. 2), and uniaxial deformation of lung strips does not allow us to distinguish two different elastic behaviors [15]. Recent structural observations have stated that to accomplish its dual structural function of scaffolding and stress-bearing, the extracellular fiber matrix has to integrate its separate components into a functional whole, the so-called integral fiber strand [16]. Instead of independent networks, collagen and elastic fibers form a macrostructure of interwoven fibers that provide the characteristic network (nylon stocking) extensibility: stretching in one direction leads to a temporary rearrangement of the fibers. Elastic fibers will restore the original arrangement upon relaxation. When this

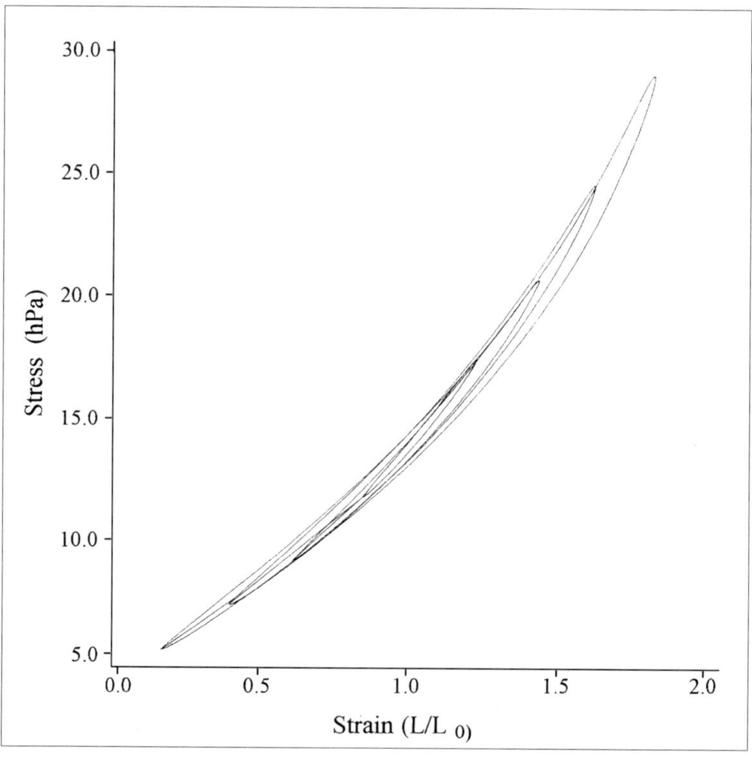

Fig. 2. Stress-strain curves obtained in a subpleural sample of rat lung (rat lung strip), submitted to uniaxial oscillatory deformation of increasing amplitudes around the operative length (obtained at 14 hPa basal stress). The smooth curvature over the entire range of deformation can be observed

system is submitted to a radial stress, it will convert the external traction into interior tension and transmit it throughout the lung via the elastic parenchymal network as in the ideal lung of Mead [2]. Under the action of a distorting force, structural intermolecular links in the proteins oppose deformation. No structural change can be performed without a remaking of interactions at the molecular level in the net. In these molecular rearrangements reside the biomechanical properties of lung parenchyma.

Nonlinearity and lung tissue structure

In vivo, alveoli are subject to finite deformation. Like many biological materials, lung tissue exhibits prominent time-dependent and frequency-dependent phenomena. Even if hysteresis and time-dependent phenomena are disregarded, the relationship between stress and strain is nonlinear over the range of physiological deformations. Many studies provide evidence that the nonlinear features of lung dynamics arise largely from elastic nonlinearities in lung tissue. Hildebrandt [17] studied the dynamic properties of excised cat lungs in a liquid plethysmograph. Lung elastic modulus and viscosity rose markedly with lung volume. Moreover, the magnitude of the unit step response fell with increasing step size and rose with lung volume. By measuring alveolar pressure to study parenchymal mechanics in mechanically ventilated rabbits, Romero et al. [18] observed an increase in both tissue elasticity and viscosity with transpulmonary pressure. As with the mechanical tissue behavior of whole lungs, several authors [19, 20, 21] have recently addressed the question of the marked dependence of the elastic modulus on the mean distending stress in isolated strips of lung parenchyma. Therefore, the elastic recoil of the lung at normal breathing is dominated by the nonlinear stress-strain characteristics of lung tissue (Fig. 2). The origin of the curvilinear stress-strain behavior is generally thought to be one of recruitment. Maksym and Bates [22] have developed a model of lung tissue based on the collagen fiber recruitment concept, by representing the collagen and elastic fibers as a series of spring-string pairs. In this model, collagen is the recruited element (string), while elastin (spring) is responsible for load-bearing at low strains when much of the collagen is "wavy" and, therefore not contributing to the tension. As strain increases, the collagen fibers become straight and so progressively take up more load, thereby stiffening the tissue. This model explains the curvilinear quasistatic stress-strain characteristics of lung tissue, but does not account for dynamic nonlinearities observed in alveolar wall preparations.

The model developed by Romero et al. [21] is represented in Fig. 3. In this model, molecular interactions presenting a linear viscoelastic behaviour are progressively recruited. Elastin and collagen interact in a more active way, and the lung behaves as a complex polymer that can be modelled as a material with two components. One is the set of all lung constituents which participate in the mechanical response in a continuous, uninterrupted way during any mechanical test. This element is known as *continuum* or matrix. The second component is formed by those elements whose participation in the mechanical response of

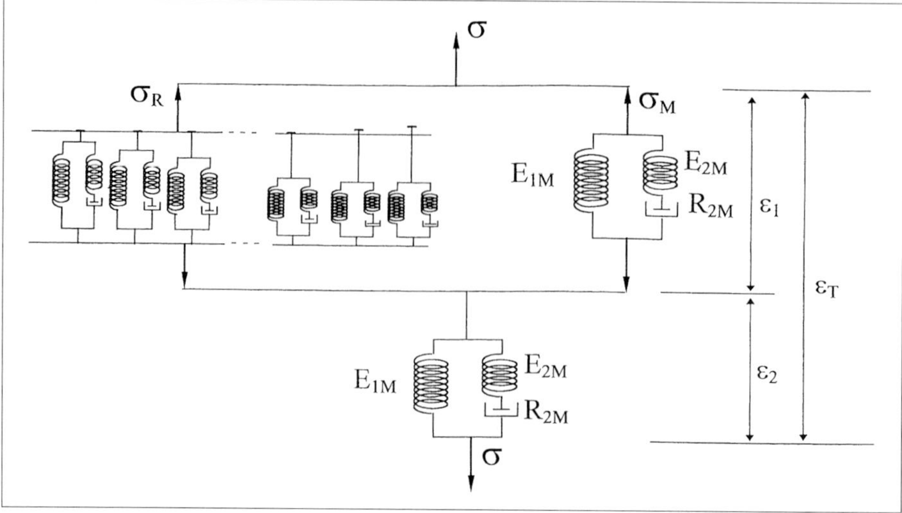

Fig. 3. Spring-dashpot scheme of the recruitment-based model of lung tissue behaviour, ordered according to Takayagashi's block diagram. The basic element is a Kelvin's element composed of elastic resistances in parallel and a viscous resistance in series with one of the elastic resistances. This Kelvin diagram represents the behaviour of the continuous part of the system or "matrix" (*M*) either in series or in parallel with the recruiting portion of the system or "filler" (*R*). This model assumes that the nonlinearity between stress and strain is due to the fact that the number of fibers with identical mechanical properties participating in the lung's mechanical response is not constant, but depends, due to recruitment, on the strain to which sample is subjected. (From [21])

the lung is dependent on the deformation to which the sample is subjected. Consequently, a given element is incorporated into the lung's mechanical response after a threshold value has been reached. This phenomenon is known as recruitment. If the sample is shortened to a deformation value lower than that at which recruitment of the element occurs, then this element will not participate in the mechanical response. This second component is assumed to be embedded in the continuum, forming a discontinuous phase and which, by analogy with compound materials is called *filler*. The mechanical behaviour of the continum+filler as a whole can be studied using the block model of Takayanagi [23] for complex polymers. This model assumes that the behaviour of the material as a whole corresponds to the behaviour of the filler material ordered in parallel with a fraction of the continuum (parallel matrix), and this set was then ordered in series with the rest of the matrix (serial matrix). Standard viscoelastic Kelvin's model has been used to represent viscoelastic behavior, both for the matrix and for each of the fiber elements composing the filler. This model assumes that the nonlinearity between stress and strain is due to the fact that the number of fibers with identical mechanical properties participating in the lung's mechanical response is not constant, but depends, due to recruitment, on the strain to which the tissue is subjected. It accounts fairly well for both static (stress relaxation, stress recovery) and dynamic (oscillatory) properties of lung tissue [21].

Alveolar stability

As a result of the interaction between surface and tissue forces in normal lungs, alveoli remain permanently opened at FRC. Only if volume is forcibly reduced to near RV (residual volume) are peripheral airways seen to close. The older, well-known arguments about the potential effects of surface forces on lung stability, based on a picture of the lung microstructure as a collection of independent bubble-like airspaces, have now been replaced by arguments that treat lung stability as a structural phenomenon. Morphological data indicate that surface tension (γ)

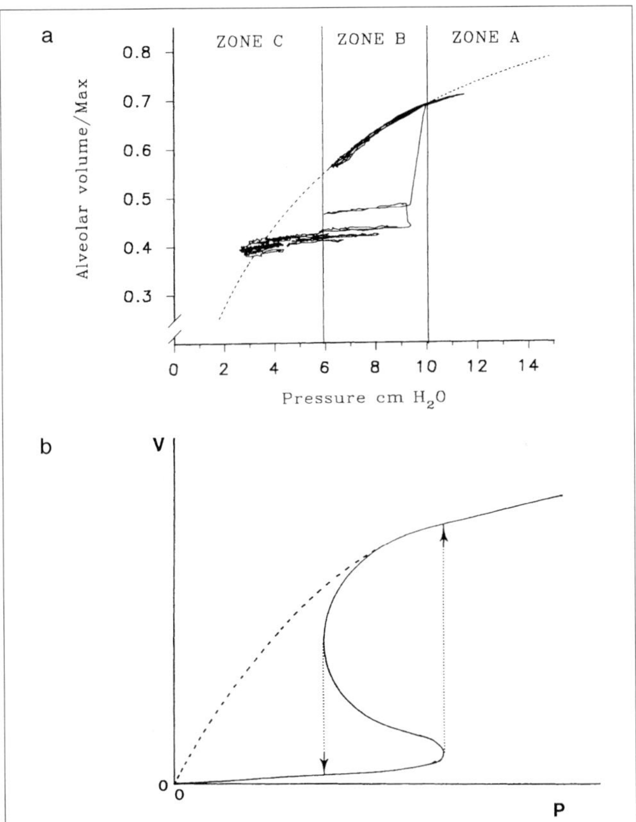

Fig. 4. (a) Experimental data of alveolar volume (derived from alveolar pressure) plotted against driving pressure in an unstable region of a rabbit lung. Rabbit was pretreated with ethchlorovynol to induce lung permeability edema; (b) pressure-volume (PV) diagram describing a uniform expansion of parenchyma with constant surface tension, according to the theoretical analysis from Stamenovic and Smith [24]. This analysis predicts that particular nonuniformities of lung expansion, representing parenchymal instability, would occur over the region where the PV curve has a negative slope. (From [26] with permission)

distorts alveolar geometry, and new models for the microstructural mechanics consider that the outward pull of γ exerted on the alveolar ducts is in equilibrium with the tissue forces of the duct structure [10]. According to Eq. 1, if surface tension were constant and high enough, the lung would be unstable at low lung volume [24, 25]. This conclusion is based on the fact that the contribution of surface tension to the transpulmonary pressure is proportional to the product of surface tension and interfacial surface-to-volume ratio and that the surface-to-volume ratio increases as the volume decreases. Therefore, if surface tension is constant and large enough, recoil pressure increases with decreasing volume and the lung is unstable. According to Stamenovic and Smith [24], alveolar pressure-volume curves from areas with constant surface tension would pass through a region of instability (Fig. 4), in agreement with the experimental observations made in rabbits after induced permeability edema [26].

Parenchymal constriction

Many studies have shown that bronchoconstrictor agents induce a substantial increase in tissue resistance (Rti) and dynamic elastance (Edyn) in several species. Several mechanisms have been invoked to induce changes in Rti and Edyn after constrictor challenge: parallel heterogeneities, lung tissue constriction, and airways-to-tissue interaction are the most relevant. Recently Romero et al. [27] have shown that pharmacologically induced changes in tissue resistance and tissue hysteresivity precede to changes in alveolar heterogeneity (Fig. 5) and are out of phase with airway resistance, whereas dynamic elastance changes are in phase with changes in the airways. Hysteresivity being an intrinsic property of the tissue dissipative behaviour at structural level [19], the authors concluded that changes in tissue resistance and tissue hysteresivity reflect the active constriction of contractile cells and smooth muscle in the parenchyma. The conclusion that parenchymal tissue is affected by bronchoconstricting agents is significant because it implies that asthma may be a disorder of lung parenchyma, not just of airways. But it has other important physiological implications in the regulation of the tensile equilibrium at the level of the acinus. At this respect, quantitative differencies between the changes in mechanical properties of lung strips submitted to pharmacological agents in vitro and the pharmacological response of the whole lung in vivo have been observed. The elastance and resistance of parenchymal strips exposed to bronchoconstrictor agents increase by less than 50%, whereas apparent lung elastance and resistance increase manifold [18, 19]. Because of this disparity between the magnitude of changes in both preparations, some authors have concluded that most of the increased impedance of the constricted lung is caused by large nonuniform airway resistance, mainly at the level of terminal bronchioles [28]. Indeed, alveolar capsule technique has allowed detection of important parallel heterogeneities once the constriction is fully established. However, the lag between the increase in tissue resistance and hysteresivity (immediate after i.v. injection of methacholine), and the increase in parallel airways inhomogeneity (Fig. 5) suggest that there is a real, not artifac-

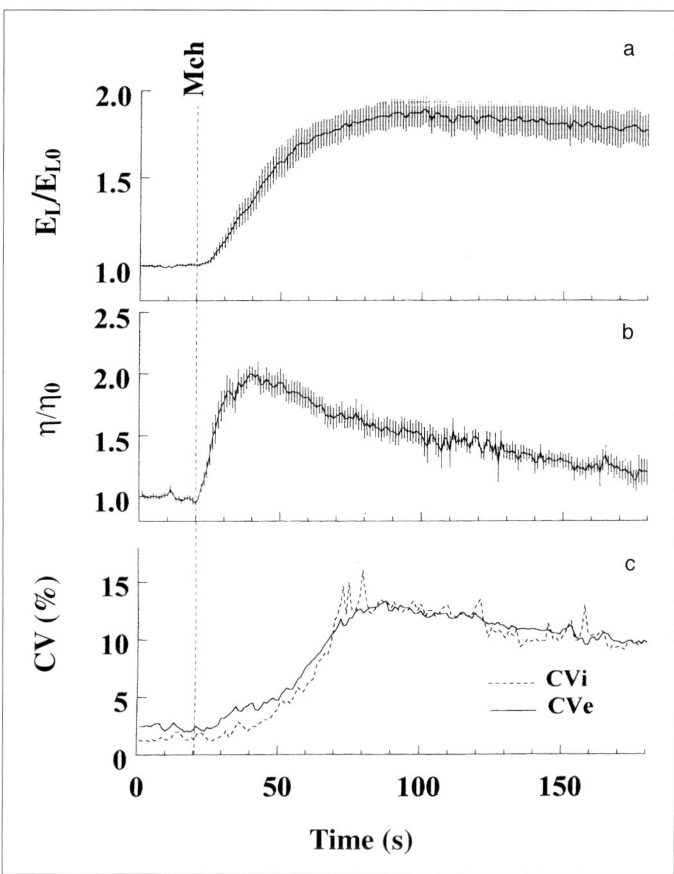

Fig. 5a-c. Time course of changes immediately after an i.v. injection of methacholine. (a) Dynamic elastance (EL); (b) lung parenchyma hysteresivity (η); (c) coefficient of variation of alveolar pressure at end expiration (CVe) and end inspiration (Cvi). A clear phase lag is observed between alveolar heterogeneity and hysteresivity changes on one hand, and between parenchyma hysteresivity and elastance on the other. (From [27] with permission)

tual increase in Rti, reflecting the activation of the contractile machinery at the level of the parenchyma. An alternative explanation of the disparity of the mechanical response to constrictor agents in the alveolar wall preparation and in the whole lung resides in the structural behavior of the acinus, and particularly in the tissue forces-surface forces interaction. Smooth muscle is distributed in the acinus in close relation with the fiber rings at the alveolar mouths. Contractile fibers have been described in the interstitial spaces in close contact with the fiberous network that forms the connective scaffold of the acinus. According to the model of interaction proposed by Wilson and Bachofen [10], if tissue tensions increase at a given alveolar volume, the interfacial pressure has to increase to keep alveolar stability. Consequently, tissue constriction would act as a regulatory mechanism of alveolar micromechanics.

References

1. Wilson TA (1981) The relations among recoil pressure, surface area and surface tension in the lung. J Appl Physiol Respirat Environ Exercise Physiol 50:921-926
2. Mead J (1961) Mechanical properties of lungs. Physiol Rev 41:281-330
3. Schürch S, Bachofen H, Weibel ER (1985) Alveolar surface tensions in excised rabbit lungs: effects of temperature. Respir Physiol 62:31-45
4. Bachofen H, Wilson TA (1991) Micromechanics of the acinus and the alveolar wall. In: Crystal RG, West JB et al (eds) The Lung: scientific foundations. Vol. I. Raven Press, New York, pp 809-819
5. Pattle RE (1955) Properties, function and origin of the alveolar lining layer. Nature 175:1125-1127
6. Von Neergard K (1929) Neue Auffassungen über einen Grundbegriff der Atemmechanik: Die Retraktionskraft der Lunge, Abhangig von der Oberflächensprannung in den Alveolen. Z Gesamte Exp Med 66:373-394
7. Hoppin FG, Hildebrandt J (1977) Mechanical properties of the lung. In: West JB (ed) Bioengineering aspects of the lung. Marcel Dekker, New York, pp 83-157
8. Schürch S, Goerke J, Clements JA (1976) Direct determination of surface tension in the lung. Proc Natl Acad Sci 73:4698-4702
9. Schürch S, Bachofen H, Goerke J, Possmayer F (1989) A captive bubble method reproduces the in situ behavior of lung surfactant monolayers. J Appl Physiol 67:2389-2396
10. Wilson TA, Bachofen H (1982) A model of mechanical structure of alveolar duct. J Appl Physiol 53:1512-1520
11. Smith JC, Stamenovic D (1986) Surface forces in the lungs. I Alveolar surface tension-lung volume relationships. J Appl Physiol 60:1341-1350
12. Setnikar I, Meschia G (1952) Propietà elastiche del polmone e di modelli meccaniche. Arch Fisiol 52:288-302
13. Karlinsky JB, Snyder GL, Franzlau C, Stone PJ, Hoppin FG Jr (1960) In vitro effects of elastase and collagenase on mechanical properties of hamster lungs. Am Rev Respir Dis 82:186-194
14. Moretto A, Dallaire M, Romero P, Ludwig M (1994) Effect of elastase on oscillation mechanics of lung parenchymal strips. J Appl Physiol 77:1623-1629
15. Romero PV, Cañete C, Lopez-Aguilar J, Romero FJ (1998) Elasticity, viscosity and plasticity in lung parenchyma. In: Milic-Emili J (ed) Applied physiology in respiratory mechanics. Springer-Verlag, Berlin Heidelberg New York, pp 57-72
16. Weibel ER, Crystal RG (1991) Structural organization of the pulmonary interstitium. In: Crystal RG, West JB et al (eds) The lung: scientific foundations. Vol I. Raven Press, New York, pp 369-380
17. Hildebrandt J (1969) Dynamic properties of air-filled excised cat lungs determined by liquid pletismograph. J Appl Physiol 27:246-250
18. Romero PV, Robatto FM, Simard S, Ludwig MS (1992) Lung tissue behavior during methacholine challenge in rabbits in vivo. J Appl Physiol 73:207-212
19. Fredberg JJ, Bunk D, Ingenito E, Shore SA (1993) Tissue resistance and the contractile state of lung parenchyma. J Appl Physiol 74:1387-1397
20. Navajas D, Maksym GN, Bates JHT (1995) Dynamic viscoelastic nonlinearity of lung parenchymal tissue. J Appl Physiol 79:348-356
21. Romero FJ, Pastor A, Lopez, J, Romero PV (1998) A recruitment-based rheological model for mechanical behavior of soft tissues. Biorheology 35:17-35
22. Maksym GN, Bates JHT (1997) A distributed nonlinear model of lung tissue elasticity. J Appl Physiol 82:32-41

23. Takayanagi M (1963) Viscoelastic properties of crystalline polymers. Mem Fac Eng Kyushu Univ 33(1):41-96
24. Stamenovic D, Smith JC (1986) Surface forces in lungs II. Microstructural mechanics and lung stability. J Appl Physiol 60:1351-1357
25. Stamenovic D, Wilson TA (1992) Parenchymal stability. J Appl Physiol 73:596-602
26. Romero PV, Lopez Aguilar J, Blanch L (1998) Pulmonary mechanics beyond peripheral airways. In: Milic-Emili J (ed) Applied physiology in respiratory mechanics. Springer-Verlag, Berlin Heidelberg New York, pp 199-210
27. Romero PV, Rodriguez B, Lopez-Aguilar J, Manresa F (1998) Parallel airways inhomogeneity and lung tissue mechanics in transition to constricted state in rabbits. J Appl Physiol 84:1040-1047
28. Hubmayr RD, Hill M, Wilson TA (1996) Nonuniform expansion of constricted dog lungs. J Appl Physiol 80:522-530

Chapter 11

Partitioning of lung responses into airway and tissue components

M.S. Ludwig

This chapter deals with the role of the lung parenchyma in contributing to the contractile response of the overall lung during induced constriction. Addressing the contribution of the parenchyma has been made easier in recent years because of the development of the alveolar capsule technique which permits direct measurement of alveolar pressure [1]. Resistive losses across the lung can, thereby, be partitioned into a component due to airway resistance (Raw) and a component due to tissue resistance (Rti). Similarly, resistance changes during induced constriction can be apportioned into the component related to changes in airway calibre and the component related to alterations in tissue mechanical behaviour. Recent studies in a number of different animal species have shown that much of the resistive pressure drop across the lung under baseline conditions is due to the resistive pressure drop at the level of the lung tissues [2-6]. Furthermore, numerous animal studies have now shown that increases in lung resistance (RL) during exogenous or endogenous constriction are due, in large part, to changes in tissue resistance [2, 5-10]. Traditionally, changes in lung resistance with induced constriction were thought to be due to changes in airway calibre. However, if increases in tissue resistance account for a large part of the increase in lung resistance, then the pathophysiology of diseases such as asthma needs to be reconsidered.

Background

The lung parenchyma was first described as a viscoelastic material by Bayliss and Robertson in 1939 [11]. Hildebrandt and colleagues [12-14] in a series of elegant studies described the hysteretic properties of the lung parenchyma in a number of different species and with lungs in the air-filled or fluid-filled state. However, the relative importance of tissue resistance in determining the overall resistive losses of the lung during cyclic ventilation has been a matter of some controversy. Contribution of tissue resistance to lung resistance has been reported to range from 15%-85% of total RL [11, 15, 16]. Some of the confusion arises because many of these measurements were made using different regimes of ventilation, i.e. different frequencies and tidal volumes or at different lung volumes; both tissue and airway resistance are sensitive to changes in these variables. Furthermore, alveolar pressure was measured indirectly in all these studies. It was only with the introduction and application of the alveolar capsule technique that direct measurement of alveolar pressure became possible.

Alveolar capsule technique

The first use of an alveolar capsule to measure alveolar pressure (PA) was reported by Takashima et al. in 1971 [17]; Fredberg et al. [1, 18] further refined this approach. Basically, a hollow capsule is glued to the pleural surface of the lung and punctures are made in the underlying pleura to bring the capsule chamber into communication with the underlying alveoli. Pressure is then measured in the chamber with a miniature transducer. Once measurement of alveolar pressure can be obtained, lung resistance can be partitioned into airway and tissue components by measuring pressure at the airway opening (Pao), PA, and flow. While alveolar pressure is measured directly with this method, regional flow is not. Rather, flow is measured at the airway opening and it is assumed that flow is homogeneously distributed throughout the lung, an assumption that is reasonable under baseline conditions [19] but can become somewhat more problematic after induced constriction [20]. The pressure drop between Pao and PA in phase with flow represents airway resistance while the pressure drop between PA and the pleural space represents tissue resistance.

Animal studies: tissue resistance at baseline

Tissue resistance is dependent on the frequency and tidal volume of oscillation as well as the lung volume at which the measurement is made [2, 3, 13]. My colleagues and I [2, 6, 21] and others [22] have shown in several different species that tissue resistance increases as the transpulmonary pressure is increased. Hence the contribution of tissue resistance to overall lung resistance will vary as the regime of ventilation varies.

In studies conducted in my laboratory, measurements were made of tissue and airway resistance at "physiologic" breathing frequencies, tidal volumes and lung volumes. Results in dogs, rabbits, guinea pigs and rats are shown in Table 1. Under baseline conditions, tissue resistance accounts for a substantial proportion of overall lung resistance.

Animal studies: tissue resistance after induced constriction

Alveolar capsules were applied to canine lungs, and airway and tissue resistances were measured before and after inhalations of histamine and prostaglandin $F_{2\alpha}$, and after vagal stimulation [2]. Increases in tissue resistance accounted for roughly half of the increase in RL after vagal stimulation and for most of the increase after histamine and $PGF_{2\alpha}$ inhalation. In subsequent experiments, concentration-response curves of airway and tissue resistance were examined after

Table 1. Values of RL, raw and rti under baseline conditions (mean ± standard error)

	Dogs ($cm\ H_2O\ s\ l^{-1}$)	Rabbits ($cm\ H_2O\ s\ ml^{-1}$)	Rats ($cm\ H_2O\ s\ ml^{-1}$)	Guinea pigs ($cm\ H_2O\ s\ ml^{-1}$)
RL	0.98±0.24	0.024±0.006	0.082±0.005	0.105±0.008
Raw	0.18±0.02	0.010±0.005	0.050±0.005	0.079±0.005
Rti	0.80±0.23	0.014±0.003	0.032±0.002	0.026±0.005

RL, lung resistance; *raw*, airway resistance; *Rti*, tissue resistance

inhalations of histamine or methacholine in dogs, rabbits, rats and guinea pigs [6, 21, 23, and unpublished data]. Although there was some interspecies variation, much of the increase in RL was attributable to the increase in Rti (Fig. 1). Several other investigators have reported similar results using alveolar capsules to partition the response to different smooth muscle agonists delivered exogenously to both mature and immature animals. Sly and Lanteri [7] showed that increases in tissue resistance accounted for most of the increase in lung resistance after methacholine nebulization in 8-10 week old mongrel puppies. Sakae et al. [24] showed that alveolar pressures increased to a greater degree than airway pressures after inhalation of methacholine in rats. Shardonofsky and collegues [22] reported increases in tissue resistance in rabbits after intravenous route can effect changes in tissue behaviour.

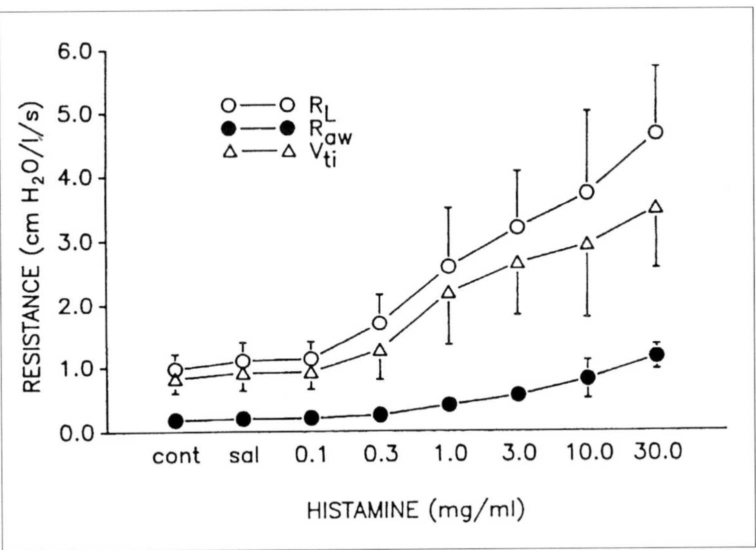

Fig. 1. Resistance values for lung resistance (RL), airway resistance (Raw) and tissue viscance or resistance (Vti) during histamine challenge in dogs (n=6). Values are mean ± standard error. *Cont*, control; *sal*, saline. (From [23] with permission)

My colleagus and I have also studied the role of the lung tissues in the allergic response in the Brown Norway rat model of intrinsic asthma [25, 26]. After inhalation of aerosols of ovalbumin in previously sensitized rats, airway and tissue resistance increased during both the early and the late response [9]. Rti accounted for roughly half of the increase in RL during the early response and 60% of the increase in RL during the late response. As expected, studies of lung morphology during the late response showed significant airway constriction (Fig. 2). In addition, the alveolar architecture was also substantially altered (Fig. 3). There was widespread tissue distortion with areas of hyperinflation adjacent to areas of atelectasis. This atelectasis was not to airway closure as none of the more than 200 airways sampled after ovalbumin exposure showed histologic evidence of airway closure.

A second model investigated is that of hyperpnea-induced constriction (HIC) in the guinea pig [10]. This model shares several common features with exercise-induced asthma, including the time course of the onset of constriction, the spontaneity of resolution, and the relationship between the amount of hyperpnea and the degree of response elicited [27]. During HIC, approximately two-thirds of the increase in RL was accounted for by the increase in Rti. Morphologic and morphometric studies of the lung tissues during the HIC response again showed substantial tissue distortion, with areas of atelectasis and relative hyperinflation.

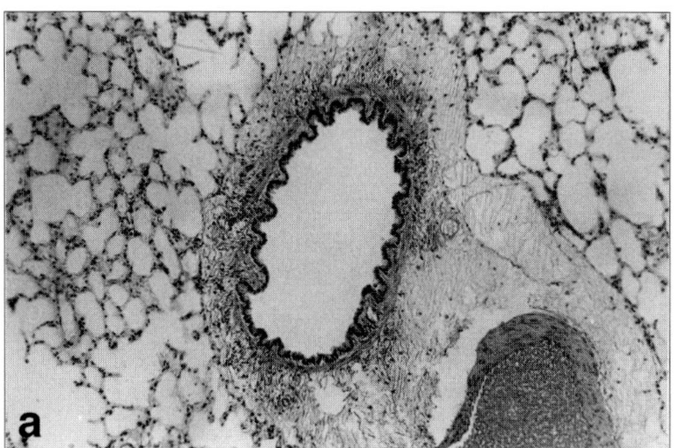

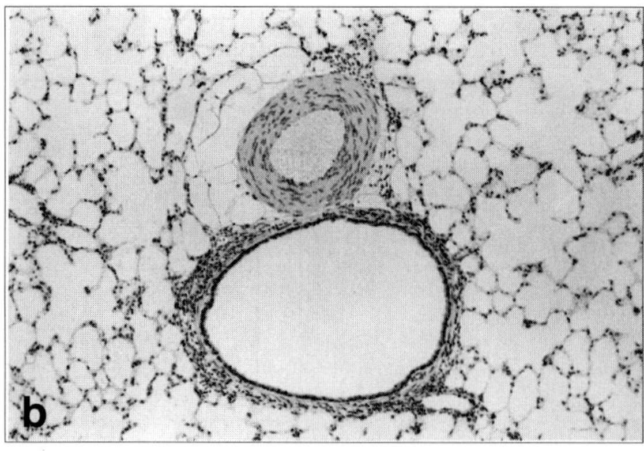

Fig. 2a,b. Photomicrographs of airway from (a) a previously sensitized, ovalbumin-challenged Brown Norway rat during the late asthmatic response (basement membrane=1.508 mm), and (b) a time-matched saline control (basement membrane=1.416 mm). Lungs fixed at 3 cm H_20 transpulmonary pressure. Hemaetoxylin-eosin stain. Magnification • 100. (From [9] with permission)

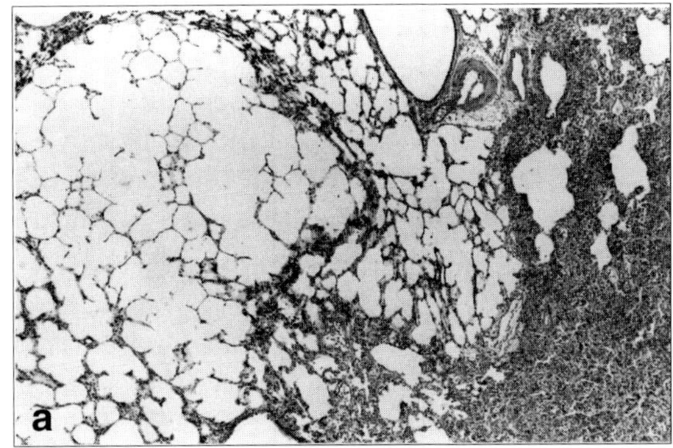

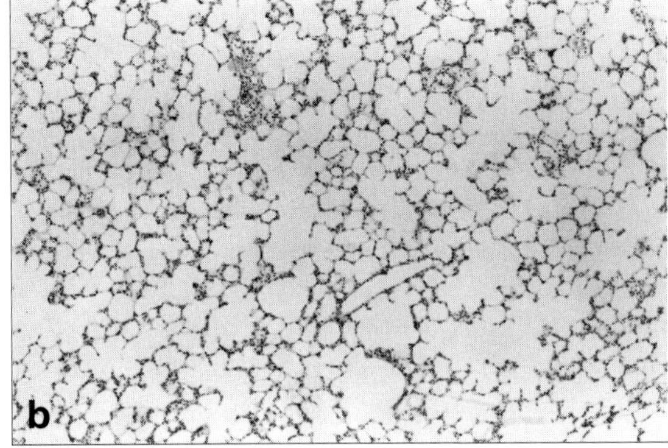

Fig. 3a,b. Photomicrographs of lung tissues from (a) a previously sensitized, ovalbumin-challenged Brown Norway rat during the late asthmatic response, and (b) a time-matched saline control. Lungs fixed at 3 cm H_2O transpu monary pressure. Hemaetoxylin-eosin stain. Magnification • 63. (From [9] with permission)

Human studies

Measurements of tissue resistance in humans have been more difficult to obtain because of the invasiveness of the alveolar capsule technique. Verbeken et al. [28, 29] made measurements in autopsy specimens, oscillating the lungs with pseudorandom noise. In normal autopsy lungs, at 4 Hz, Rti accounted for 36% of total resistance at distending pressures of 6 cm H_2O, and 74% of total resistance at distending pressures of 20 cm H_2O. In lungs from patients with emphysema, the proportion of RL attributable to Rti decreased; in patients with fibrosis the proportion remained the same. More recently investigators made measurements of complex impedence to partition resistance into airway and tissue components. Kaczka and colleagues [30] used the optimal ventilator waveform technique, whereby a complex signal was simultaneously delivered to a subject along with tidal volume ventilation. Data were fit to a model which included an airway resistance component and a tissue damping or resistance component. Their data showed that, at typical breathing frequencies, Rti accounted for roughly 60% of intrathoracic RL. After induced constriction, however, most of the increase in RL was due to a change in the airway component. Similarly, Peslin and Duvivier [31] made measurements of airway and tissue impedence during pressure oscillations in normal subjects seated in a body plethysmograph. They showed that Raw and Rti were of a similar magnitude under baseline conditions. Induced constriction caused a change primarily in the airway component. Whether similar responses would be seen in patients with asthma is not known. A recent study in chronic stable asthmatics showed that much of the inflammation present in the lung occurs at the level of the alveolar tissue [32]. To the extent that inflammation would alter the viscoelastic properties of the alveolar tissues, one might expect a change in the tissue resistance.

Mechanisms contributing to increased tissue resistance during induced constriction site of response

Contractile element

Kapanci et al. first described "contractile interstitial cells" which bound anti-actin antibodies in the alveolar wall [33]. Subsequently other investigators described myoepithelial cells which contain molecules of actin and myosin [34] (Fig. 4). It is possible that constriction of the contractile elements in these cells leads to the increase in Rti seen during exogenous and endogenous constriction. The contractile element responding may be at the level of the alveolar duct. Lai et al. [35], in a preliminary study of parenchymal strips in an organ bath, used confocal microscopy to show changes in alveolar duct geometry in response to histamine. Alternately, the responding element could be at the level of the terminal or respiratory bronchiole or even reflect a response in more proximal airways [36]. Because of the mechanical interdependence between airways and surrounding parenchyma, airway smooth muscle constriction could cause changes in the stress on the tethered parenchymal attachments and thereby affect local parenchymal mechanics [37].

Alterations in alveolar geometry and the air-liquid interface

The collagen-elastin-proteoglycan matrix may be responsible for the hysteretic or resistive pressure losses at the level of the lung parenchyma. Individual colla-

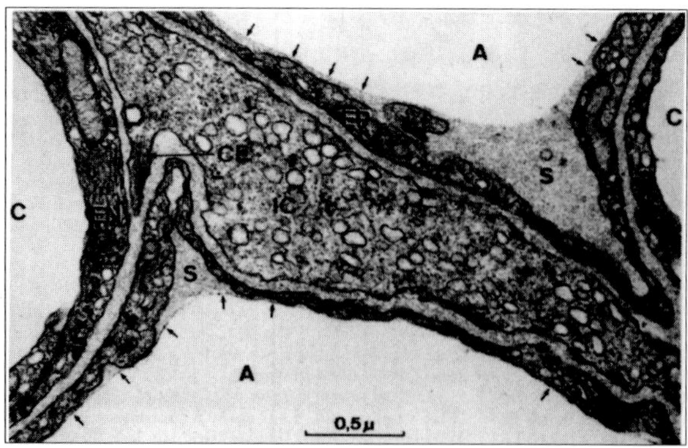

Fig. 4. Detail of alveolar septum from adult rabbit fixed at 0.4 total lung capacity. Interstitial cell (IC) with contractile element (CE). *A*, alveolar air space; *C*, capillary; *S*, small pool of alveolar lining layer; *EN*, endothelium; *EP*, epithelium. (From [34] with permission)

gen and elastic fibres demonstrate little hysteresis; however, when fibres are organized into a network, the behaviour of the network may be different from that of the individual constituents [38]. Proteoglycans, molecules which constitute the ground substance of the matrix, are highly hydrophilic and can alter the tissue turgor and thereby, its viscoelastic properties. Constriction of contractile elements can cause distortion of alveolar geometry which would result in changes in the hysteretic or resistive behaviour of the lung of the tissues. Furthermore, microvascular leak caused by the agonists employed or by release of mediators during allergen or hyperpnea challenge [39] could alter the water content of the tissues. The surface film (surfactant) is highly hysteretic [40]. Changes in the surface layer could also occur as a consequence of microvascular leak. Finally, the interactions between the matrix and the surface film could be altered once the lung is constricted.

Regional heterogeneities and microatelectasis

In addition to the mechanisms described above, regional heterogeneities can cause alterations in the dynamic mechanical behaviour of the lung tissues. Frequency dependence of compliance, i.e. changes in compliance due to heterogeneous distribution of airflow, has been well described, but heterogeneous distribution of airflow could also affect tissue resistance. For example, if the tidal volume is distributed primarily to regions of the lung where the alveoli are relatively hyperinflated, then Rti will increase because it is related to lung volume [2]. If the tidal volume is distributed to areas of the lung where atelectasis is present, then Rti will increase on the basis of the energy required to recruit and derecruit atelectatic airspaces [41]. Finally, constriction-induced airway heterogeneties can contribute to the measured increase in tissue resistance [42].

Conclusions

This chapter describes the important role of tissue resistance in determining the overall resistance of the lung in both animals and humans. Tissue resistance increases during induced constriction and in different animal models of asthma. While preliminary data suggest that the parenchymal tissues in normal humans respond modestly to inhaled constrictors, studies in human asthmatics or in tissue from asthmatics are necessary to define the role of the tissue response in asthmatic disease. The mechanism of the tissue resistance response is unclear at the present time, but may involve a response of contractile myoepithelial cells, constriction-induced changes in alveolar geometry and in the air-liquid interface, or alterations in dynamic mechanical behaviour because of prominent tissue distortion and mechanical heterogeneities. Understanding the mechanisms giving rise to the tissue resistance response may have important implications for understanding the underlying pathophysiology of obstructive lung diseases.

References

1. Fredberg JJ, Keefe DH, Glass GM, Castile RG, Frantz III ID (1984) Alveolar pressure nonhomogeneity during small-amplitude high-frequency oscillation. J Appl Physiol 57:788-800
2. Ludwig MS, Dreshaj I, Solway J, Munoz A, Ingram Jr RH (1987) Partitioning of pulmonary resistance during constriction in the dog: effects of volume history. J Appl Physiol 62:807-815
3. Brusasco V, Warner DO, Beck KC, Rodarte JR, Rehder K (1989) Partitioning of pulmonary resistance in dogs: effect of tidal volume and frequency. J Appl Physiol 66:1190-1196
4. Warner DO, Vettermann J, Brusasco V, Rehder K (1989) Pulmonary resistance during halothane anesthesia is not determined only by airway caliber. Anesthesiology 70:453-460
5. Romero PV, Ludwig MS (1991) Maximal methacholine-induced constriction in rabbit lung: interactions between airways and tissue? J Appl Physiol 70:1044-1050
6. Nagase T, Ito T, Yanai M, Martin JG, Ludwig MS (1993) Responsiveness of and interactions between airways and tissue in guinea pigs during induced constriction. J Appl Physiol 74:2848-2854
7. Sly PD, Lanteri CJ (1991) Partitioning of pulmonary responses to inhaled methacholine in puppies. J Appl Physiol 71:886-891
8. Martins MA, Dolhkinoff M, Zin WA, Saldiva PHN (1993) Airway and pulmonary tissue responses to capsaicin in guinea pigs assessed with the alveolar capsule technique. Am Rev Respir Dis 147:466-470
9. Nagase T, Moretto A, Dallaire MJ, Eidelman DH, Martin JG, Ludwig MS (1994) Airway and tissue responses to antigen challenge in sensitized Brown Norway rats. Am J Respir Crit Care Med 150:218-226
10. Nagase T, Dallaire MJ, Ludwig MS (1994) Airway and tissue responses during hypnea-induced constriction in guinea pigs. Am J Respir Crit Care Med 149:1342-1347
11. Bayliss LE, Robertson GW (1939) The viscoelastic properties of the lungs. Q J Exp Physiol 29:27-47
12. Hildebrandt J (1969) Dyamic properties of air-filled excised cat lung determined by liquid plethysmograph. J Appl Physiol 27:246-250
13. Bachofen H, Hidebrandt J (1971) Area analysis of pressure-volume hysteresis in mammalian lung. J Appl Physiol 30:493-497
14. Bachofen H, Hildebrandt J, Bachofen M (1970) Pressure-volume curves of air- and liquid-filled excised lungs - Surface tension in situ. J Appl Physiol 29:422-431
15. Marshall R, Dubois AB (1956) The measurement of the viscous resistance of the lung tissues in normal man. Clin Sci 15:161-170
16. Loring SH, Drazen JM, Smith JC, Hoppin Jr FG (1981) Vagal stimulation and aerosol histamine increase hysteresis of lung recoil. J Appl Physiol 51:477-484
17. Takashima T, Ishikawa T, Sasaki T, Nakamura T (1971) Measurement of collateral flow at quasialveolar levels in excised dog lung. Tohuku J Exp Med 105:405-406
18. Fredberg JJ, Ingram Jr RH, Castile RG, Glass GM, Drazen JM (1985) Nonhomogeneity of lung response to inhaled histamine assessed with alveolar capsules. J Appl Physiol 58:1914-1922
19. Bates JHT, Ludwig MS, Sly PD, Brown K, Martin JG, Fredberg JJ (1988) Interrupter resistance elucidated by alveolar pressure measurement in open-chested normal dogs. J Appl Physiol 65:408-414

20. Lauzon AM, Dechman G, Bates JHT (1995) On the use of alveolar capsule technique to study bronchoconstriction. Respir Physiol 99:139-146
21. Romero PV, Robatto FM, Simard S, Ludwig MS (1992) Lung tissue behaviour during methacholine challenge in rabbits in vivo. J Appl Physiol 73:207-212
22. Shardonofsky FR, McDonough JM, Grunstein MM (1993) Effects of positive end-expiratory pressure on lung tissue mechanics in rabbits. J Appl Physiol 75:2506-2513
23. Ludwig MS, Romero PV, Bates JHT (1989) A comparison of the dose-response behaviour of canine airways and parenchyma. J Appl Pysiol 67:1220-1225
24. Sakae RS, Martins MA, Criado PMP, Zin WA, Saldiva PHN (1992) In vivo evaluation of airway and pulmonary tissue response to inhaled methacholine in the rat. J Appl Toxic 12:235-238
25. Eidelman DH, Bellofiore S, Martin JG (1988) Late airway response to antigen challenge in sensitized inbred rats. Am Rev Respir Dis 137:1033-1037
26. Sapienza S, Du T, Eidelman DH, Wang NS, Martin JG (1991) Structural changes in the airways of sensitized Brown Norway rats after antigen challenge. Am Rev Respir Dis 144:423-427
27. Ray DW, Hernandez C, Munoz N, Leff AR, Solway J (1988) Bronchoconstriction elicitated by isocapnic hyperpnea in guinea pigs. J Appl Physiol 65:934-939
28. Verbeken EK, Cauberghs M, Mertens I, Lauweryns JM, Van de Woestijne KP (1992) Tissue and airway impedence of excised normal, senile, and emphysematous lungs. J Appl Physiol 72:2343-2353
29. Verbeken EK, Cauberghs M, Lauweryns JM, Van de Woestijne KP (1994) Structure and function in fibrosing alveolitis. J Appl Physiol 76:731-742
30. Kaczka D, Ingenito EP, Suki B, Lutchen KR (1997) Partitioning airway and lung tissue resistance in humans: effects of bronchoconstriction. J Appl Physiol 82:1531-1541
31. Peslin R, Duvivier C (1998) Partitioning of airway and respiratory tissue mechanical impedences by body plethysmography. J Appl Physiol 84:553-561
32. Kraft M, Djukanovic R, Wilson S, Holgate ST, Martin RJ (1996) Alveolar tissue inflammation in asthma. Am J Respir Crit Care Med 154:1505-1510
33. Kapanci Y, Assimacopoulos A, Irle C, Zwahlen A, Gabbiani G (1974) "Contractile interstitial cells" in pulmonary alveolar septa: a possible regulator of ventilation/perfusion ratio. J Cell Biol 60:375-392
34. Gil J, Bachofen JGH, Gehr P, Weibel ER (1979) Alveolar volume-surface area relation in air- and saline-filled lungs fixed by vascular perfusion. J Appl Physiol 47:990-1001
35. Lai J, Rogers RA, Ekstein BA, Fredberg JJ (1994) Dynamic changes in alveolar duct geometry in response to 10^{-3} M histamine. Am J Respir Crit Care Med 149:A539
36. Mitzner W, Blosser S, Yager S, Wagner E (1992) Effect of bronchial smooth muscle contraction on compliance. J Appl Physiol 72:158-167
37. Mead J, Takishima T, Leith D (1970) Stress distribution in lungs: a model of pulmonary elasticity. J Appl Physiol 28:596-608
38. Bull HB (1957) Protein structure and elasticity. In: Remington JW (ed) Tissue elasticity. Waverly Press, Washington, pp 33-42
39. Erjefalt I, Greiff L, Alkner U, Persson CGA (1993) Allergen-induced biphasic plasma exudation responses in guinea pig large airways. Am Rev Respir Dis 148:695-701
40. Schurch S, Bachofen H, Goerke J, Green F (1992) Surface properties of rat pulmonary surfactant studied with the captive bubble method: adsorption, hysteresis, stability. Biochim Biophys Acta 1103:127-136

41. Smaldone GC, Mitzner W, Itoh H (1983) Role of alveolar recruitment in lung inflammation: influence on pressure-volume hysteresis. J Appl Physiol 55:1321-1332
42. Lutchen KR, Hantos Z, Petak F, Adamicza A, Suki B (1996) Airway inhomogeneities contribute to apparent lung tissue mechanics during constriction. J Appl Physiol 80:1841-1849

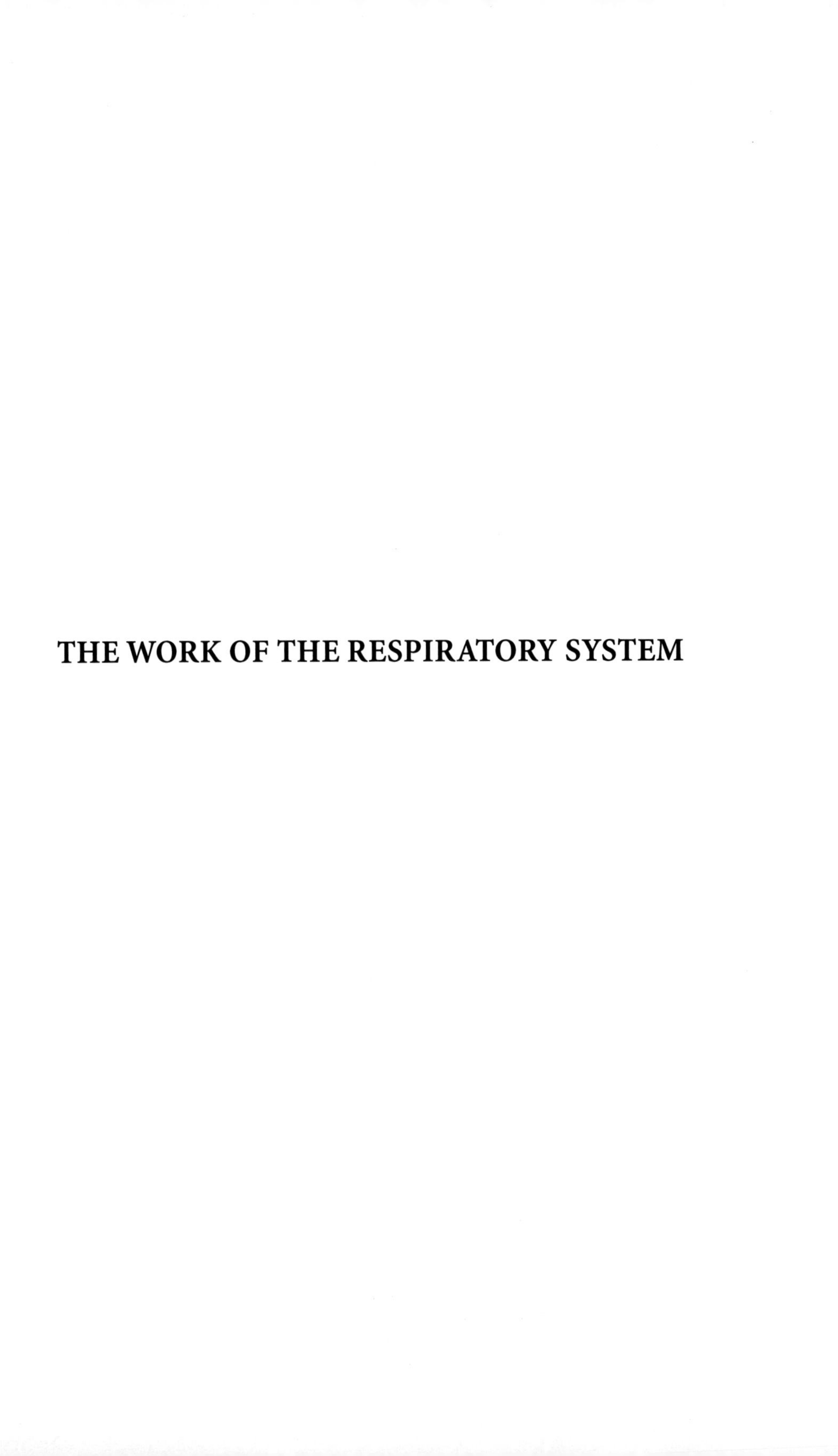

THE WORK OF THE RESPIRATORY SYSTEM

Chapter 12

How the diaphragm works in normal subjects

N.B. Pride

About 25 years ago, it was proposed that the diaphragm was the only inspiratory muscle active in quiet breathing, but subsequent work has shown that this is not the case. Indeed most recent developments have been in understanding the inter relations between the actions of the diaphragm and the muscles acting on the rib cage and abdominal muscles. Thus, while the diaphragm plays the major role in sustaining ventilation, it is not absolutely essential for life; other muscles can sustain ventilation - albeit with little reserve capacity for use on exercise - when there is undoubted bilateral diaphragm paralysis [1].

Resting breathing

Contraction of the diaphragm (Fig. 1) enlarges the lungs by two actions: caudal movement of the dome, and elevation and expansion of the lower rib cage. Enlargement of the lungs by diaphragm contraction usually leads to outward movement of the anterior abdominal wall on inspiration. On inspiration pres-

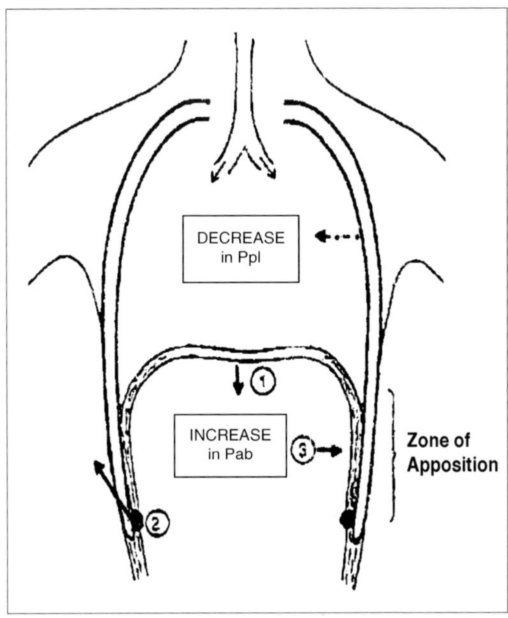

Fig. 1. Mechanisms of lung inflation by contraction of the diaphragm. Contraction of the diaphragm muscle fibres leads to shortening of the zones of apposition (ZOA) and results in: (1) descent of the dome (piston-like action); (2) elevation and lateral expansion of the lower rib cage (insertional action); (3) lateral expansion of the lower rib cage by increase in abdominal pressure (appositional action). These actions reduce pleural surface and hence alveolar pressure leading to inspiratory flow. The reduction in pleural pressure potentially can reduce lateral dimensions of the pulmonary-apposed rib cage: in practice this does not occur because of co-activation of muscles acting on the upper rib cage

sure in the abdomen tends to rise while pressure in the thoracic cavity falls. Increased tension in diaphragmatic muscle fibres moves the dome caudally; this piston-like action shortens the zone of apposition (ZOA) where the costal diaphragm lies apposed to the internal surface of the rib cage. Contraction of the diaphragm also results in elevation and expansion of the lower rib cage by a combination of its insertional action and its appositional action [2]. The costal diaphragm inserts into the lower six ribs close to the lower margin of the rib cage. Because the muscle fibres run in a cranial-caudal orientation in the ZOA, contraction results in elevation of the lower ribs. Because of the oblique position of the long axis of rotation of the lower rib neck-vertebral articulations, elevation of these ribs is accompanied by the "bucket handle" action expanding the lateral rib cage dimension. The latter action is amplified by the appositional action, the inspiratory increase in abdominal pressure being transmitted as an increase in the pressure in the pleural recess internal to the rib cage in the ZOA. In the upright, normal subject the ZOA at functional residual capacity (FRC) is approximately at the level of the xiphoid process and moves caudally 1.5-2.0 cm during a tidal inspiration [3]. Hence, about 25%-30% of the rib cage during tidal breathing is exposed to abdominal pressure rather than pleural pressure; potentially, this means that the rib cage is exposed to distorting forces on inspiration when the diaphragm contracts alone, the lower rib cage being expanded while the upper rib cage could be pulled in by the reduction in pleural surface pressure. In practice, such distortions do not occur in healthy subjects, because during tidal breathing there is also inspiratory tidal activation of scalene muscles (which insert into the top two ribs) and parasternal internal intercostal muscles which insert into the sternum and the costochondrial junctions of the upper ribs close to the sternum [2, 4]. Contraction of these two sets of rib cage muscles elevates the upper rib cage and sternum; because of the more horizontal angle of the rib neck-vertebral articulations and the restrictions imposed anteriorly by the insertion of the upper ribs into the manubrium sternum, the action of these muscles is to elevate the upper rib cage with an increase in its anterior posterior dimensions ("pump-handle" action) without expanding its lateral diameters.

Exercise

During exercise, the abdominal muscles as well as rib cage muscles and diaphragm are active. Increase in tidal volume in normal subjects is achieved by a reduction in end-expired lung volume as well as by an increase in end-inspired lung volume. The former change is achieved by contraction of abdominal muscles and aids the diaphragm by increasing its resting length at the beginning of inspiration [5]. The increase in end-inspired lung volume is accommodated by an increase in rib cage volume. Studies in animals have shown that the optimum length for force generation by the diaphragm is slightly below functional residual capacity (FRC), and for the parasternal intercostal muscles slightly above FRC [6]. If this is the case in upright humans, these changes in rib cage and abdominal dimensions could optimize action of the parasternal muscles and diaphragm. A recent analysis of respiratory muscle activation during exercise has confirmed and elaborated these findings using a more sophisticated analysis of chest wall movement which follows the movement of 86 markers [7, 8] on the chest wall during vigorous exercise. This analysis demonstrated that there was remarkably little distortion of the upper and lower rib cage which was attributed to subtle interactions between the three active muscle groups [7]. But the most interesting finding was that immediately on commencing cycle exercise, "programming" of the diaphragm, rib cage and abdominal muscles switches from that appropriate for rest [8]. With increase in exercise intensity, activation of all three muscle groups increased proportionately but with rib cage muscle activation being 180° out of phase in the ventilatory cycle with activation of the abdominal muscles [8]. This enabled the rib cage and abdominal muscles to develop the pressures to displace the rib cage and abdomen, respectively, leaving the diaphragm to act predominantly as a flow generator with only a modest increase in tidal change in transdiaphragmatic pressure (Pdi) even during strenuous exercise. Hence, ventilation during exercise is achieved by sharing the increased work amongst all the available muscle groups.

Force-generating capacity

In general, diaphragm performance is not regarded as limiting exercise in normal subjects, but information on the normal range of force-generating capacity and how this is altered by changes in lung volume is relevant to its functioning in severe respiratory disease which is characterized by increases in mechanical load which are often accompanied by hyperinflation. The diaphragm is largely "hidden" from the direct assessments of force, length and velocity of shortening made in limb muscles, and surrogate measurements are usually necessary. Measuring Pdi is the surrogate for direct measurements of diaphragm force but the force-Pdi relationship is influenced by the radius of curvature of the dome of the diaphragm which in turn varies with the size of the individual [9]. Further factors influencing the absolute pressures generated in the thoracic and abdominal cavities - and the partitioning of Pdi between the two cavities - are their compliance which is altered by activation of other respiratory muscles. Most knowledge of muscle strength comes from measurements of mouth pressure generated during attempted maximum inspiratory efforts (PI max) at FRC or at residual volume [9-11]. PI max indicates the intrathoracic pressure developed by all the inspiratory muscles; there is much less information on Pdimax during such efforts. There is a wide range of normal values of Pimax but it is clear that, as expected from studies in limb muscles, the inspiratory muscles are stronger in men than in women and that strength declines with increasing age. This implies that the inspiratory muscles of the elderly, particularly women, are more likely to have problems in coping with the increased mechanical loads of severe respiratory disease. It is unclear how much of the wide range of values of PI max in normal subjects is due to true differences in strength and how much to incomplete activation of the muscles during the procedure. Methodological details are important; the type of mouthpiece affects values [12] and more negative inspiratory pressure may be achieved in some subjects during a dynamic sniff manoeuvre measured either in the oesophagus [13] or in an occluded naris [14] rather than during the standard method of making the inspiratory effort against a closed airway (or an airway with a very small leak to prevent pressure being generated by cheek muscles [9]). If activation was complete in both the static and the sniff manoeuvre, inspiratory pressure would be smaller in the sniff manoeuvre which is associated with greater muscle shortening. Even in efforts against a closed airway which prevents gas movement into the lungs, the inspiratory muscles shorten due to expansion of alveolar gas caused by the development of a subatmospheric alveolar pressure. Activation of a muscle during a voluntary effort can be assessed by superimposing a twitch activation of the supplying nerve; if this results in an additional force then activation is submaximal. This "twitch interpolation" test has been used occasionally in the diaphragm [15, 16] but until recently its invasive nature (requiring at least oesophageal intubation) and bilateral electrical phrenic nerve stimulation precluded its wider use. Twitch stimulation of the phrenic nerves is now obtained much more easily and painlessly with magnetic stimulation, either posteriorly over the phrenic nerve roots [17] or anteriorly in the neck [18]. Furthermore, in carefully controlled circumstances, the resulting twitch pressure can be measured at the mouth rather than in the oesophagus [19], making twitch occlusion potentially a much more widely applicable test [20]. A major source of variability in limb muscle strength is the bulk of the muscles and this is also the case for the diaphragm. The thickness of the costal diaphragm in vivo can be measured using ultrasound at least in the right ZOA [21, 22]. In trained weight lifters large values of Pdimax are associated with considerable increase of diaphragm thickness [22].

Compared with the difficulties of establishing the range of diaphragmatic strength in different individuals, there has been no difficulty in establishing that as lung volume is increased above about 50% vital capacity in an individual $P_i$max becomes less negative and Pdimax is reduced [9, 23]. Furthermore twitch Pdi developed with electrical [24] or magnetic [25] stimulation of the relaxed diaphragm shows a similar reduction as lung volume is increased. These changes are consistent with the findings in limb muscles, which develop less force when shortened beyond an optimum length and are of obvious relevance to the enforced hyperinflation accompanying severe intrathoracic airflow obstruction.

Sustainable loads

Implicit in the use of assisted mechanical ventilation to relieve respiratory distress or "exhaustion" in severe respiratory disease is the idea that the respiratory muscles may be unable to cope with the increased mechanical load. This has stimulated a great deal of work on the effects of increased loads on the normal diaphragm in the last two decades [26-29]. Most often the load used has been an imposed, external mechanical load, but the ability to sustain a high target ventilation and, less frequently, exercise carried to exhaustion have also been studied. Highly motivated subjects are required. A variety of endpoints have been used; at one extreme inability to maintain or repeat the required or imposed force - that is overt exhaustion or task failure [26]. But muscle fatigue has been defined as "reduction in force-generating capacity of the muscle resulting from muscle activity under load which is reversible by rest" [30] and so can be detected before task failure occurs by reductions in volitional mouth, oesophageal or transdiaphragmatic pressures during maximum inspiratory efforts or by reductions in twitch pressure produced by phrenic nerve stimulation. Even earlier changes in the fatiguing process are a reduction in the maximum relaxation rate (MRR) of the inspiratory muscles (usually measured by the decay of oesophageal pressure in a sniff manoeuvre [31]), or in the high-low (H/L) ratio of the frequency spectrum of the diaphragm electromyogram (EMG) [32]. Both these changes develop soon after a heavy load is applied and probably represent normal adaptive mechanisms in a muscle under load, which allow preservation of force-generating capacity and precede overt contractile failure.

In the early 1980s Bellemare and Grassino [27, 28] attempted to quantify the sustainable load on the diaphragm in terms of a tension (strictly pressure)-time index (TTdi), which equals the target tidal Pdi, expressed as a % of Pdimax, multiplied by the proportion of the breathing cycle spent on inspiration ("duty cycle"). To define a critical TTdi, a range of target pressures were imposed using a variable inspiratory resistance, and the time each could be sustained (up to a maximum of 45 min) was measured. Bellemare and Grassino found that as TTdi was increased above 0.15, the time a given load could be sustained was reduced; TTdi at rest was about 0.02, implying a considerable reserve of pressure generating capacity in these normal subjects. Reductions in H/L ratio occurred when TTdi was >0.15 [28]. Another approach is to study how long isocapnic maximum voluntary ventilation (MVV) can be sustained, comparing later values to the value of MVV that can be generated over 15 s in a rested subject ("sprint" MVV) [33]. On average in normal subjects MVV falls to about 70% of sprint MVV over the first 2 to 3 minutes and can be sustained thereafter [33]. MRR is prolonged but recovers after about a 10 min of rest [34]. True low-frequency fatigue of the diaphragm, shown by a lower twitch Pdi, also develops after sustained MVV and persists for most of the following hour [35].

Both these changes can also be found when exercise is carried out to exhaustion at least when extremely high ventilations - 150 l min^{-1} - are sustained [36]. It is doubtful if reductions in twitch Pdi would be found in less fit normal subjects because they normally cease exercise at much lower levels of maximum ventilation. These studies therefore provide convincing evidence that the inspiratory muscles, and specifically the diaphragm, can show fatigue when exposed to heavy load – a characteristic they share with skeletal limb muscles; but judged by the resting TTdi there is a very large reserve of diaphragm function and fatigue is only likely to be reached in exceptional physiological circumstances in normal subjects. The major insights in these studies lie in comparisons with disease where loads are increased and pressure-generating capacity is often reduced.

Future developments

Most of the features of normal diaphragm function summarised above were described in the 1980s. They often required complex experiments, invasive procedures and elaborate analysis and so were not easily transferable outside the few highly specialised laboratories. Recent research has used several simpler techniques. Twitch stimulation of the phrenic nerves has been greatly simplified by the development of magnetic rather than electrical excitation [17], while mouth rather than oesophageal pressure can sometimes be used to assess responses [19]. This makes measurement of twitch pressure a much more practical proposition, even in the intensive care unit. Twitch interpolation might be used on a wider scale to assess diaphragm activation during attempted maximum inspiratory efforts. Estimates of diaphragm movement and thickness in the ZOA can be made with ultrasound; they have already been used to show the thicker diaphragm of weight-lifters [22] and thinning with unilateral paralysis [37] and perhaps might be used to show detraining (as in the intensive care unit). Ultrasound measurements can also be used to measure tidal changes in length of the ZOA and, in combination with measurement of rib cage diameter using magnetometers, can estimate tidal changes in length of the diaphragm in the coronal plane [3]. Ultrasound also aids inserting needle electrodes into the costal diaphragm, parasternal or abdominal muscles to obtain electrical information about neural drive to individual motor units [38, 39]. Developments in computer processing now allow chest wall movements to be analysed in much more detail from an array of markers [7, 8]. Three-dimensional reconstructions of diaphragm shape can be made from computed tomography (CT) [40] or magnetic resonance imaging (MRI) [41] scans. As a result of these developments the ability to make direct, rather than surrogate, measurements of diaphragm function has considerably improved in the last few years.

Conclusions

Co-ordinated activation of diaphragm and other inspiratory muscles acting on the upper rib cage are required to produce undistorted expansion of the rib cage during quiet tidal breathing. During exercise phasic activation of rib cage and abdominal muscles share the ventilatory load with the diaphragm, greatly assisting its flow-generating capacity. Pressure generation by the inspiratory muscles is less in women than in men and declines with increasing age and within an individual, with increase in lung volume. The normal diaphragm fatigues when exposed experimentally to heavy loads, but fatigue is only likely to develop in exceptional physiological circumstances. New techniques have expanded the ability to examine diaphragm function directly.

References

1. Laroche CM, Carroll N, Moxham J, Green M (1988) Clinical significance of severe isolated diaphragm weakness. Am Rev Respir Dis 138:862-866
2. De Troyer A, Loring SH (1995) Actions of the respiratory muscles. In: Roussos CH (ed) The Thorax, 2nd ed. Marcel Dekker, New York, pp 535-563
3. McKenzie DK, Gorman RB, Pride NB, Tolman JF, Gandevia SC (1998) Diaphragm contribution to tidal volume in patients with severe chronic airflow limitation. Am J Resp Crit Care Med 157:A359
4. De Troyer A, Estenne M (1984) Coordination between rib cage muscles and diaphragm during quiet breathing in humans. J Appl Physiol 57:899-906
5. Grimby G, Elgefors B, Oxhoj H (1973) Ventilatory levels and chest wall mechanics during exercise in obstructive lung disease. Scand J Respir Dis 54:45-52
6. Farkas GA, Decramer M, Rochester DF, De Troyer A (1985) Contractile properties of intercostal muscles and their functional significance. J Appl Physiol 59:528-535
7. Kenyon CM, Cala SJ, Yan S, Aliverti A, Scano G, Duranti R, Pedotti A, Macklem PT (1997) Rib cage mechanics during quiet breathing and exercise in humans. J Appl Physiol 83:1242-1255
8. Aliverti A, Cala SJ, Duranti R, Ferrigno G, Kenyon CM, Pedotti A, Scano G, Sliwinski P, Macklem PT, Yan S (1997) Human respiratory muscle actions and control during exercise. J Appl Physiol 83:1256-1269
9. Ringqvist T (1966) The ventilatory capacity in healthy subjects. Scand J Clin & Lab Invest 18(Suppl 88):8-179
10. Black LF, Hyatt RE (1969) Maximal respiratory pressure: normal values and relationships to age and sex. Am Rev Respir Dis 99:698-702
11. Enright PL, Kronmal RA, Manolio TA, Schenker MB, Hyatt RC (1994) Respiratory muscle strength in the elderly: correlates and reference values. Am J Respir Crit Care Med 149:430-438
12. Koulouris N, Mulvey D, Laroche CM, Green M, Moxham J (1988) Comparison of two different mouthpieces for the measurement of PI max and PE max in normal and weak subjects. Eur Respir J 1:863-866
13. Koulouris N, Mulvey D, Laroche CM, Sawicka E, Green M, Moxham J (1989) The measurement of inspiratory muscle strength by sniff oesophageal, nasopharyngeal and mouth pressures. Am Rev Respir Dis 139:641-646
14. Heritier F, Rahm F, Pasche P, Fitting J-W (1994) Sniff nasal pressure. A non invasive assessment of inspiratory muscle strength. Am J Respir Crit Care Med 150:1678-1683
15. Bellemare F, Bigland-Ritchie B (1984) Assessment of human diaphragm strength and activation using phrenic nerve stimulation. Respir Physiol 58:263-277
16. Similowski T, Yan S, Gauthier AP, Macklem PT, Bellemare F (1991) Contractile properties of the human diaphragm during chronic hyperinflation. N Eng J Med 325:917-923
17. Similowski T, Fleury B, Launois S, Cathala HP, Bouche P, Derenne JP (1989) Cervical magnetic stimulation: a new painless method for bilateral nerve stimulation in conscious humans. J Appl Physiol 67:1311-1318
18. Mills GH, Kryoussis D, Hamnegård CH, Polkey MI, Green M, Moxham J (1996) Bilateral magnetic stimulation of the phrenic nerves from an anterolateral approach. Am J Respir Crit Care Med 154:1099-1105
19. Yan S, Gauthier AP, Similowski T, Macklem PT, Bellemare F (1992) Evaluation of human diaphragm contractility using mouth pressure twitches. Am Rev Respir Dis 145:1064-1069

20. De Bruin PFC, Watson RA, Khalil N, Pride NB (1998) Use of mouth pressure twitches induced by cervical magnetic stimulation to assess voluntary activation of the diaphragm. Eur Respir J 12:672-678
21. Ueki J, De Bruin PF, Pride NB (1995) In vivo assessment of diaphragm contraction by ultrasound in normal subjects. Thorax 50:1157-1161
22. McCool FD, Benditt JO, Conomos P, Anderson L, Sherman CB, Hoppin Jr FG (1997) Variability of diaphragm structure among healthy individuals. Am J Respir Crit Care Med 155:1323-1328
23. Gibson GJ, Clark E, Pride NB (1981) Static transdiaphragmatic pressures in normal subjects and in patients with chronic hyperinflation. Am Rev Respir Dis 124:685-689
24. Smith J, Bellemare F (1987) Effect of lung volume on in vivo contraction characteristics of human diaphragm. J Appl Physiol 62:1893-1900
25. Hamnegård C-H, Wragg S, Mills GH et al (1995) The effect of lung volume on transdiaphragmatic pressure. Eur Respir J 9:241-247
26. Roussos C, Macklem PT (1977) Diaphragmatic fatigue in man. J Appl Physiol 43:189-197
27. Bellemare F, Grassino A (1982) Evaluation of human diaphragm fatigue. J Appl Physiol 53:1196-1206
28. Bellemare F, Grassino A (1982) Effect of pressure and timing of contraction on human diaphragm fatigue. J Appl Physiol 53:1190-1195
29. Clanton TL (1995) Respiratory muscle endurance in humans. In: Roussos CH (ed) The Thorax, 2nd ed. Marcel Dekker, New York, pp 1199-1230
30. NHLBI Workshop Summary (1990) Respiratory muscle fatigue. Am Rev Respir Dis 142:474-480
31. Esau SA, Bellemare F, Grassino A, Permutt S, Roussos C, Pardy RL (1983) Changes in relaxation rate with diaphragmatic fatigue in humans. J Appl Physiol 54:1353-1360
32. Gross D, Grassino A, Ross D, Macklem PT (1979) The EMG pattern of diaphragmatic fatigue. J Appl Physiol 46:1-7
33. Freedman S (1970) Sustained maximum voluntary ventilation. Respir Physiol 41:230-244
34. Mulvey DA, Koulouris NG, Elliott MW, Laroche CM, Moxham J, Green M (1991) Inspiratory muscle relaxation rate after voluntary maximal isocapnic ventilation in humans. J Appl Physiol 70:2173-2180
35. Hamnegård C-H, Wragg S, Kyroussis D et al (1996) Diaphragm fatigue following maximal ventilation in man. Eur Respir J 9:241-247
36. Johnson BD, Babcock MA, Suman OE, Dempsey JA (1993) Exercise-induced diaphragmatic fatigue in healthy humans. J Physiol 460:385-405
37. Gottesman E, McCool FD (1997) Ultrasound evaluation of the paralyzed diaphragm. Am J Respir Crit Care Med 155:1570-1574
38. Gandevia SC, Leeper JB, McKenzie DK, De Troyer A (1996) Discharge frequencies of parasternal intercostal and scalene motor units during breathing in normal and COPD subjects. Am J Respir Crit Care Med 153:622-628
39. De Troyer A, Leeper JB, McKenzie DK, Gandevia SC (1997) Neural drive to the diaphragm in patients with severe COPD. Am J Respir Crit Care Med 155:1335-1340
40. Pettiaux N, Cassart M, Paiva M, Estenne M (1997) Three dimensional reconstructions of human diaphragm with the use of spiral computed tomography. J Appl Physiol 82:998-1002
41. Gauthier AP, Verbanck S, Estenne M, Segebarth C, Macklem PT, Paiva M (1994) Three-dimensional reconstruction of the in vivo human diaphragm shape at different lung volumes. J Appl Physiol 76:495-406

Chapter 13

How the diaphragm works in respiratory disease

N.B. PRIDE

The strength of the diaphragm may be reduced by a wide range of primary neurological or muscular diseases and, more subtly, by endocrine or metabolic disorders including many acute abnormalities that may develop in critically ill patients. In respiratory disease, the major problem is usually not loss of strength but impairment of mechanical action of the diaphragm. The commonest cause of impaired diaphragm function is the symmetrical hyperinflation of chronic obstructive pulmonary disease (COPD) and acute, severe asthma. Diaphragm-lung coupling is also impaired by deformity of the chest wall (i.e., kyphoscoliosis, thoracoplasty) or pleural disease (i.e., pneumothorax, pleural effusion, fibrosis). Of course with advanced chronic respiratory disease, true weakness and loss of muscle strength may develop due to cachexia, metabolic abnormalities [1] or glucocorticosteroid treatment [2].

Almost nothing is known about how diaphragm performance adapts to asymmetrical chest wall or intrathoracic disease (e.g. single lung transplant) or indeed how it is affected by unilateral disease in the central nervous system, such as stroke [3]. Investigation of the diaphragm in respiratory disease has concentrated on COPD and, to a lesser extent, asthma.

COPD

In patients with COPD, the inspiratory muscles have to generate greater force (and greater reductions in pleural pressure) than in normal subjects during tidal breathing to overcome the increased airflow resistance and dynamic pulmonary elastance; however, comparable intrapulmonary loads occur in severe fibrosing alveolitis, and are well tolerated when imposed in healthy subjects. The most important factor compromising diaphragm performance in patients with COPD appears to be hyperinflation [1].

The extent of the hyperinflation and the consequent caudal movement of the diaphragm are functions of the severity of COPD. Most clinical assessments are based on chest radiographs taken at full inspiration (total lung capacity, TLC) when the domes may be flat (particularly in lateral radiographs) and the diaphragm insertions into the lateral rib cage may be seen, indicating the absence of a zone of apposition (ZOA) of the costal diaphragm to the rib cage. This has led to the assertion that (at least in upright postures) the diaphragm may have completely lost its inspiratory action and tidal contraction may only have the effect of narrowing the lower rib cage on inspiration (Hoover's sign).

It is more relevant to look at the diaphragm at functional residual capacity (FRC) and during tidal breathing. A few measurements have been made using static posterior-anterior chest radiographs at FRC, but dynamic measurements of right-sided ZOA can be made more effectively using an ultrasound probe placed cranial-caudally over the lateral rib cage, usually in the anterior axillary line. With this technique the upper limit of the ZOA can be recognized by the level at which the diaphragm image (actually produced by reflections not from the muscle but from the lining of pleural and peritoneal membranes) is lost due to the intervention of aerated lung between the internal surface of the rib cage and the diaphragm. Ultrasound measurements can be made at TLC and at full expiration (residual volume, RV) as well as at FRC and during tidal breathing. The absolute length of the ZOA can be estimated with reference to its origin on the lowest rib at TLC. In 10 patients with COPD who had low FEV_1 (mean 23% predicted, 0.71 l) and severe hyperinflation (mean FRC 199% predicted, FRC/TLC 0.82), my colleagues and I found the expected shortening of the right ZOA at FRC. Estimates of tidal change in total length of the diaphragm made using measurements of rib cage diameter from magnetometers and length of ZOA showed that fractional shortening and volume displaced was similar in control and COPD subjects (Table 1) [4]. Hence, tidal movement of the diaphragm was normal in these patients with severe COPD.

Furthermore, studies in some of these patients by Gandevia et al. [5] and De Troyer et al. [6] showed that the neural drive to motor units of the diaphragm during tidal breathing was increased [6] to a greater extent than drive to the parasternal or scalene muscles [5], a pattern found in stimulated breathing in normal subjects. Hence tidal movement and activation of the diaphragm was maintained in these patients with COPD; of course this does not reveal how effective the diaphragm is in lowering pleural pressure and expanding the lungs. The reduced ZOA and hence area of the rib cage potentially exposed to abdominal pressure may be responsible for the reduced lateral expansion of the lower rib cage during inspiration.

Table 1. Length of right zone of apposition at functional residual capacity and during tidal breathing. (Modified from [4])

	Normals (n=10)	**COPD (n=10)**
Age (years)	65.4	65.8
FRC/TLC	0.58	0.82
Vt (l)	0.85	0.77
Zone of apposition		
• Length at FRC (mm)	72.5	32.5
• Change in length over Vt (mm)	18.0	20.0

Vt, Tidal volume

Studies of pressures above and below the diaphragm (oesophageal and gastric) consistently suggest that for a given fall in oesophageal pressure, the rise in abdominal pressure is smaller in COPD than in normal subjects [7, 8]. This in part may be due to the low diaphragm position at FRC-presumably with a completely flat diaphragm, contraction results in little change in pressure in thorax or abdomen. However, the change in oesophageal/gastric pressure pattern probably is also related to increased recruitment of parasternal and scalene muscles (but usually not sternocleidomastoid muscles) during tidal breathing [9]. This is similar to the pattern of recruitment when the ventilatory requirement is increased during exercise in a normal subject. Unfortunately, it is difficult to apportion the precise contributions of the diaphragm and other inspiratory muscles to the generation of pleural pressure during tidal breathing without reliable relaxation curves of the chest wall [7].

Measuring the transdiaphragmatic pressure (Pdi) generated by twitch stimulation of the phrenic nerves shows a strong dependence of twitch Pdi on lung volume in both normal subjects and patients with COPD. Although twitch Pdi is smaller at the increased FRC in COPD than at FRC in normal subjects, if lung volume is expressed as % predicted TLC, twitch Pdi is larger in COPD patients than in control subjects [10, 11]. However, the fraction converted into negative oesophageal pressure in COPD is disputed. During voluntary maximum inspiratory efforts, pressures generated at residual volume (RV) and FRC in most patients with COPD are also normal, or even slightly supranormal when allowance is made for the increase in FRC [1, 12]. Indeed, it can be argued that the ability of COPD patients to continue to generate negative pressures at a TLC which has presumably increased from its original adult volume as disease progresses indicates adaptation to hyperinflation. In chronic animal models of emphysema, the diaphragm loses sarcomeres in series, so optimizing its force-length characteristics to the new shorter resting length of the diaphragm [13]. All these results suggest retention of diaphragm strength in COPD but some uncertainty about how effectively contraction is transformed into an inspiratory action on the lungs.

A more controversial area is how close to "task failure" or fatigue the diaphragm is in COPD. Bellemare and Grassino in the early 1980s showed that normal subjects could not sustain indefinitely a tension-time product of the diaphragm (TTdi) which exceeded 0.15 of the available pressure-generating capacity [14]. A subsequent study of 20 patients with stable COPD showed TTdi could be as high as 0.12 at rest, suggesting that exacerbations could easily precipitate such patients into task failure of the diaphragm [15]. Because of the obvious difficulties in studying acute exacerbations, the usual methods to study endurance of the inspiratory muscles have been to impose repetitive pressure tasks [14, 16, 17], or to study function after maximum voluntary ventilation (MVV) [18] or exercise carried to the point of exhaustion [19, 20]. The last two procedures lead to an increase in end-expired lung volume above that at rest in patients with COPD. Perhaps surprisingly, the diaphragm in COPD appears to perform remarkably well in all three types of task [17-20]. Thus, although exhaustive exercise reduces the high-low ratio of the electromyogram (EMG) of the costal diaphragm during exercise, and slows the maximum relaxation rate of the inspiratory muscles for a few minutes after stopping exercise [19], it does not cause any fall in twitch Pdi [20] which would occur if there was low frequency muscle fatigue. Two minutes of MVV reduces maximum relaxation rate [21] and twitch Pdi [22] in normal subjects, but does not cause a reduction in twitch Pdi in patients with COPD [18]. The reasons for this paradox are not clear. Absolute values of MVV are considerably lower in COPD than in normal subjects and it has been known for many years that patients with COPD are able to sustain MVV much more effectively than normal subjects [23]. One suggestion has been that shortening of the diaphragm while reducing potential force output actually *protects* against fatigue [18].

Measurements of the weight and thickness of the diaphragm in COPD at post-mortem have given variable results [1]. A major confounding factor is that weight loss and malnutrition are common in the end-stages of disease, resulting in a general muscular weakness affecting limb and expiratory muscles as well as the diaphragm; the balance of evidence suggests the mass of the diaphragm remains normal when allowance is made for weight [24], but the results are too crude to provide useful information on whether there is adaptation in the number of sarcomeres.

Unfortunately, it is difficult to assess thickness of the costal diaphragm in vivo with ultrasound in patients with emphysema, because corrections have to be made for the increased FRC and thickness appears to vary considerably at different points around the rib cage, which is not the case in normal subjects [25]. The advent of lung volume reduction surgery (LVRS) – for which one of the main benefits claimed is an improvement in the mechanical performance of the diaphragm [26-28] – also allows biopsy of the diaphragm in advanced COPD. A recent biopsy study found a higher than normal percent of slow-twitch (type I) fibres and a lower percent of fast myosin heavy chain (type II ab) fibres than in age-matched controls [29]. LVRS also provides a direct opportunity to assess the results of reducing hyperinflation on diaphragm function. Improvements have been consistently found and these have appeared to be larger than can be explained by the observed reduction in FRC [28]. Potentially, examination of diaphragm function before and after LVRS could provide new insights into the effects of hyperinflation, although concurrent improvements in pulmonary mechanics will need to be taken into account.

From the point of view of intensive care specialists, the most important question is whether there is task failure by the diaphragm in acute exacerbations of COPD associated with hypercapnia [15]. An alternative is that central processes prevent the diaphragm being worked into task failure. Currently, direct evidence of diaphragm performance in the acute crisis is restricted to a few studies of voluntary maximum inspiratory pressures or of maximum relaxation rate [30], or analysis of the frequency spectrum of the EMG, because non-volitional tests have been impractical. The development of magnetic stimulation of the phrenic nerves or nerve roots [11, 18, 20] has greatly improved the possibility of measuring twitch pressures in intensive care and should soon provide an answer to this question which, despite extensive research, has eluded solution for the last 20 years.

Asthma

Severe hyperinflation also develops in acute, severe asthma and is associated with more dramatic increases in total minute ventilation than in exacerbations of COPD. Inability to sustain ventilation is the usual reason for initiating mechanical ventilation in severe asthma, although it is difficult to dissect out the specific roles of "central" processes, inspiratory muscle performance and airflow obstruction. There is surprisingly little information on respiratory muscle performance in asthma. In young asthmatic subjects, studied at a time of moderate airway obstruction and hyperinflation, strength and endurance of the inspiratory muscles is normal or enhanced [31, 32]. However diaphragm strength declines with age, is less in women than men, and may be reduced by chronic treatment with oral glucocorticosteroids [2, 33, 34]; since the mechanical load imposed by asthma remains as great as in younger subjects, the older subject would be expected to be at greater risk of reaching the limits of diaphragm performance. Middle aged subjects with chronic, incompletely reversible asthma have slightly reduced inspiratory muscle strength [35]; imaging of the costal diaphragm in the zone of apposition shows slight thickening compared to normal, conceivably a "training" effect [35]. An intriguing finding is that some asthmatic subjects have difficulty in fully activating the diaphragm [36]; this volitional difficulty is related to depression, providing a possible explanation for the known link between depression and increased risk of death from asthma [37]. But such interval measurements cannot compensate for the absence of data in acute asthma; maximum inspiratory pressure produced by voluntary efforts declines rapidly as volume is increased above 75% of total lung capacity, while the elastic load on the diaphragm and other inspiratory muscles at such large volumes is greatly augmented by the effects of intrinsic positive end-expired pressure (PEEP), let alone the increases in intrapulmonary resistance and elastance. It seems inevitable that with extreme hyperinflation, the decreased capacity to develop inspiratory pressures and the increased demand must eventually lead to inspiratory muscle failure, regardless of whether or not there is a decline in force generation at a given lung volume or diaphragm length ("peripheral fatigue"). Volitional tests such as attempted maximum inspiratory efforts and inspiratory capacity can give some information. but, as with COPD, real progress requires non-volitional tests that can be applied during severe asthma.

Conclusions

Although the proposition that the diaphragm must be close to the limits of performance in acute severe asthma or in COPD remains entirely reasonable, experiments imposing considerable pressure, ventilatory or exercise tasks on stable patients have not resulted in the development of diaphragm fatigue. Simpler non-volitional tests are now becoming available which should enable diaphragm performance to be assessed during the spontaneous acute crisis.

References

1. DeTroyer A, Pride NB (1995) The chest wall and respiratory muscles in chronic obstructive pulmonary disease. In: Roussos C (ed) The Thorax, 2nd ed. Dekker, New York, pp1975-2006
2. Decramer M, Lacquet LM, Fagard R, Rogiers P (1994) Corticosteroids contribute to muscle weakness in chronic airflow obstruction. Am J Respir Crit Care Med 150:11-16
3. Cohen E, Mier A, Heywood P, Murphy K, Boultbee J, Guz A (1994) Diaphragmatic movement in hemiplegic patients measured by ultrasonography. Thorax 49:890-895
4. McKenzie DK, Gorman RB, Pride NB, Tolman JF, Gandevia SC (1998) Diaphragm contribution to tidal volume in patients with severe chronic airflow limitation. Am J Resp Crit Care Med 157:A359.
5. Gandevia SC, Leeper JB, McKenzie DK, De Troyer A (1996) Discharge frequencies of parasternal intercostal and scalene motor units during breathing in normal and COPD subjects. Am J Respir Crit Care Med 153:622-628
6. De Troyer A, Leeper JB, McKenzie DK, Gandevia SC (1997) Neural drive to the diaphragm in patients with severe COPD. Am J Respir Crit Care Med 155:1335-1340
7. Levine S, Gillen M, Weiser P, Feiss G, Goldman M, Henson D (1988) Inspiratory pressure generation: comparison of subjects with COPD and age-matched normals. J Appl Physiol 65:888-899
8. Martinez FJ, Couser JL, Celli BR (1990) Factors influencing ventilatory muscle recruitment in patients with chronic airflow obstruction. Am Rev Respir Dis 142:276-282
9. De Troyer A, Peche R, Yernault J-C, Estenne M (1994) Neck muscle activity in patients with severe chronic obstructive pulmonary disease. Am J Respir Crit Care Med 150:41-47
10. Similowski T, Yan S, Gauthier AP, Macklem PT, Bellemare F (1991) Contractile properties of the human diaphragm during chronic hyperinflation. N Engl J Med 325:917-923
11. Polkey MI, Kyroussis D, Hamnegård C-H, Mills GH, Green M, Moxham J (1996) Diaphragm strength in chronic obstructive pulmonary disease. Am J Respir Crit Care Med 154:1310-1317
12. Rochester DF, Braun NMT (1985) Determinants of maximal inspiratory pressure in chronic obstructive pulmonary disease. Am Rev Respir Dis 132:42-47
13. Farkas GA, Roussos C (1983) Diaphragm in emphysematous hamsters: sarcomere adaptability. J Appl Physiol 54:1635-1640
14. Bellemare F, Grassino A (1982) Effects of pressure and timing of contraction on human diaphragm fatigue. J Appl Physiol Respirat Environ: Exercise Physiol 53:1190-1195
15. Bellemare F, Grassino A (1983) Force reserve of the diaphragm in patients with chronic obstructive pulmonary disease. J Appl Physiol 55:8-15
16. Esau SA, Bellemare F, Grassino A, Permutt S, Roussos C, Pardy RL (1983) Changes in relaxation rate with diaphragmatic fatigue in humans. J Appl Physiol 54:1353-1360
17. Newell SZ, McKenzie DK, Gandevia SC (1989) Inspiratory and skeletal muscle strength and endurance and diaphragmatic activation in patients with chronic airflow limitation. Thorax 44:903-912
18. Polkey MI, Kyroussis D, Hamnegård C-H, Mills GH, Hughes PD, Green M, Moxham J (1997) Diaphragm performance during maximal voluntary ventilation in chronic obstructive pulmonary disease. Am J Respir Crit Care Med 155:642-648
19. Kyroussis D, Polkey MI, Keilty SEJ, Mills GH, Hamnegård CH, Moxham J, Green M

(1996) Exhaustive exercise slows inspiratory muscle relaxation rate in chronic obstructive pulmonary disease. Am J Crit Care Med 153:787-793

20. Polkey MI, Kyroussis D, Keilty SEJ, Hamnegård CH, Mills GH, Green M, Moxham J (1995) Exhaustive treadmill exercise does not reduce twitch transdiaphragmatic pressure in patients with COPD. Am J Respir Crit Care Med 152:959-964
21. Mulvey DA, Koulouris NG, Elliott MW, Laroche CM, Moxham J, Green M (1991) Inspiratory muscle relaxation rate after voluntary maximal isocapnic ventilation in humans. J Appl Physiol 70:2173-2180
22. Hamnegård CH, Wragg S, Kyroussis D, Mills GH, Polkey MI, Moran J, Road J, Bake B, Green M, Moxham J (1996) Diaphragm fatigue following maximal ventilation in man. Eur Respir J 9:241-247
23. Freedman S (1970) Sustained maximum voluntary ventilation. Respir Physiol 8:230-244
24. Arora NS, Rochester DF (1987) COPD and human diaphragm muscle dimensions. Chest 91:719-724
25. Ueki J, Obata K, Takahashi H, Dambara T, Fukuchi Y (1998) Assessment of the unevenness in diaphragm thickness in patients with chronic moderate to severe pulmonary emphysema by using ultrasound. Am J Resp Crit Care Med 157:A666
26. Teschler H, Stamatis G, Farhat AA, El-Raouf F, Meyer FJ, Costabel U, Konietzko N (1996) Effect of surgical lung volume reduction on respiratory muscle function in pulmonary emphysema. Eur Respir J 9:1779-1784
27. Martinez FJ, Montes de Oca M, Whyte RI, Stetz K, Gay SE, Celli BR (1997) Lung-volume reduction improves dyspnea, dynamic hyperinflation, and respiratory muscle function. Am J Respir Crit Care Med 155:1984-1990
28. Laghi F, Jubran A, Topeli A, Fahey PJ, Garrity ER Jr, Arcidi JM, de Pinto DJ, Edwards LC, Tobin MJ (1998) Effect of lung volume reduction surgery on neuromechanical coupling of the diaphragm. Am J Respir Crit Care Med 157:475-483
29. Levine S, Kaiser L, Leferovich J, Tikunov B (1997) Cellular adaptations in the diaphragm in chronic obstructive pulmonary disease. N Engl J Med 337:1799-1806
30. Goldstone JC, Green M, Moxham J (1994) Maximum relaxation rate of the diaphragm during weaning from mechanical ventilation. Thorax 49:54-60
31. McKenzie DK, Gandevia SC (1986) Strength and endurance of inspiratory, expiratory and limb muscles in asthma. Am Rev Respir Dis 134:999-1004
32. Gorman RB, McKenzie DK, Gandevia SC, Plassman BL (1992) Inspiratory muscle strength and endurance during hyperinflation and histamine induced bronchoconstriction. Thorax 47:922-792
33. Picado C, Fiz JA, Montserrat JM, Grau JM, Fernandez-Sola J, Luengo MT, Casademont J, Agusti-Vidal A (1990) Respiratory and skeletal muscle function in steroid-dependent bronchial asthma. Am Rev Respir Dis 141:14-21
34. Perez T, Becquart L-A, Stach B, Wallaert B, Tonnel A-B (1996) Inspiratory muscle strength and endurance in steroid-dependent asthma. Am J Respir Crit Care Med 153:610-615
35. De Bruin PF, Ueki J, Watson A, Pride NB (1997) Size and strength of the respiratory and quadriceps muscles in patients with chronic asthma. Eur Respir J 10:59-64
36. Allen GM, McKenzie DK, Gandevia SC, Bass S (1993) Reduced voluntary drive to breathe in asthmatic subjects. Respir Physiol 93:29-40
37. Allen GM, Hickie I, Gandevia SC, McKenzie DK (1994) Impaired voluntary drive to breathe: a possible link between depression and unexplained ventilatory failure in asthmatic patients. Thorax 49:881-884

Chapter 14

Evaluation of the inspiratory muscle mechanical activity during Pressure Support Ventilation

M.C. Olivei, C. Galbusera, M. Zanierato, G. Iotti

Pressure Support Ventilation (PSV) is a ventilatory mode designed to unload the respiratory muscles, while preserving the spontaneous respiratory activity of the patient [1]. PSV has been used both as a weaning technique and as a stand-alone ventilatory support mode in patients with acute respiratory failure [2, 3].

In order to maximise the efficacy of PSV, it is essential to correctly set the Pressure Support (PS) level: this should be high enough to prevent excessive work of breathing, and low enough to avoid depression of the respiratory drive activity. Generally, the setting of the PS level is based on the evaluation of respiratory pattern and clinical tolerance, thus requiring a certain amount of clinical experience. The assessment of the patient inspiratory effort could considerably simplify the operation (both manual and automatic) of setting the PS level.

This presentation focuses on the techniques for measuring the inspiratory effort of the patient in terms of total mechanical activity of the respiratory muscles. Such a measurement is the basis for the calculation of the work of breathing performed by the patient, and is particularly valuable in patients assisted with PSV.

The direct measurement of the respiratory muscles activity requires the measurement of oesophageal pressure, which is known to reflect pleural pressure. Even if this method has been simplified by technological developments, it is not yet common in the clinical setting. Rather, the measurement of oesophageal pressure is considered a valuable technique for scientific studies.

Considerable effort has been recently performed in order to develop simple, clinically applicable techniques for measuring the mechanical activity of the respiratory muscles in mechanically ventilated patients.

The methods proposed as an alternative to the measurement of oesophageal pressure have a common feature: their basis is represented by the analysis of airway pressure, airflow, and volume. The monitoring of such signals is noninvasive, and is commonly performed in clinical practice.

Iotti et al. have demonstrated the possibility to assess the instantaneous net pressure applied by the respiratory muscles (P_{musc},(t)) using an entirely noninvasive procedure [4]. According to this procedure, the P_{musc},(t) signal is obtained from measurements of airway pressure, airflow and volume change, with the input of data for the compliance and the resistance of the respiratory system. A similar approach has been recently applied for proportional assist ventilation (PAV), a new mode of mechanical ventilation designed for the separate compensation of the resistive and the elastic load of the respiratory system [5].

Another interesting approach for the breath-by-breath evaluation of the inspiratory work is represented by the measurement of P0.1. In principle, this parameter is just an index of respiratory drive [6]. However, it has been shown that, in mechanically ventilated patients, P0.1 is also well correlated with the inspiratory work performed by the patient [7-9]. Iotti et al. have developed a method for breath-by-breath monitoring of P0.1 [10]. This method, designed for pressure-trigger ventilation, evaluates the airway pressure drop at the start of inspiration, identifies the maximum slope, and provides an estimate of P0.1 on each cycle. A practical application of this method is represented by the P0.1 monitoring-function which is presently available on the new Hamilton® Galileo ventilator.

The above mentioned P0.1 monitoring system has also been used as a basis for a closed-loop control which, by automatically adjusting pressure support level, stabilizes P0.1, and hence patient inspiratory activity, at a desired target [10].

However, the method proposed by Iotti for continuous P0.1 monitoring has a great disadvantage, since it provides a reliable breath-by-breath evaluation of P0.1 only during pressure-trigger ventilation without flow-by. In this regard, we report the data of a study in which we evaluated the reliability of the above described method of P0.1 monitoring during PSV, while using a pressure-trigger without flow-by, or a flow-trigger with flow-by. We studied 24 patients ventilated in PSV for acute respiratory failure. Of the patients, 11 were ventilated with a pressure-triggered ventilator and 13 with a flow-by ventilator. The P0.1 data evaluated automatically breath-by-breath, (P0.1calc), were compared with standard measurements of P0.1, (P0.1ref), which were obtained by means of end-expiratory occlusion manoeuvers. In patients ventilated with a pressure-triggered ventilator the relationship between P0.1calc and P0.1 ref was near to identity: $P0.1calc=0.89 \cdot P0.1ref+0.35$; $r^2=0.93$); mean error±SD: -0.10±0.66 cmH_2O. On the contrary, in patients ventilated with a flow-by ventilator, P0.1calc considerably understimate P0.1ref:$P0.1calc=0.28 \cdot P0.1ref+0.57$; $r^2=0.77$; mean error±SD: 1.55±1.76 cmH_2O. This underestimate increased with increasing P0.1 values.

The use of flow-by ventilators is becoming increasingly widespread. Therefore, besides being simple and noninvasive, the ideal method for measuring the respiratory muscles activity should be applicable also in patients ventilated with flow-by ventilators.

In this regard, an interesting approach has been recently proposed by Foti et al. [11]. This method is designed for PSV and based on the intermittent application of an end-inspiratory occlusion. The difference between the end-inspiratory occlusion plateau pressure and the airway pressure before the occlusion provides an estimate of the mechanical activity of the inspiratory muscles. Even if this method is theoretically suitable also for flow-by mechanical ventilation, its reliability has been so far investigated only in patients ventilated in PSV without flow-by.

We propose a new method for the noninvasive evaluation of the instantaneous mechanical activity of the respiratory muscles, indicated as "Delta-inst"

[12]. Contrarily to the methods so far described in the literature, the "Delta-inst" method has been specifically designed for application during PSV with a flow-by ventilator. The basis of this method is the calculation of coefficients for total respiratory resistance (Rrs-coeff) and compliance (Crs-coeff) by multiple regression analysis of differences in instantaneous airway pressure, flow and volume between the inspiratory phases of two consecutive cycles at different pressure support level. It is assumed that a change in PS for one breath does not affect respiratory muscles activity. Rrs-coeff and Crs-coeff are used to calculate the instantaneous pressure applied by the respiratory muscles (Pmusc) [4], and hence, work of breathing.

The "Delta-inst" method was tested on 12 patients ventilated in PSV for acute respiratory failure with a flow-by ventilator. Three different levels of PS were used to progressively unload the respiratory muscles. At all PS levels, one "special cycle" was applied every 1 sec, for 5 times: this "special cycle" corresponded to the total withdrawal of PS, whenever the PS level was ≥6 cmH_2O, and to a 5 cmH_2O increase, whenever the PS level was <6 cmH_2O. Each "special cycle", together with the respective previous normal cycle, was analysed for Rrs-coeff and Crs-coeff. Rrs-coeff and Crs-coeff data, expressed as the mean of 5 manoeuvers, were compared with the total compliance (Crs-ref) and resistance (Rrs-ref) data obtained with the oesophageal balloon technique. On the basis of Rrs-coeff and Crs-coeff, we calculated instantaneous Pmusc, from which we further calculated inspiratory work (Wcalc). Wcalc was compared with standard measurements of inspiratory work (Wref).

The difference between Rrs-coeff and Rrs-ref averaged 2.3±3.3 $cmH_2O/L/s$, and the one between Crs-coeff and Crs-ref averaged -6.9±10 ml/cmH_2O. Wcalc agreed well with Wref:Wcalc=1.38•Wref+0.06, r^2=0.77; mean difference between Wcalc and Wref: 0.15±0.14 J. Crs-coeff and Rrs-coeff, although based on a simple model, enable acceptable estimates of the inspiratory loads, and can be used for noninvasive calculation of Pmusc and, thus, for continuous evaluation of the respiratory work.

In conclusion, the "Delta-inst" method demonstrates the possibility to perform noninvasive evaluation of the respiratory muscles mechanical activity during delivery of PSV with a flow-by ventilator.

The model on which the "Delta-inst" method is based deserves further investigation. Indeed, other studies made by our group indicate that this model can be used with different approaches, in order to noninvasively evaluate the mechanical activity of the respiratory muscles in patients ventilated with flow-by ventilators [13].

References

1. Brochard L (1991) Pressure Support Ventilation. In: Marini JJ and Roussos C (eds) Ventilatory failure. Springer-Verlag, Berlin Heidelberg New York, pp 381-391
2. Esteban A, Frutos F, Tobin MJ, Alia I, Solsona JF, Valverdú I, Fernandez R, De La Cal MA, Benito S, Tomas R, Carriedo D, Macias S, Blanco J (1995) A comparison of four

methods of weaning patients from mechanical ventilation. N Engl J Med 332:345-350

3. MacIntyre MR (1991) Pressure support ventilation in contemporary management in critical care. In: Grenvik A, Downs JB, Rasanen J, Smith R (eds) Mechanical ventilation and assisted respiration. Vol 1:1. Contemporary management in critical care. Churchill Livingstone, New York, pp 51-62
4. Iotti G, Braschi A, Brunner JX, Palo A, Olivei M (1995) Noninvasive instantaneous evaluation of total mechanical activity of the respiratory muscles during pressure support ventilation. Chest 108:208-215
5. Younes M (1992) Proportional assist ventilation, a new approach to ventilatory support. Am Rev Respir Dis 145:114-120
6. Milic-Emili J, Whitelaw WA, Derenne JP (1975) Occlusion pressure: a simple measurement of respiratory's center output. N Engl J Med 292:1029-1030
7. Galbusera C, Iotti G, Palo A, Olivei M et al (1993) Relationship between P0.1 and inspiratory work of breathing during pressure support ventilation (PSV). Am Rev Respir Dis 147:A876
8. Foti G, Cereda M, Banfi G, Pelosi P, D'Andrea L, Pesenti A (1993) Simple estimate of patient inspiratory effort (PE) at different levels of pressure support (PS). Am Rev Respir Dis 147:A876
9. Alberti A, Gallo F, Fongaro A, Valenti S, Rossi A (1995) P0.1 is a useful parameter in setting the level of pressure support ventilation. Intensive Care Med 21:547-553
10. Iotti G, Brunner JX, Braschi A, Laubscher T, Olivei M, Palo A, Galbusera C, Comelli A (1996) Closed loop control of airway occlusion pressure at 0.1 second (P0.1) applied to pressure support ventilation: Algorithm and application in intubated patients. Crit Care Med 5:771-779
11. Foti G, Cereda M, Banfi G, Pelosi P, Fumagalli R, Pesenti P (1997) A method to assess the pressure developed by inspiratory muscles in patients with acute lung injury undergoing pressure support. Am J Respir Crit Care Med 156:1210-1216
12. Cortis G, Olivei M, Hannemann U, Brauer M, Zanierato M, Palo A, Galbusera C, Klein U, Reinhart K, Iotti G, Braschi A (1998) New method "Delta-inst" for noninvasive, continuous assessment of the instantaneous mechanical activity of the respiratory muscles. Am J Respir Crit Care Med 157:A684
13. Palo A, Hannemann U, Olivei M, Galbusera C, Toscani M, Cortis G, Tosi PF, Grande C, Brunner JX, Klein U, Reinhart K, Iotti G, Braschi A (1998) Automatic method for noninvasive, intermittent evaluation of inspiratory muscles activity. Intensive Care Med 24(Suppl 99):A307

Chapter 15

Work of breathing

J. Milic-Emili, E. Rocca, E. D'Angelo

Breathing is a form of muscular exercise. The work of breathing may be assessed by two different, but complementary, approaches: a) by measuring the mechanical work done by the respiratory muscles (or by a ventilator substituting for them); b) by estimating the total energy cost of breathing by measurement of the oxygen consumption of the respiratory muscles. The ratio of mechanical work to energy cost yields mechanical efficiency.

Until the 1950s, respiratory muscle energetics occupied a quiet spot in the field of physiology. The early work on the subject was reviewed by Otis [1], whose succinct publication is still a classic. Since then, several detailed reviews of respiratory mechanics and energetics have been provided [2-4]. Although in the last 50 years there has been growing interest in respiratory muscle energetics, relatively little progress has been made, as witnessed by the great variability in estimates of oxygen cost. On the other hand, substantial advances have been made in assessment of the mechanical work of breathing. The present account will focus on assessment of work of breathing during passive mechanical ventilation.

Mechanical work and power

Definitions

In a fluid system, the mechanical work (W) is the integral of the pressure applied (P) and the resulting volume change (V):

$$W = \int P \cdot dV \tag{1}$$

Indeed, since pressure is force per unit area (F/A) and volume is area times length (A•l), the above equation is equivalent to $W=\int F \cdot dl$.

Mechanical work is performed by a contracting muscle only if there is displacement: the work is positive if the muscle shortens and hence does external work (myometric contraction), whereas the work is negative when the muscle lengthens as a result of the applied force (pliometric contraction). When no change in length occurs during contraction (isometric contraction), no external work is done. The work per unit time is termed *power* ($\dot{W}$=W•f, where f respiratory frequency).

Positive work involves several factors:

a. volume-dependent static elastic forces within the lung and chest wall;
b. flow-dependent resistive forces offered by the airways and chest wall to flow of gas;
c. time-dependent viscoelastic forces due to stress adaptation units within the thoracic tissues (lung and chest wall);
d. plastoelastic forces within the thoracic tissues, as reflected by differences in static recoil pressure of the lung and chest wall between inflation and deflation, i.e. "quasi-static hysteresis";
e. inertial forces that depend on the mass of gases and tissues;
f. time constant inequality;
g. compressibility of thoracic gas;
h. distortion of the chest wall from its passive (relaxed) configuration.

At rest and with moderately increased spontaneous ventilation, the configuration of the chest wall remains in normal subjects similar to that obtained with respiratory muscles relaxed. However, as ventilation increases, distortions from passive thoracoabdominal configuration occur, and these distortions imply additional work, which can be estimated from the separate volume pressure (V-P) diagrams of the abdomen and ribcage [5]. In patients with respiratory diseases, work due to distortion of the chest wall may be important even at rest.

Negative work is relatively large during resting expiration and is caused by persistent activity of the diaphragm and other inspiratory muscles during early expiration [6, 7]. However, it becomes relatively small with increasing ventilation [6]. Negative work is commonly neglected because the mechanical efficiency during pliometric work is considerable greater than during myometric work [8], and hence the oxygen cost of negative work is negligible.

Measurement of mechanical work

In relaxed or anesthetized/paralyzed subjects, the total mechanical work done to inflate the respiratory system can be obtained by simultaneous plots of the volume change versus the pressure applied by the ventilator across the respiratory system. The area subtended by the resulting V-P curve is equal to the total mechanical work done during inspiration. Since under these conditions it is also possible to determine the relaxation curve of the total respiratory system, the total work can further be partitioned into its elastic and nonelastic components. In this context it should be noted that with relaxed respiratory muscles there is little change in thoracoabdominal configuration during passive lung inflation and deflation [9], and hence the work due to distortion of the chest wall is negligible. Although measurements on relaxed or anesthetized/paralyzed subjects have provided useful insights into respiratory mechanics, the results are not representative of spontaneous breathing because a) anesthesia/paralysis alters the mechanical properties of the respiratory system [10]; b) the breathing pattern is set by the ventilator; and c) during active breathing there may be substantial distortion of the chest wall, at least in patients with respiratory disease. In contrast to passive ventilation, assessment of the total mechanical work of breathing during spontaneous ventilation is problematic [2, 4].

Theoretical estimation of mechanical power

In the present model analysis we predict the effects of the various inspiratory flow waveforms which are commonly used during mechanical ventilation on inspiratory work in normal subjects: C, constant flow; S, sinusoidal flow; and $D_{1/3}$ and D_0, decelerating flow from a maximal initial value ($\dot{V}$ max) to one-third $\dot{V}$ max and zero, respectively. The analysis is based on the viscoelastic model of the respiratory system described in the Chapter 9, which takes into account both viscoelastic behavior and non-linearities of resistance. A full account of the derivation of the equations used in our predictions is provided elsewhere [10]. The model has been validated in experiments on anesthetized/paralyzed normal humans [11, 12]. Table 1 provides the average values of respiratory mechanics parameters obtained in these studies.

The viscoelastic model used in our predictions does not take into account: a) inertial factors; b) time constant inequality, and (c) quasi-static hysteresis. Inertial factors are not considered because under the conditions examined they are trivial [13]. Similarly, in normal lungs time constant inequality plays a negligible role [14]. Quasi-static hysteresis also appears negligible during mechanical ventilation of normal lungs with normal tidal volumes [15].

Figure 1 depicts the time-courses of the inspiratory flow ($\dot{V}$) and inflation volume (V) with the four flow waveforms explored. In all instances passive inflation started from the elastic equilibrium volume of the respiratory system, and tidal volume (VT) and duration of inspiration (TI) were fixed (0.6 l and 0.8 s, respectively).

Table 1. Average values (± SD) of respiratory mechanics parameters in normal anesthetized paralyzed subjects

Est,rs (cm $H_2O \cdot l^{-1}$)	Raw (cm $H_2O \cdot s \cdot l^{-1}$)	Rint,w (cm $H_2O \cdot s \cdot l^{-1}$)	Evisc (cm $H_2O \cdot s \cdot l^{-1}$)	Rvisc (cm $H_2O \cdot s \cdot l^{-1}$)	τvisc (s)
14.5±2.1[a]	1.2±0.4[b]	0.4±0.1[b]	4.5±0.9[a]	5.9±1.8[a]	1.3±0.3[a]

Est,rs, static elastance of respiratory system; *Raw*, airway resistance; *Rint,w*, interrupter resistance of chest wall; *Evisc*, *Rvisc*, and *τvisc*, viscoelastic elastance, resistance and time constant of respiratory system

[a] Values of 16 subjects from [11]

[b] Values of 12 subjects from [12]

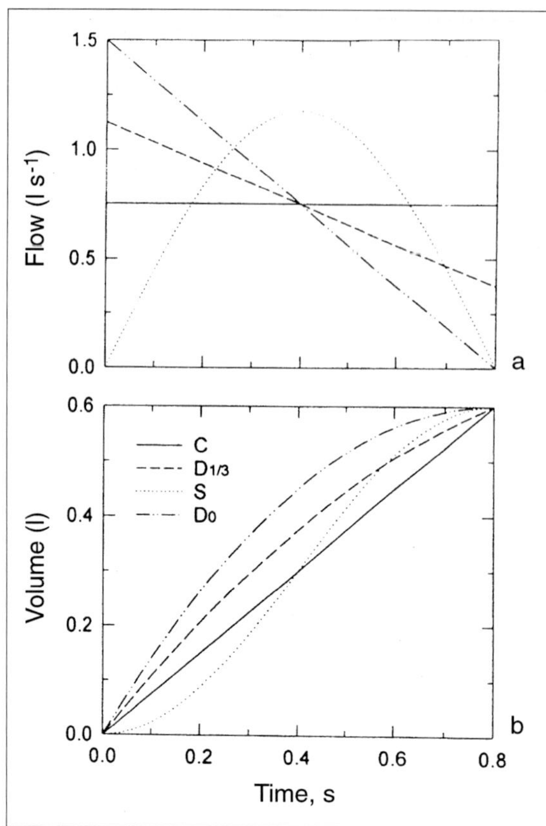

Fig. 1a,b. Flow patterns (a) and corresponding volume-time courses; (b) for standard lung inflation of 0.6 l and 0.8 s duration. *C*, constant flow; *S*, sinusoidal flow; D1/3 and D0, decelerating flow from a maximal initial value ($\dot{V}max$) to one-third $\dot{V}max$ and zero, respectively. (From [10] with permission)

Inspiratory work

Static inspiratory work

The static inspiratory work ($W_{I,st}$), which is independent of the flow pattern, is given by:

$$W_{I,st} = 0.5 \cdot Est \cdot V_T^2 \tag{1}$$

where Est,rs is static elastance of the respiratory system.

Resistive inspiratory work

The resistive inspiratory work ($W_{I,res}$) is given by:

$$W_{I,res} = V_T \cdot [a \cdot (Raw + Rint,w + K_1) \cdot (V_T/T_I) + b \cdot K_2 \cdot (V_T/T_I)^2] \tag{2}$$

where Raw is airway resistance, Rint,w is interrupter resistance of the chest wall, K_1 and K_2 are Rohrer's constants of the endotracheal tube, and a and b are factors which depend on the inspiratory flow waveform [10]. Table 2 provides

Table 2. Values of constants *a* and *b* in Eq. 2 for various inspiratory flow patterns

Flow pattern	**a**	**b**
Constant (C)	1.00	1.00
Sinusoidal (S)	1.23	1.64
Decelerating to one-third Vmax ($D_{1/3}$)	1.08	1.25
Decelerating to zero flow (D_0)	1.33	2.00

Vmax, flow at the onset of lung inflation

the values of these shape-dependent constants while Table 3 gives the values of K_1 and K_2 for three different endotracheal tubes. The K_1 and K_2 values of the ET tubes vary with the prevailing gas mixture and temperature. The flow pattern affects both right-hand terms of Eq. 2: WI,res is larger with D_0 than S, larger with S than $D_{1/3}$, and lowest with C. Moreover, the ratio of WI,res with S, $D_{1/3}$, and D_0 to that with C increases with increasing VT/TI, until it approaches the corresponding value of *b*.

Table 3. Values constant K_1 and K_2 in Eq. 2 for endotracheal tubes (including connectors) of different internal diameters (ID) and standard length[a]

ID (mm)	**K_1 ($cm\ H_2O \cdot s \cdot l^{-1}$)**	**K_2 ($cm\ H_2O \cdot Ol^{-2}$)**
7	0.75	8.75
8	0.52	4.32
9	0.31	2.42

[a] Values determined by P. Navalesi and S. Gottfried (unpublished observations) during flow of air at room temperature. ET tubes manufactured by Mallinckrodt Medical (Athlow, Ireland)

Viscoelastic inspiratory work

The viscoelastic inspiratory work (WI, visc) is given by:

$$W_{I,visc} = R_{visc} \cdot (V_T/T_I)V_T \cdot f\ (\tau_{visc}, T_I) \quad (3)$$

where Rvisc and τvisc are viscoelastic resistance and time constant (Table 1), and *f* is a function that depends on the flow pattern and τvisc/TI [10].

Total inspiratory work

Figure 2 depicts the total inspiratory work per breath (W_I) and its components for fixed V_T (0.6 l) and T_I (0.8 s) with the four flow patterns and the three ET tubes. In all instances, W_I is lowest with C, and highest with D_0. With S,W_I exceeds that with $D_{1/3}$. With ET tube #7, $W_{I,tot}$ with D_0 and S markedly exceeds that with C and $D_{1/3}$. Note that virtually all the discrepancy in W_I among the different flow patterns is due to differences in $W_{I,res}$. Indeed, $W_{I,st}$ is independent of flow pattern (Eq. 1) and though $W_{I,visc}$ changes slightly with the flow pattern (Eq. 3), its contribution to W_I is small. As shown in Figure 2, the relative changes of W_I with flow pattern increase with decreasing the size of the ET tube. According to Eq. 2 the relative difference of W_I among the various flow patterns should become more pronounced with increasing V_T/T_I.

In normal anesthetized paralyzed subjects, airway resistance (Raw) is essentially constant, i.e. there is no appreciable K_2 within the range of flows commonly used during mechanical ventilation [12]. As a result, the changes in flow pattern affect only the "laminar" term in Eq. 2. The same applies to the resistive pressure losses within the chest wall, because $R_{int,w}$ is also independent of flow [12]. Patients with severe chronic obstructive pulmonary disease (COPD), however, are characterized by relatively high K_2 values (2.7 ± 0.6 cm $H_2O \cdot s^2 \cdot l^{-2}$) [16]. Accordingly, in these patients the changes in $W_{I,res}$ with changing inspiratory flow pattern should be more pronounced than in normal subjects. The present analysis indicates that for comparative purposes, measurements of W_I need to be made at fixed V_T, V_T/T_I, and inspiratory flow pattern.

Although measurement of work of breathing in mechanically ventilated

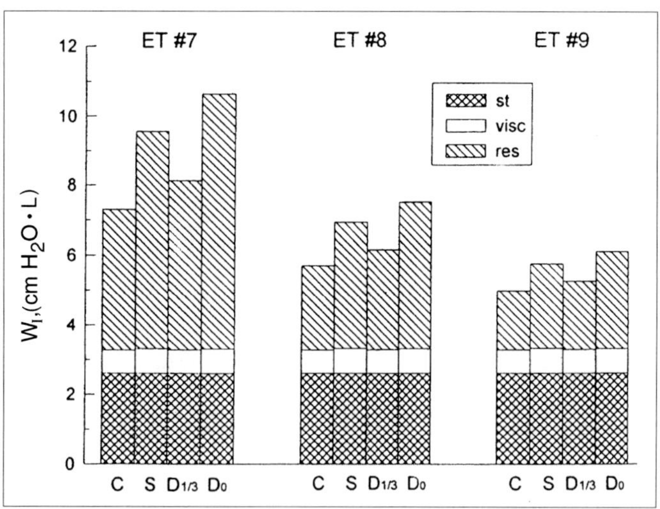

Fig. 2. Total inspiratory work per breath (W_I) and its components for V_T of 0.6 l and T_I of 0.8 s in normal anesthetized/paralyzed subjects inflated with different flow patterns and endotracheal tubes. *st*, static; *visc*, viscoelastic; *res*, resistive. (From [10] with permission)

patients has been long advocated as a useful global measure of the abnormalities in respiratory mechanics [17], relatively few measurements have been reported in subjects with respiratory disease, mainly COPD and adult respiratory distress syndrome (ARDS). Furthermore, most measurements have been made during constant flow inflation. In line with the predictions in Figure 2, however, a recent report indicated that in patients after open heart surgery, WI was smaller with C compared to S and $D_{1/3}$ [18].

Work of breathing in COPD

In 1954, McIlroy and Christie [19] observed that WI was increased in stable COPD patients; this they attributed to increased airway and "viscous" resistance of the lung. In later studies [20, 21] it was shown that in COPD patients there is an increase of work of breathing also as a result of: a) time constant inequality within the lung which causes an increase in effective dynamic pulmonary elastance and flow resistance, and b) intrinsic positive end-expiratory pressure (PEEPi).

Recently, detailed comprehensive measurements of WI have been made in mechanically ventilated COPD patients [22, 23]. The average values of total inspiratory work of the respiratory system (WI,rs) and its components of 10 mechanically ventilated sedated/paralyzed COPD patients with acute respiratory failure (ARF) are shown in Figure 3, together with the corresponding values

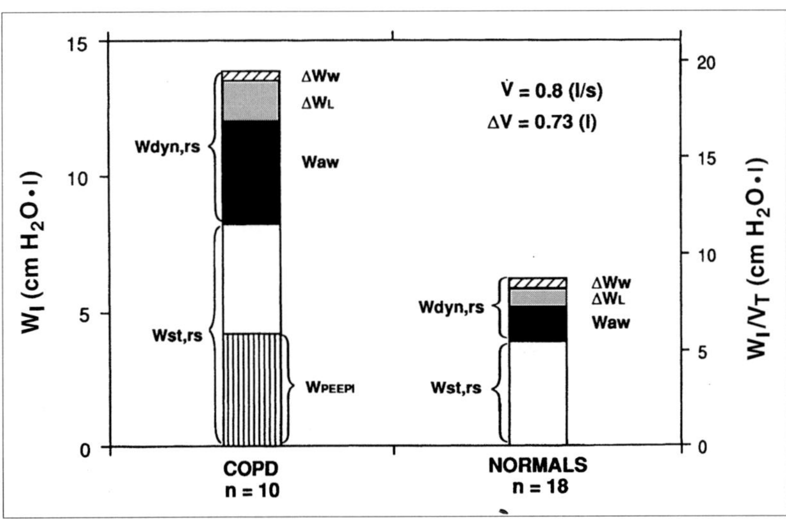

Fig. 3. Average values of inspiratory work (WI) done on the respiratory system and its components in COPD patients and normal anesthetized/paralyzed subjects with inflation flow of 0.8 l/s and tidal volume of 0.73 l. *Wst,rs*, Total static work of respiratory system; *WPEEPi*, static work due to intrinsic PEEP; *Wdyn,rs*, Total dynamic work of respiratory system; *Waw*, airway resistive work; *ΔWw*, viscoelastic work of chest wall; *ΔWL*, work on lung due to time constant inequality and/or viscoelastic pressure dissipations. Work per litre of inspired volume (WI/VT) is shown on right ordinate. (From [22] with permission)

of 18 anesthetized/paralyzed normal subjects. The measurements were obtained during constant flow inflation with tidal volume of 0.73 l, frequency of 12.5 bpm and inspiratory duration of 0.92 s. $W_{I,rs}$ was two-fold greater in COPD patients than in normal subjects, the difference reflecting an increase of both static ($W_{st,rs}$) and dynamic ($W_{dyn,rs}$) work. The latter was due both to an increase in airway resistive work (W_{aw}) and in the additional work done on the lung (ΔW_L) as a result of pressure dissipations caused by time constant inequality and viscoelastic behavior of pulmonary tissue. The dynamic work due to the tissues of the chest wall (ΔW_w) was similar in COPD patients to that of normal subjects. The increase in $W_{st,rs}$ in the COPD patients was caused entirely by the work due to P_{PEEPi} (W_{PEEPi}). On average, W_{PEEPi} represented 57% of the overall increase in W_I exhibited by the COPD patients relative to normal subjects, while the corresponding increases for W_{aw} and ΔW_L were 34% and 9%, respectively.

The values of W_I in Figure 3 do not include the resistive work done on the endotracheal tubes which is relatively high, particularly if tubes of small size are used [22]. In COPD patients, for a given ventilation and breathing pattern, W_I during spontaneous ventilation should be higher than during passive mechanical ventilation because during active breathing there is distortion of the chest wall from its passive configuration [24]. Furthermore, the data in Figure 3 pertain to mechanical ventilation with "normal" resting tidal volume whereas spontaneously breathing COPD patients with ARF virtually always exhibit rapid shallow breathing [21, 25]. Nonetheless, the data in Figure 3 are useful because the measurements were made under similar conditions, and hence the discrepancies between COPD patients and normal subjects are due entirely to differences in respiratory mechanics. Since the data in Figure 3 pertain to COPD patients with ARF, it reflects extreme abnormality of respiratory mechanics.

Work of breathing in ARDS

The adult respiratory distress syndrome (ARDS) is known to adversely affect the mechanical properties of the respiratory system, with reduced compliance as hallmark [26]. Recent reports, however, have shown that ARDS is also characterized by increased pulmonary and thoracic tissue flow resistance [27, 28]. Furthermore, ARDS patients commonly exhibit intrinsic PEEP. As a result, in ARDS patients $W_{I,rs}$ is increased as a result of increased $W_{I,st}$, W_{PEEPi}, and Wdyn due to both increased airway resistance and viscoelastic resistance (Fig. 4) [29]. While in COPD patients the increase in $W_{I,rs}$ is mainly due to increased W_{PEEPi} (Fig. 3), in ARDS patients it is due mainly to increased $W_{I,st}$ as a result of increased lung elastance (Fig. 4). In both COPD and ARDS patients, however, there is a substantial increase in dynamic work due to increased airway resistance and viscoelastic resistance.

Although measurement of $W_{I,rs}$ in mechanically ventilated patients has long been suggested as a useful index to assess the status and follow the progress of intensive care unit (ICU) patients [17, 21], there are no reports in which $W_{I,rs}$ has been measured serially in ICU patients. Similarly, although $W_{I,rs}$ has been long proposed as a useful potential weaning index [17], it has been seldomly

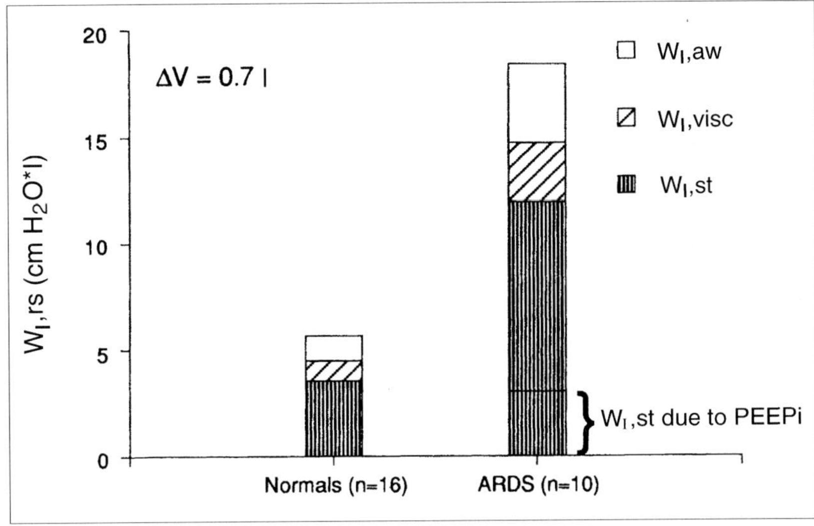

Fig. 4. Average values of total inspiratory work (WI) done on the respiratory system and its components in ARDS patients and normal anesthetized/paralyzed subjects with inflation flow of 1 l•s^{-1} and tidal volume of 0.7 l. *WI,st*, total static work of respiratory system; *WI,aw*, airway resistive work; *WI,visc*, total viscoelastic work and work due to time constant inequality. (From [29] with permission)

used as such. Nevertheless, WI,rs and its components are potentially useful for assessing the status and progress of ICU patients. Clearly, however, serial measurements of WI,rs should be made under standardized conditions of mechanical ventilation, i.e. with fixed inspiratory flow pattern and ventilatory settings (VT, TI, TTOT and PEEP). Furthermore, allowance should be made for the work due to the resistance of the endotracheal tubes [10, 22].

Acknowledgement The authors thank Ms. Angie Bentivegna for secretarial work.

References

1. Otis AB (1954) The work of breathing. Physiol Rev 34:449-458
2. Roussos C, Campell EJM (1986) Respiratory muscle energetics. In: Macklem PT, Mead J (eds) The respiratory system. Mechanics of breathing. Handbook of physiology. Vol 3. American Physiological Society, Washington DC, pp 481-509
3. D'Angelo E, Milic-Emili J (1995) Dynamics of respiratory system. In: Roussos C (ed) The thorax. Marcel Dekker, New York, pp 495-513
4. Otis AB (1964) The work of breathing. In: Fenn WO, Rahn H (eds) Handbook of Physiology. Vol I. Respiration American Physiological Society, Washington DC, pp 436-476
5. Goldman MD, Grimby J, Mead J (1976) Mechanical work of breathing derived from rib cage and abdominal V-P partitioning. J Appl Physiol 41:752-763

6. Petit JM, Milic-Emili J, Delhez L (1960) Role of the diaphragm in breathing in conscious normal man: an electromyographic study. J Appl Physiol 15:1001-1106
7. Shee CD, Ploy-Song-Sang Y, Milic-Emili J (1985) Decay of inspiratory muscle pressure during expiration in conscious humans. J Appl Physiol 58:1859-1865
8. Abbott BC, Bigland-Richie B (1953) The effects of force and speed changes on the rate of oxygen consumption during negative work. J Physiol 120:319-325
9. Barnas GM, Yoshiro K, Loring STL, Mead J (1987) Impedance and relative displacements of relaxed chest wall up to 4 Hz. J Appl Physiol 62:71-81
10. D'Angelo E, Rocca E, Milic-Emili J (1998) Inspiratory flow pattern and work of breathing. In: Milic Emili J (ed) Respiratory mechanics. Eur Respir Monograph, Sheffield (in press)
11. D'Angelo E, Robatto FM, Calderini E, Tavola M, Bono D, Torri G, Milic-Emili J (1991) Pulmonary and chest wall mechanics in anesthetized paralyzed humans. J Appl Physiol 70:2602-2610
12. D'Angelo E, Prandi E, Tavola M, Calderini E, Milic-Emili J (1994) Chest wall interrupter resistance in anesthetized paralyzed humans. J Appl Physiol 77:883-887
13. Mead J (1956) Measurement of intertia of the lungs at increased ambient pressure. J Appl Physiol 9:208-212
14. Bates JHT, Ludwig MS, Sly PD, Brown K, Martin JG, Fredberg JJ (1988) Interrupter resistance elucidated by alveolar pressure measurement in open-chest normal dogs. J Appl Physiol 65:408-414
15. Shardonofsky FR, Sato J, Bates JHT (1990). Quasi-static pressure-volume hysteresis in the canine respiratory system in vivo. J Appl Physiol 68:2230-2236
16. Guérin C, Coussa ML, Eissa NT, Corbeil C, Chassé M, Braidy J, Matar N, Milic-Emili J (1993) Lung and chest wall mechanics in mechanically ventilated COPD patients. J Appl Physiol 74:1571-1580
17. Henning RJ, Shubin H, Weil MH (1977) The measurement of the work of breathing for the clinical assessment of ventilator dependence. Crit Care Med 5:264-268
18. Polese G, Lubli P, Poggi R, Luzzani A, Milic-Emili J, Rossi A (1997) Effects of inspiratory flow waveforms on arterial blood gases and respiratory mechanics after open heart surgery. Eur Respir J 10:2820-2824
19. McIlroy MB, Christie RV (1954) The work of breathing in emphysema. J Clin Sci 13:147-154
20. Otis AB, McKerrow CB, Bartlett RA, Mead J, McIlroy MB, Selverstone NJ, Radford EP (1956) Mechanical factors in distribution of pulmonary ventilation. J Appl Physiol 8:427-443
21. Fleury B, Murciano D, Talamo C, Aubier M, Pariente R, Milic-Emili J (1985) Work of breathing in patients with chronic obstructive pulmonary disease in acute respiratory failure. Am Rev Respir Dis 131:822-827
22. Coussa ML, Guérin C, Eissa NT, Corbeil C, Chassé M, Braidy J, Matar N, Milic-Emili J (1993) Partitioning of work of breathing in mechanically ventilated COPD patients. J Appl Physiol 75:1711-1719
23. Guérin C, LeMasson S, DeVarax R, Milic-Emili J, Fournier G (1997) Small airway closure and positive end-expiratory pressure in mechanically ventilated patients with chronic obstructive pulmonary disease. Am J Respir Crit Care Med 155:1949-1956
24. Sharp JT (1985) The chest wall and respiratory muscles in airflow limitation. In: Roussos C, Macklem PT (eds) The thorax. Marcel Dekker, New York, pp 1155-1202
25. Aubier M, Murciano D, Fournier M (1980) Central respiratory drive in acute respiratory failure of patients with chronic obstructive pulmonary disease. Am Rev Respir Dis 122:191-199

26. Ashbaugh DG, Biglow DB, Petty TL, Levine BE (1967) Acute respiratory distress in adults. Lancet ii:319-323
27. Broseghini C, Brandolese R, Poggi R, Polese G, Manzin E, Milic-Emili J, Rossi A (1988) Respiratory mechanics during the first day of mechanical ventilation in patients with pulmonary edema and chronic airway obstruction. Am Rev Respir Dis 138:355-361
28. Eissa NT, Ranieri VM, Corbeil C, Chassé M, Braidy J, Robatto M, Braidy J, Milic-Emili J (1991) Analysis of behavior of the respiratory system in ARDS patients: Effects of flow, volume, and time. J Appl Physiol 70:2719-2729
29. Eissa NT, Ranieri VM, Corbeil C, Chassé M, Braidy J, Milic-Emili J (1992) effects of positive end-expiratory pressure on the work of breathing in adult respiratory distress syndrome patients. J Crit Care 7:142-149

ARTIFICIAL VENTILATION - PRINCIPLES, TECHNIQUES, CLINICAL APPLICATIONS

Chapter 16

Respiratory mechanics in ARDS

P. Pelosi, M. Resta, L. Gattinoni

Diagnostic and prognostic value of the assessment of respiratory mechanics in patients with adult respiratory distress syndrome (ARDS) has been extensively investigated and clearly defined [1-3]. Most studies have investigated the role of compliance and resistance of the total respiratory system in ARDS patients, but only few studies separately considered the relative contributions of the lung and the chest wall. Partitioning of the respiratory mechanics into its lung and chest wall components, in fact, needs the use of an esophageal balloon which is considered, by the majority of physicians, a waste of time and a tedious technique. However, it may allow better definition of the pathophysiology of ARDS in order to improve the consequent clinical management.

The aim of this chapter is to briefly review several studies which investigated respiratory mechanics in patients with ARDS and to give a selected list of references that can be useful in clinical practice. Finally, we discuss possible ARDS etiologies and alterations in chest wall mechanics, and their role on the therapeutic management in such patients.

Literature review

We reviewed 40 studies (published from 1976 to 1998) performed in 568 mechanically ventilated patients with acute respiratory failure, and dealing with respiratory mechanics. Some of these studies considered only ARDS patients [1-37], while others [38-45] investigated subjects with acute respiratory failure of different etiologies, including ARDS, cardiogenic pulmonary edema and chronic airway obstruction. In our review we took into account only ARDS patients to better define their clinical characteristics, average data of respiratory mechanics (compliance, resistance, functional residual capacity) and the most commonly used methods of measurement.

Characteristics of the patients

Various studies (43%) investigated only a limited number (<10) of ARDS patients [4-7, 9-15, 38-40, 43, 44] and clinical characteristics have not been always accurately described [1, 11, 12, 14-22, 42-44]. In fact, several studies did not report the level of oxygenation (25%) [1, 12, 14, 16-18, 20, 21, 42, 44], the clinically adopted levels of inspired oxygen fraction (FiO_2) (17%) [1, 14, 16, 18, 21, 22, 42], or the positive end-expiratory pressure (PEEP) (30%) [1, 11, 14, 16-

19, 21, 42, 43, 45]. Moreover, in each study, different etiopathological events leading to ARDS (i.e., hemorrhage, sepsis, trauma, pneumonia) were considered together. These factors are included in the "magic" classification of ARDS, hypothesizing that different causes of ARDS produce similar derangements in respiratory mechanics. Many studies (32%) [1-3, 12, 14, 16, 18-20, 23, 34, 35, 45] did not report the number of days from onset of respiratory failure or intubation. Except for three studies [11, 24, 36], all the others had been performed in the early stages of ARDS (within 8 days from onset).

Investigators dealing with respiratory mechanics in ARDS should better define the clinical characteristics of the patients to obtain comparable data among studies. Moreover, most physiopathological considerations about respiratory mechanics in ARDS are drawn from, and thus may be applied to, only the early phases of this syndrome, while the later phases are almost completely neglected.

Functional residual capacity

Functional residual capacity (FRC) is an important clinical parameter since it can be considered the "true" value of ventilable lung volume. FRC also represents the major O_2 reservoir (thereby minimizing the fluctuations in PaO_2) and determines the resting lenght of the respiratory muscles (thereby influencing their capacity to generate force).

FRC was measured in 30% of the studies [11, 13, 15-17, 19, 22, 23, 35, 37, 42]. As shown in Table 1, the average value of FRC is 1.17±0.44 l with great variability between the studies (range, 0.7-2.07 l). This difference is probably due to the diverse clinical conditions of the patients and the various adopted methods of measurement: in 8 studies FRC was measured with a helium dilution technique [13, 15, 16, 19, 22, 23, 35, 37], while in 3 it was measured with argon or nitrogen wash-out [11, 17, 42]. Moreover, in a recent study [15], the reduction in FRC was shown to be an interesting tool to evaluate the stage of disease severity, together with compliance values.

FRC therefore allows an estimation of the ventilable lung and the severity of disease, which can also be easily obtained in clinical practice both during controlled mechanical ventilation and spontaneous or partially assisted breathing.

Compliance

Many investigators are interested in measuring the elastic properties of the respiratory system in mechanically ventilated ARDS patients. In fact, compliance provides useful information on the condition of the diseased lung and may be a good indicator of the evolution of disease [1-3, 15, 24].

As shown by Gattinoni et al. [23], the measurement of respiratory compliance in ARDS patients explores only the ventilable lung regions which are approximately one-third in size compared to those of healthy subjects (Fig. 1).

Several methods have been proposed to measure respiratory compliance. In clinical practice the most commonly used methods appear to be the end-inspi-

Table 1. Compliance and functional residual capacity in normal subjects and in ARDS patients. Mean ± SD

	TV (l)	TV (ml/kl)	Cst,rs (ml/cm H_2O)	Cst,l (ml/cm H_2O)	Cst,w (ml/cmH_2O)	FRC (l)
Normals[a]	0.54±0.1	–	68.1±11.3	110.1±19.0	205.5±74.8	1.43±0.3
ARDS[b]	0.74±0.3	12.8 ± 3.8	39.3±9.5	49.3±17.6	128.9±35.8	1.17±0.4

TV, tidal volume; *Cst,rs*, static compliance of the respiratory system; *Cst,l*, static compliance of the lung; *Cst,w*, static compliance of the chest wall; *FRC*, functional residual capacity

[a] Data obtained from [15] and compared to [26, 27]

[b] Data obtained from [1-3, 4-21, 23-25, 32-37, 39-43, 45]

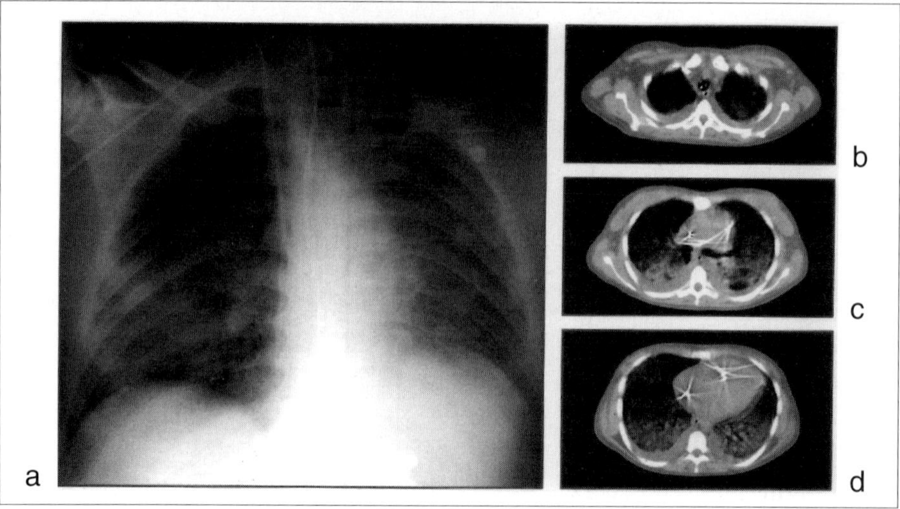

Fig. 1a-d. Typical chest of X-ray of a patients with ARDS (a); computed tomography of an ARDS lung at APEX (b), HILUM (c), and BASE (d). Note the prevalent dependent distribution of the lung lesions (approximately one-third of the entire section)

ratory occlusion (73%) [1, 4-10, 12, 14-17, 19, 20, 25, 32-44] and the syringe (25%) [2, 3, 11, 13, 18, 22-24, 45]. Some studies reported the amount of insufflated gas volume (60%) [1, 4-10, 12-15, 17, 32, 34-41, 44], while others reported the gas volume standardized for body weight (48%) [2, 3, 5-7, 10, 13, 14, 16, 18-20, 22-25, 43-45]. On average, the volume at which respiratory compliance was measured is about 10-15 ml/kg. In Table 1, average data of compliance of the total respiratory system (Cst,rs), lung (Cst,L) and chest wall (Cst,w) in ARDS patients [1-3, 11-21, 23-25, 32-37, 42, 43, 45] are compared to those obtained in 8 anesthetized, paralyzed, healthy subjects [16]. In spite of the great variability in ARDS patients (range, Cst,rs 21.5-57 ml/cm H_2O; Cst,L 27-94 ml/cm H_2O; Cst,w 80-204 ml/cm H_2O), respiratory, lung and chest wall compliance appeared markedly lower than those reported in normal subjects.

The presence of an "inflection point" (Pflex) in the pressure-volume (P-V) curve has been considered by some Authors to be a useful tool to set the optimal PEEP level during mechanical ventilation [15]. The Pflex should indicate the pressure necessary to reopen the atelectatic lung regions compressed by increased lung weight [28]. For this reason, when a level of PEEP above Pflex is selected, the P-V relationship becomes more favorable, i.e. equal increments in tidal volume generate smaller increases in airway pressure. Whenever PEEP level has been set to 0 cm H_2O, an "inflection point" has been always found during the early phases of ARDS [5, 10, 11, 13, 23, 45] but not in the later ones [11], suggesting an evolution of the disease with time of mechanical ventilation [24]. However, in the 44% of the studies on Pflex, it was not possible to find Pflex in all the examined patients [10, 11, 25, 35]. In spite of its possible clinical meaning, only two studies investigated the effect of PEEP on Pflex [10, 13]. The mean Pflex of the respiratory system in these studies was 9.8±3.8 cm H_2O.

Various Authors reported the effects of PEEP on respiratory compliance with conflicting results: five studies [8, 10, 13, 19, 37] did not find any modification, four studies [15, 17, 41, 42] found a decrease in respiratory compliance only at PEEP levels >10 cm H_2O and two studies [12, 16] found an improvement in respiratory compliance at 5-10 cm H_2O of PEEP and a reduction at PEEP levels >10 cm H_2O. This spreading of PEEP effects on respiratory compliance could be due to the different methods of measurement adopted (end-inspiratory occlusion vs. syringe), to the variability of inflated volume (from 6 to 15 ml/kg), or to the different ARDS etiopathologies. In fact, at high PEEP levels, low tidal volumes may increase compliance preventing overdistension otherwise common adopting high tidal volumes.

Although the compliance of the total respiratory system has been extensively investigated, relatively few studies (23%) examined separately the role of the lung and the chest wall [4, 12, 15, 16, 25, 34, 35, 37, 42]. In fact, although respiratory system mechanics are used as a surrogate measure of the degree of alveolar inflation and recruitment, the correlation of lung mechanics to respiratory system mechanics has not been much questioned.

Interestingly all these studies found that, in general, ARDS patients are characterized not only by a marked reduction in lung compliance (as previously supposed), but also by a significant decrease in chest wall compliance (Tab. 1). The reduction in lung compliance may be attributed to a decrease in lung volume or to intrinsic modifications of the mechanical properties of lung tissues. A separation between these two factors may be obtained computing the "specific lung compliance", i.e. relating the lung compliance to the end-expiratory lung volume. Specific lung compliance has been seldomly investigated [15, 23]; its value always ranges between normal limits (50-100 ml/cm H_2O/l^1) indicating that, at least in early ARDS, decreased lung volume rather than intrinsic mechanical alterations of lung tissues could be the major determinant of the reduction in lung compliance.

However, these studies [11, 15, 16, 23] have all been performed in early ARDS and different results might have been obtained if patients were examined in successive stages of the disease, because of remarkable modifications in lung structure (emphysema-like lesions or bullae) occurring during the period of mechanical ventilation [24].

Resistance

In the past several years, increasing attention has been given to respiratory resistance. In ARDS patients respiratory resistance is markedly increased, but the underlying physiopathological cause and its effective clinical relevance are not clear. Total resistance of the respiratory system (Rmax,rs) may be partitioned into its "ohmic" (Rmin,rs) and "additional" (ΔR,rs), components [29]. Rmin,rs represents the airway resistance, while ΔR,rs represents viscoelastic phenomena or time constant inequalities ("pendelluft") within the respiratory tissues (lung and chest wall). Both Rmin,rs and ΔR,rs are increased in ARDS [4-9, 14, 15, 39-41]. Average values of total respiratory system, lung and chest wall resistance in normal subjects [15] and in ARDS patients [4, 5, 7-9, 14, 15, 39-41] are shown in Table 2. High airway resistance in ARDS has been attributed to several factors such as airway flooding, airway hyperactivity, vagal reflexes and reduced lung volume.

In a recent study, we standardized airway resistance to absolute lung volume, thus obtaining "specific airway resistance", which was found not different from normal [15]. This indicated that the increase in airway resistance in ARDS was probably due not to anatomical narrowing, but only to reduced lung volume and possibly to a reduced amount of ventilated lung ("baby lung") [24, 28]. In spite of this, in specific cases bronchodilators might be useful in ARDS patients [41].

Few studies have investigated the effects of PEEP on respiratory resistance [6, 8, 15, 37, 41]. In two studies [15, 41], a significant unexpected increase in respiratory resistance with PEEP was found. PEEP is generally assumed to reduce airway resistance by inducing bronchodilatation either directly or as a result of increasing lung volume. Actually, high PEEP levels (>10 cm H_2O) decrease airway resistance according to the lung volume [6, 15], but markedly increase the "additional" resistance [15, 42]. This suggests that significant alterations in viscoelastic properties of the lung tissues or alveolar inhomogeneities occur when high PEEP levels are applied in ARDS. However, the etiology of ARDS may also influence the behavior of resistances responding to PEEP [37].

The role of the chest wall

As already described, ARDS patients are characterized by marked derangements in respiratory mechanics (high resistance, low compliance and FRC). These alterations cause an increase in the elastic and resistive load during spontaneous or partially assisted breathing with a marked increase in the respiratory work. It is commonly believed that alterations of respiratory system mechanics are due to derangements in lung rather than in chest wall mechanics. Nevertheless, nine studies [4, 12, 15, 16, 27, 34, 35, 37, 42] reported a marked alteration in chest wall mechanics, at least in selected groups of patients.

In Figure 2, the average compliance of the lung and chest wall in patients with moderate or severe ARDS is presented. A marked reduction in chest wall compliance in diseased patients compared to normal subjects is evident.

Alterations of chest wall mechanics may be attributed to: 1) decreased functional residual capacity, which may produce a reduction in the volume of the thoracic cage, moving it to a less compliant portion of its pressure-volume (P-V) curve; or 2) intrinsic alteration of the chest wall due to abdominal distension, edema, or pleural effusions. The first hypothesis may be ruled out since a direct relationship between FRC and intrathoracic value does not apply in ARDS. In fact, a significant portion of the intrathoracic volume is occupied by blood, exudate, edema and pleural fluid [30]. Moreover, by increasing lung volume with PEEP, chest wall compliance does not change significantly as it would

Table 2. Resistance in normal subjects and ARDS patients. Mean ± SD

	Vi (l/s)	Rmax,rs (cm H_2O s l^{-1})	ΔR,rs (cm H_2O s l^{-1})	Rmax,L (cm H_2O s l^{-1})	Rmin,L (cm H_2O s l^{-1})	ΔR,L (cm H_2O sl^{-1})	Rmax,w (cm H_2O s l^{-1})
Normals[a]	0.51±0.1	4.2±1.4	2.1±0.8	3.2±1.4	2.1±0.9	1.01±0.6	1±0.4
ARDS[b]	0.70±0.2	9.6±3.5	5.1±1.8	8.2±1.0	4.5±2.1	3.7±1.3	1.3±0.4

Vi, inspiratory flow; *Rmax,rs*, total resistance of the respiratory system; *ΔR,rs*, "additional" resistance of the respiratory system; *Rmax,L*, total resistance of the lung; *Rmin,L*, "airway" resistance; *ΔR,L*, "additional" resistance of the lung; *Rmax,w*, total resistance of the chest wall

[a] Data obtained from [15] and compared to [26, 27]

[b] Data obtained from [4, 5, 7-9, 14, 15, 39-41]

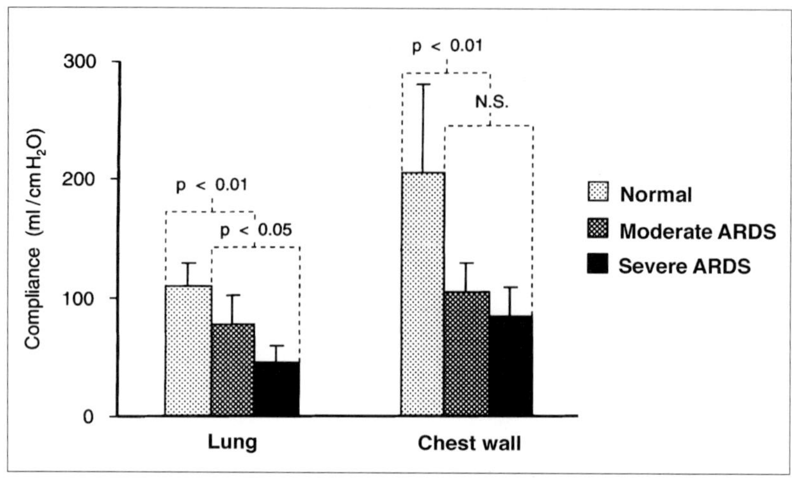

Fig. 2. Lung and chest wall compliance in normal subjects and in patients with moderate or severe ARDS. (Modified from [22])

be expected if the decrease in intrathoracic volume was the main cause of the reduction in chest wall compliance [15]. Thus, in ARDS patients, the chest wall is probably structurally altered. Presently, factors affecting chest wall compliance are unknown, but some considerations might be suggested.

During mechanical ventilation, patients are often sedated with oppioids, hence gut pathophysiology is affected and abdominal distention results, which may markedly affect chest wall mechanics [31]. Moreover in ARDS, positive fluid balances and pleural effusions are often present and may significantly modify chest wall properties [1, 42].

Recently, we found that the etiology of ARDS may deeply influence respiratory mechanics and response to PEEP. Patients with ARDS due to a "direct" insult to the lung (pulmonary ARDS) showed lower lung compliance, higher chest wall compliance and similar resistance when compared to patients with ARDS due to an "indirect insult" to the lung (extrapulmonary ARDS). The lower chest wall compliance has been ascribed to an increased intra-abdominal pressure in patients with extrapulmonary ARDS. The mechanical response to PEEP was also different in the two groups. In fact, patients with pulmonary ARDS markedly deteriorated their respiratory and lung compliance with PEEP, while patients with extrapulmonary ARDS improved. Moreover, patients with extrapulmonary ARDS recruited with PEEP much more than did patients with pulmonary ARDS.

Ranieri et al. [25] compared patients with ARDS consequent to major abdominal surgery "surgical ARDS" to patients with "medical ARDS". In surgical ARDS, the static inspiratory P-V relationship of the respiratory system and lung showed a downward concavity indicating that compliance decreased with tidal volume, and suggesting alveolar over-distention. Patients with ARDS consequent to medical conditions had an upward concavity, indicating an increase in compliance and alveolar recruitment during inflation.

Mangoni et al. [34] showed in a subset of patients with ARDS that the lower inflection point of the static P-V curve of the respiratory system was due to the shape of the P-V curve of the chest wall and not of the lung. Therefore, the etiology of ARDS is an important determinant of the mechanical characteristics of the respiratory system [37].

Conclusions

Many studies have dealt with alterations in total respiratory system mechanics in ARDS patients. However, few informations is available regarding the relative contribution of the lung and the chest wall in determining respiratory mechanics. It appears that not only lung mechanics, but also chest wall mechanics are affected in a subset of ARDS patients. Thus, interpretation of data deriving from the respiratory system alone is limited. Finally, the etiology of ARDS should always be considered when respiratory mechanics are measured.

References

1. Bone RC (1976) Diagnosis of causes for acute respiratory distress by pressure-volume curves. Chest 70:740-746
2. Mancebo J, Benito S, Net A (1988) Value of static pulmonary compliance in predicting mortality in patients with acute respiratory failure. Intensive Care Med 14:110-114
3. Gattinoni L, Pesenti A, Caspani ML et al (1984) The role of static lung compliance in the management of severe ARDS unresponsive to conventional treatment. Intensive Care Med 10:121-126
4 Polese G, Rossi A, Appendini L, Brandi G, Bates JHT, Brandolese R (1991) Partitioning of respiratory mechanics in mechanically ventilated patients. J Appl Physiol 71:2425-2433
5. Eissa NT, Ranieri VM, Corbeil C et al (1991) Analysis of behavior of the respiratory system in ARDS patients: effects of flow, volume, and time. J Appl Physiol 70:2719-2729
6. Eissa NT, Ranieri VM, Corbeil C, Chassé M, Braidy J, Milic-Emily J (1991) Effects of positive end-expiratory pressure, lung volume and inspiratory flow on interrupter resistance in patients with adult respiratory distress syndrome. Am Rev Respir Dis 144:538-543
7. Tantucci C, Corbeil C, Chassé M et al (1992) Flow and volume dependence of respiratory system flow resistance in patient with adult respiratory distress syndrome. Am Rev Respir Dis 145:355-360
8. Brandolese R, Broseghini C, Polese G et al (1993) Effects of intrinsic PEEP on pulmonary gas exchange in mechanically ventilated patients. Eur Respir J 6:358-363
9. Pesenti A, Pelosi P, Rossi N, Aprigliano M, Brazzi L, Fumagalli R (1993) Respiratory mechanics and broncodilatory responsiveness in patients with the adult respiratory distress syndrome. Crit Care Med 21:78-83
10. Ranieri VM, Eissa NT, Corbeil C et al (1991) Effects of positive end-expiratory pres-

sure on alveolar recruitment and gas exchange in patients with the adult respiratory distress syndrome. Am Rev Respir Dis 144:544-551
11. Matamis D, Lemaire F, Harf A, Brun-Guisson C, Ansquer JC, Atlan G (1984) Total respiratory pressure-volume curves in adult respiratory distress syndrome. Chest 86:58-66
12. Jardin F, Genevray B, Brun-Ney D, Bourdarias JP (1985) Influence of lung and chest wall compliances on transmission of airway pressure to the pleural space in critically ill patients. Chest 88:653-658
13. Benito S, Lemaire F (1990) Pulmonary pressure-volume relationship in acute respiratory distress syndrome in adults: role of positive end expiratory pressure. J Crit Care 5:27-34
14. Auler JOC, Salvida PHN, Martins MA et al (1990) Flow and volume dependence of respiratory system mechanics during constant flow ventilation in normal subjects and in adult respiratory distress syndrome. Crit Care Med 18:1080-1086
15. Pelosi P, Cereda M, Foti G, Giacomini M, Pesenti A (1995) Alterations of lung and chest wall mechanics in patients with acute lung injury: effects of positive end-expiratory pressure. Am J Respir Crit Care Med 152:531-537
16. Suter IM, Fairley HB, Isenberg MD (1978) Effect of tidal volume and positive end-expiratory pressure on compliance during mechanical ventilation. Chest 73:158-162
17. Katz JA, Ozanne GM, Zinn SE, Fairley HB (1981) Time course and mechanisms of lung-volume increase with PEEP in acute pulmonary failure. Anesthesiology 54:9-16
18. Benito S, Lemaire F, Mankikian B, Harf A (1985) Total respiratory compliance as a function of lung volume in patients with mechanical ventilation. Intensive Care Med 11:76-79
19. Suter PM, Fairley HB, Schlobohm RM (1975) Shunt, lung volume and perfusion during short periods of ventilation with oxygen. Anesthesiology 43:617-627
20. Mancebo J, Calaf N, Benito S (1985) Pulmonary compliance measurement in acute respiratory failure. Critical Care Med 13:589-591
21. Wrigh PE, Bernard GR (1989) The role of airflow resistance in patients with the adult respiratory distress syndrome. Am Rev Respir Dis 139:1169-1174
22. Mancebo J, Benito S, Calaf N, Net A (1988) Simplified syringe procedures for the estimation of functional residual capacity. J Crit Care 3:180-189
23. Gattinoni L, Pesenti A, Avalli L, Rossi F, Bombino M (1987) Pressure-volume curve of total respiratory system in acute respiratory failure. Computed tomographic scan study. Am Rev Respir Dis 136:730-736
24. Gattinoni L, Bombino M, Pelosi P et al (1994) Lung structure and function in different stages of severe adult respiratory distress syndrome. JAMA 271:1772-1779
25. Ranieri VM, Brienza N, Santostasi S et al (1997) Impairment of lung and chest wall mechanics in patients with ARDS. Am J Respir Crit Care Med 156:1082-1091
26. D'Angelo E, Calderini E, Torri G, Robatto F, Bono D, Milic-Emili J (1988) Respiratory mechanics in anesthetized paralyzed humans: Effect of flow, volume and time. J Appl Physiol 64:441-450
27. D'Angelo E, Robatto FM, Calderini E et al (1991) Pulmonary and chest wall mechanics in anesthetized paralyzed humans. J Appl Physiol 70:2602-2610
28. Gattinoni L, D'Andrea L, Pelosi P, Vitale G, Pesenti A, Fumagalli R (1993) Regional effects and mechanism of positive end-expiratory pressure in early adult respiratory distress syndrome. JAMA 269:2122-2127
29. Bates JHT, Rossi A, Milic-Emili J (1985) Analysis of the behavior of the respiratory system with constant inspiratory flow. J Appl Physiol 58:1840-1848
30. Pelosi P, D'Andrea L, Vitale G, Pesenti A, Gattinoni L (1994) Vertical gradient of

regional inflation in adult respiratory distress syndrome. Am J Respir Crit Care Med 149:8-13

31. Mutoh T, Lamm WJE, Hidebrandt J, Albert RK (1991) Abdominal distention alters regional pleural pressures and chest wall mechanics in pigs in vivo. J Appl Physiol 70:2611-2618
32. Morina P, Herrera M, Venegas J, Mora D, Rodriguez M, Pino E (1997) Effects of nebulized salbutamol on respiratory mechanics in ARDS. Intensive Care Med 23:58-64
33. Servillo G, Svantesson C, Beydon L et al (1997) Pressure-volume curves in acute respiratory failure. Am J Respir Crit Care Med 155:1629-1636
34. Mergoni M, Martelli A, Volpi A, Primavera S, Zuccoli P, Rossi A (1997) Impact of positive end-expiratory pressure on chest wall and lung pressure-volume curve in acute respiratory failure. Am J Respir Crit Care Med 156:846-854
35. Pelosi P, Tubiolo D, Mascheroni D et al (1998) Effects of the prone position on respiratory mechanics and gas exchange during acute lung injury. Am J Respir Crit Care Med 157:387-393
36. Blanch L, Mancebo J, Perez M (1997) Short term effects of prone position in critically ill patients with acute respiratory distress syndrome. Intensive Care Med 23:1033-1039
37. Gattinoni L, Pelosi P, Suter OM, Pedoto A, Vercesi P, Lissoni A (1998) Acute respiratory distress syndrome caused by pulmonary and extrapulmonary disease. Different syndromes? Am J Respir Crit Care Med (in press)
38. Rossi A, Gottfried SB, Zocchi L et al (1985) Measurement of static compliance of total respiratory system in patients with acute respiratory failure during mechanical ventilation. Am Rev Respir Dis 131:672-677
39. Bernasconi M, Ploysongsang Y, Gottfried SB, Milic-Emili J, Rossi A (1988) Respiratory compliance and resistance in mechanically ventilated patients with acute respiratory failure. Intensive Care Medicine 14:547-553
40. Broseghini C, Brandolese R, Poggi R et al (1988) Respiratory mechanics during the first day of mechanical ventilation in patients with pulmonary edema and chronic airway obstruction. Am Rev Respir Dis 138:355-361
41. Pesenti A, Pelosi P, Rossi N, Virtuani A, Brazzi L, Rossi A (1991) The effects of positive end-expiratory pressure on respiratory resistance in patients with the adult respiratory distress syndrome and in normal anesthetized subjects. Am Rev Respir Dis 144:101-107
42. Katz JA, Zinn SE, Ozanne GM, Fairley HB (1981) Pulmonary, chest wall, and lung-thorax elastances in acute respiratory failure. Chest 80:304-311
43. Connors AF, McCaffree DR, Gray BA (1991) Effect of inspiratory flow rate on gas exchange during mechanical ventilation. Am Rev Respir Dis 124:537-543
44. Gottfried SB, Rossi A, Higgs BD et al (1985) Noninvasive determination of respiratory system mechanics during mechanical ventilation for acute respiratory failure. Am Rev Respir Dis 131:414-420
45. Gattinoni L, Mascheroni D, Basilico E, Foti G, Pesenti A, Avalli L (1987) Volume/pressure curve of total respiratory system in paralyzed patients: Artifacts and correction factors. Intensive Care Med 13:19-25

Chapter 17

Altered elastic properties of the respiratory system

R. Brandolese, U. Andreose

The lungs can be expanded by downward or upward movements of the diaphragm to lengthen or shorten the chest cavity, and by elevation or depression of the ribs to increase and decrease the anteroposterior diameter of the chest cavity [1]. The lung is an elastic structure; at any time of the respiratory cycle, the inspiratory muscles have to overcome the elastic recoil pressure of the total respiratory system to inflate the lungs. The muscular pressure generated by the respiratory muscles is dependent on the elastic and resistive properties of the respiratory system at any value of tidal volume. Between the lung pleura and the chest wall there is a slight suction that maintains a moderate subatmospheric (negative) pressure in the pleural space. During inspiration, the expansion of the chest wall creates a greater negative pressure. Therefore, the lungs can be inflated by the tidal volume [2].

The alveolar pressure is the pressure inside the alveoli of the lung. When the glottis is open and there is no flow of inspiratory gas to the lungs, the alveolar pressure equals the atmospheric pressure, considered to be 0 cm H_2O. To initiate inspiration, the pressure in the alveoli falls to a subatmospheric value; this slight negative alveolar pressure is sufficient to move about 500 ml air into the lungs. The difference between alveolar pressure and pleural pressure is called transpulmonary pressure and it is a measure of the elastic forces in the lungs that tend to collapse the lung at any point of expansion and regulate the diameter of the alveoli at different heights of the lung. This pressure is also termed recoil pressure [3, 4].

The extent to which the respiratory system expands for each unit increase in transpulmonary pressure is called compliance [5]. Normal lung compliance in adults is approximately of 200 ml/cm H_2O. That is, if the transpulmonary pressure increases by 1 cm H_2O, the lungs expand by 200 ml. Recording the changes in transpulmonary pressure at different values of tidal volume permits computation of the inspiratory compliance curve with its characteristics due to elastic forces of the lungs [3, 7]: the greater the slope of the volume-pressure (V-P) relationship, the smaller the compliance of the respiratory system. The elastic forces of the lung tissue and those caused by the surface tension of the fluid-film lining of the inside walls of the alveoli are determinants of the shape of the respiratory compliance curve. The surface tension elastic forces of the lungs represent two-thirds of the total elastic forces that tend to collapse the lungs. Surfactant is an active surface agent that is able to dramatically reduce the pulmonary surface tension to 5-30 dyn/cm (70-80 dyn/cm is the value of surface tension when surfactant is absent) [6].

If the air spaces of the lungs are blocked, the surface tension tends to collapse the alveoli and create a positive pressure in the alveoli. The amount of the pressure generated in this way, can be calculated using the Laplace law:

$$\text{Pressure} = 2T/\text{ radius}$$

where T is surface tension. For an alveolus of about 100 μm in diameter, the pressure is about 4 cm H_2O, which is the pressure needed to keep an alveolus open. The pressure required to maintain the lungs inflated is inversely related to the radius of the alveolus, and therefore the smaller the alveolus the greater this pressure will be [3]. The phenomenon for which the smaller alveoli tend to collapse is termed *alveolar instability.* This condition is not very important in the normal lung, but it assumes relevance in those conditions in which surfactant is poor e.g. in adult respiratory distress syndrome (ARDS).

The thoracic cage has viscous and elastic properties similar to those of the lung. Even if the lungs were not present in the thoracic cavity, a remarkable muscular effort would have to be made to expand the chest wall. Chest wall compliance equals lung compliance in the normal adult but, because the lung and the chest wall are linked in series, the compliance of total respiratory system reaches a value that is half (100 ml/cm H_2O) of the compliances measured separately [7].

The respiratory muscles perform work during inspiration that can be divided into three different components:

- that required to expand the lungs against their elastic recoil forces;
- that required to overcome the viscoelastic component of the lung and chest wall;
- that required to overcome the airway resistance during the movement of gas from the mouth to the alveoli.

The work of breathing (WOB) is expressed by the following equation:

$$WOB = 0.5\,(VT)^2\,E + 0{,}25\,\pi\,(VT)^2\,Rf$$

where VT is tidal volume, E is elastance of total respiratory system, R is resistance of total respiratory system, and f is respiratory rate.

In pulmonary diseases, all three types of work are frequently vastly increased. Compliance work and tissue resistance work are increased by diseases (i.e. adult respiraory distress syndrome (ARDS)) that cause fibrosis of the lungs and a reduction in the amount of aerated pulmonary parenchyma. Airway resistance work is increased by diseases that cause a reduction of airway caliber, such as happens during asthmatic attacks.

Lung mechanism in pulmonary diseases

Emphysema is characterized by enlargement of the airspaces distal to the terminal bronchiole. The most characteristic feature in lung mechanics is marked loss of elastic recoil pressure of the lung which determines an increase of total lung capacity (TLC). In emphysematous patients, the elastic equilibrium volume of total respiratory system is changed to a position in the relaxation curve of respiratory system which is higher than that in normal subjects; functional residual volume (FRC) is increased and a state of static hyperinflation is present [8, 10]. The combined effect of increased respiratory resistance, (usually present in emphysematous patients), decreased dynamic lung compliance because of hyperinflation, and increased FRC has a fundamental role in stressing the inspiratory muscles. The most obvious requirement in these patients is an increased swing in pleural pressure to overcome inspiratory workload (increased airflow resistance and decreased dynamic lung compliance). Hyperinflation decreases the resting length of inspiratory muscles fibers which have to work at a mechanical disadvantage based on the length-tension relationship [8]. During these conditions, the efficiency of the respiratory muscles is markedly reduced and the muscular oxygen consumption may be as high as 30% of total oxygen consumption [11]. Moreover, during inspiration, these patients must overcome an added elasic load termed auto-positive end expiratory pressure due to dynamic hyperinflation from rapid, shallow breathing. Therefore the inspiratory muscles reduce their capacity to lower surface pleural pressure.

The inspiratory muscles can partially adapt to chronic hyperinflation [9]. In normal subjects the ability to decrease mouth and pleural pressure (more negative pressure) during maximum inspiratory effort declines close to TLC. Therefore, comparison between normal subjects and patients with chronic obstractive pulmonary disease (COPD) allows appreciation of the differences in lung inflation. Despite any compensatory adaptation in the inspiratory muscles, their capacity is reduced in COPD patients compared to that of with normal subjects. As more negative pressure is required of the inspiratory muscles in COPD patients to perform tidal ventilation, the inspiratory muscles must work at a higher percentage of their maximum inspiratory pressure than those of normal subjects. In addition, the Campbell diagram (which shows the relation between tidal volume and the elastic recoil pressure of the lung and chest wall) underestimates the total respiratory work performed because it takes no account of the distortion and hysteresis of the chest wall during tidal breathing [9]. There is less movement of the abdomen and a greater displacement of the rib cage so that the chest wall is distorted from its relaxation position. Moreover there is an inward movement, during inspiration, of the lateral portion of the rib cage (Hoover's sign) indicating that the patient is not utilizing the diaphragm to perform tidal breathing. In COPD patients the diaphragm, because of hyperinflation, is flattened, so that its curvature radius is greatly augmented.

The force generated by the diaphragm fits the equation of Laplace: $P=2T/r$.

If the curvature radius is infinite, the force generated is null. In other words the diaphragm is motionless. As a result of these changes, the O_2 consumption of the respiratory muscles is greatly increased out of proportion to the mechanical workload. In normal subjects, the expiration is completely passive and no electric muscular activity is recorded other than the early phase of expiration during which the post-inspiratory activity of the inspiratory muscles is present. The elastic recoil pressure at end inflation is the driving pressure of the expiration (Pel,rs=Pres,rs).

In many COPD patients observed an abdominal muscular contraction is what truly affects the behaviour of the respiratory system and is responsible, in part, for the positive end-expiratory pressure (PEEPi). PEEP can be overestimated if the value of abdominal pressure reflected by gastric pressure (Pga) is not taken into account for its computation [12, 13].

Emphysema is a progressive disease that leads to disabling dyspnea and to great exercise limitation. The symptoms are related to the gravity of obstruction, to static and dynamic hyperinflation, and consequently to the increased mechanical workload for the respiratory muscles [14]. These mechanical constraints are associated with an increased central neural respiratory drive measured during exercise and at rest. The inability of the fatigued respiratory muscles to perform a predictable task leads to hypercapnia, acidosis, hypoxemia, and ventilatory failure requiring mechanical ventilatory support with a poor prognosis.

Lung volume reduction

In recent years, surgical lung volume reduction procedures to improve pulmonary status in COPD patients have been widely investigated [15]. Lung volume reduction surgery involves resection of 20%-30% of the tissue of each lung and has been reported to produce short-term improvement in lung function and in 6-min walk distance. Lung volume reduction decreases dynamic hyperinflation because it decreases flow limitation due to an increased elastance of the lung after surgery. The normalization of lung and chest wall elastic recoil should decrease respiratory impedence and consequently also decrease central respiratory drive [16].

Lung volume reduction also ameliorates the dyspnea score by reducing the mechanical workload resulting from breathing at lower lung volume. The reduction in hyperinflation improves inspiratory muscle action because of a better operational length. The radius of the diaphragm is decreased so that it is able to produce an increased maximum transdiaphragmatic pressure. In spite of encouraging results, further investigations are needed to define selection criteria regarding optimal surgical candidates [18].

The opposite form of obstructive lung disease is restrictive pulmonary disease in which all pulmonary static and dynamic volumes are regularly reduced. There are many causes which determine a reduction in lung compliance so that total lung capacity is reduced (i.e. bronchopneumonia, adult respiratory distress syndrome, lobectomy). Lung expansion may be inhibited by extrapulmonary causes such as diseases of the pleura or chest wall and muscular fatigue of inspiratory muscles that reduces their force distending the lung and chest wall. In restrictive pulmonary diseases due to intrapulmonary causes the static V-P curve is displaced to right in a Cartesian diagram, indicating that compliance is reduced and lung recoil pressure is augmented at a given lung volume.

Lung resection and atelectasis cause a loss of gas volume without an increase in tissue volume [17].The static V-P curve is shifted to the right in proportion to the amount of pulmonary tissue lost. Total lung capacity and functional residual capacity both depend on interactions between chest wall and lung that are able to generate opposite recoil pressure. Therefore, if gas volume is lost, the reduction of TLC and FRC is not proportional to the loss of alveoli. The chest wall tends to prevent FRC reduction by distending the surviving alveoli; thus the reduction in FRC will depend on the shape of the V-P curve of the chest wall: the less compliant chest wall, the less the net loss of intrapulmonary gas.

In acute lung injury, as in both cardiogenic pulmonary edema (CPE) and non-cardiogenic pulmonary edema (i.e. ARDS), airspaces are flooded by blood, edema liquid, and inflammatory cells. The liquids compete with air in the alveoli. If the alveoli are filled by liquid there will be a lesser amount of gas in the lung with a reduction in the amount of normally ventilated tissue. Consequently, compliance of the respiratory system is reduced proportionally to the amount of diseased lung [19, 20, 22].

Pulmonary edema

We have investigated the mechanical properties of the respiratory system in patients mechanically ventilated because acute respiratory failure due to pulmonary edema (cardiogenic and not) [21]. We found that PEEPi (a hallmark of altered respiratory mechanics in COPD patients) was present in all patient with cardiogenic and non-cardiogenic pulmonary edema. Average values were 3.0 and 3.8 cm H_2O, respectively. The presence of PEEPi has implications in terms of the mode of mechanical ventilation. In fact, to trigger the ventilator, PEEPi has to be counterbalanced by the respiratory muscles before initiating inspiratory flow. This isometric contraction of inspiratory muscles determines an increased oxygen cost of breathing which in these patients (CPE and ARDS) is already high because of increased elastance. Average values of compliance in CPE and ARDS patients were 0.044 l/cm H_2O and 0.035 l/cmH_2O, respectively. The lower value in ARDS probably reflects more severe air-space flooding than in CPE. Acute respiratory failure (ARF) (including ARDS and CPE) is a disease in which the elastic lung tissue is compromised [22-24]. Nevertheless respiratory resistance is also increased. Both maximum and minimum respiratory resistances are increased. Rmin which reflects bronchial resistance, has increased because of the narrowing of bronchial caliber due to vagal reflexes, airway flooding and decreased lung volume. Rmin was higher in ARDS than in CPE patients. The higher difference in maximum and minimum resistances in ARDS than in CPE patients reflects the higher degree of time constant inequalities within the lung, probably indicating that ARDS is a more severe disease than CPE. In our study, the PaO_2/PAO_2 oxygenation index correlated with a decrease in compliance due to reduction of lung gas volume [21].

Measurement of respiratory mechanics of total respiratory system is important to define the gravity of the disease and its progress. Nevertheless partitioning of respiratory system mechanics into lung and chest wall components provides a better understanding of the disease underlying ARF. Therefore we have studied ten mechanically ventilated patients because of ARF due to pulmonary edema (PE) and acute exacerbation of chronic airway obstruction (CAO) [25]. We found that PEEPi was present in all CAO patients, and in line with other studies, in some patients affected by pulmonary edema. PEEPi was due almost entirely to end-expiratory elastic recoil of the lung (Table 1). The presence in a CAO patient of PEEPi due to elastic recoil of the chest wall, (Table 1) indicated that the chest wall is inwardly recoiling because of hyperinflation, providing a possible explanation for the flow limitation observed in mechanically ventilated COPD patient, during the expiration period.

Both lung and chest wall elastances are increased in COPD patients with ARF, perhaps because of hyperinflation, and in PE patients [26, 27]. Table 2 shows that chest wall elastances were not substantially different between patients with pulmonary edema and those with COPD. Lung elastances were markedly increased, reflecting the underlying disease, in PE patients. Partitioning of respiratory mechanics in mechanically ventilated patients with ARF due to intrapulmonary causes, has demonstrated that chest wall mechanics were slightly different from

Table 1. Intrinsic PEEP of total respiratory system, lung and chest wall and δ EELV

Subject	PEEPi,rs,[a] (cm H_2O)	PEEPi,L[b] (cm H_2O)	PEEPi,W[c] (cm H_2O)	δEELV[d] (l)
COP patients				
1	9.8	7.5	2.3	0.56
2	6.6	5.5	1.1	1.48
3	7.7	6.9	0.8	0.66
4	9.2	8.5	0.7	0.44
5	3.8	2.7	1.1	0.18
6	6.5	5.4	1.1	0.18
–	–	–	–	–
Mean±SD	7.3±2.2	6.1±2.0	1.2±0.6	0.60±0.46
PE patients				
1	0	0	0	0
2	0	0	0	0
3	1.1	0.9	0.2	0
4	2.1	2.0	0.4	0.27
	–	–	–	–
Mean±SD	0.8±1.0	0.7±1.0	0.2±0.2	0.07±0.13

COPD, chronic obstructive lung disease; *PE*, pulmonary edema
[a] Intrinsic positive end-exiratory pressure (elastic recoil) of total respiratory system
[b] Intrinsic positive end-exiratory pressure of lung
[c] Intrinsic positive end-exiratory pressure of chest wall
[d] Difference between end-expiratory lung volume (EELV) and relaxation volume

Table 2. Dynamic and static elastances of total respiratory system, lung, and chest wall in COPD and PE patients

Subject	Edyn,rs ($cm\ H_2O/l$)	Edyn,L ($cm\ H_2O/l$)	Edyn,W ($cm\ H_2O/l$)	Est,rs ($cm\ H_2O/l$)	Est, L ($cm\ H_2O/l$)	Est, W ($cm\ H_2O/l$)
COPD patients						
1	24.7	16.0	8.7	16.4	9.4	7.0
2	18.7	14.8	3.9	11.0	6.8	4.2
3	30.9	16.2	14.7	22.4	11.4	11.3
4	23.0	11.9	11.1	16.1	7.7	8.4
5	17.4	9.9	7.5	13.3	5.8	7.5
6	17.5	11.9	5.7	12.7	6.5	6.2
–	–	–	–	–	–	–
Mean±SD	22.0±5.3	13.5±2.6	8.6±3.9	15.3±4.0	7.9±2.1	7.4±2.4
PE patients						
1	28.3	20.7	7.6	25.6	18.8	6.8
2	28.4	22.7	5.7	25.6	15.6	10.0
3	36.1	32.4	3.7	33.4	28.8	4.3
4	21.9	12.7	9.2	17.5	10.0	7.5
	–	–	–	–	–	–
Mean±SD	28.7±5.8	22.1±8.1	6.6±2.4	25.5±6.5	18.3±7.9	7.2±2.3

Edyn, dynamic elastance; *Est*, static elastance; *rs*, total respiratory system; *L*, lung; *W*, chest wall; *COPD*, chronic obstructive lung disease; *PE*, pulmonary edema

those of normal subjects, and that alteration in respiratory mechanics is due mainly to lung components [25].

Volume-pressure curves

Respiratory system volume-pressure (V-P) curves have been widely used in patients with adult respiratory distress syndrome for optimization of mechanical ventilation settings and staging of disease [28]. From the slope of the V-P curve it is possible to quantify compliance at any given pressure and volume range. The shape of V-P curve is not linear; changes in the measured parameters depend on the arbitrary pressure and volume used. Moreover, accurate estimation of these parameters requires the collection of data at precise points along the V-P curve and extrapolation of data. [28]. The relaxation curve of respiratory system characteristically presents three different portions (Fig. 1):

1. lower inflexion point;
2. linear part;
3. upper inflexion point.

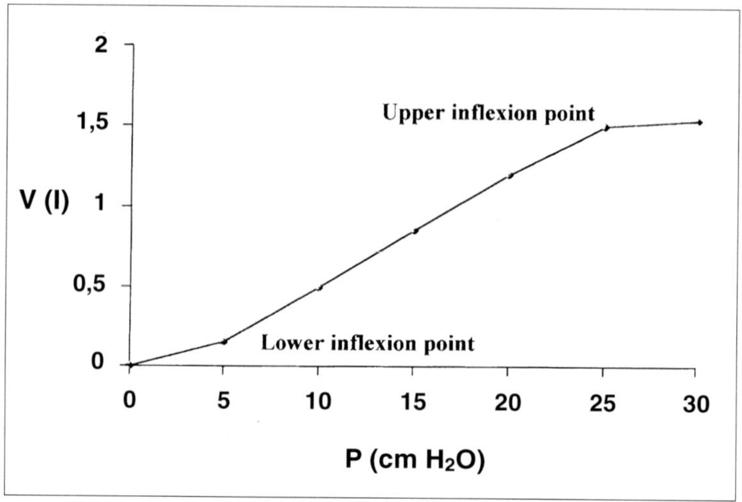

Fig 1. Inspiratory volume-pressure curve determined by the supersyringe method, from a representative ARDS patient who was paralyzed and mechanically ventilated with zero end-expiratory pressure (ZEEP)

The inflation limb of the V-P curve defines a safe range of ventilatory pressures during mechanical ventilation of ARDS patients [29]. Ventilator-induced lung injury is caused by overdistension of the alveoli or by share forces that occur by the repetitive recruitment and derecruitment of alveolar units. The lower inflexion point in V-P curves corresponds to the point of rapid change in curvature and is referred to as the pressure at which maximal alveolar recruitment occurs. The upper inflexion point corresponds to the pressure at which overdistension of parenchyma occurs with risk of barotrauma (pneumothorax, pneumomediastinum, gas embolism).

Evaluation of the critical points of V-P curves i.e the lower and upper points, is made by eye: a method that is too imprecise and subjective. It is possible obviate this by using an equation to fit the V-P curve. Thus, it becomes possible to derive more definite parameters of respiratory mechanics in ARDS patients [28]. We suggest the following equation as proposed by Venegas et al [28]:

$$V = a + \frac{b}{(1+e^{-(P-c)/d})}, \lambda$$

where V is the inflation volume, a is the volume that approximates FRC, e is Neper's number, b is vital capacity, P is the pressure at airway opening, c is the pressure at the point of highest compliance, and d is related to pressure range between lower and upper inflexion point. From the equation, it is possible to obtain the lower inflexion point as c -2d, and the upper inflexion point as c+2d.

References

1. Fishman AP(1980) Assessment of pulmonary function. McGraw-Hill, New York, pp 18-51
2. Forster RE (1987) Introduction to respiratory physiology. Annu Rev Physiol 49:555
3. Levitzky MG (1982) Pulmonary physiology. Mc Graw-Hill, New York pp 5-38
4. Murray JF (1986) The normal lung, 2nd ed. WB Saunders, Philadelphia pp 87-11
5. Rahn H et al (1946) The pressure volume diagram of the thorax and the lung. Am J Physiol 146:161-163
6. Weibel ER, Bachofen H (1987) How to stabilize the pulmonary alveoli Surfactant or fibers? New Physiol Sci 2:72-74
7. West JB (1987) Pulmonary pathophysiology: the essentials, 3rd ed. William and Wilkins, Baltimore, pp 85-113
8. Mahler DA (1993) Chronic obstructive pulmonary disease. In: Mahler D (ed) Pulmonary diseases of the elderly patient. Marcel Dekker, New York, pp 159-163
9. O'Connel JM, Campbell AH (1976) Respiratory mechanics in airway obstruction with inspiratory dyspnoea. In: Roussos C (ed) Thorax. Marcel Dekker, New York, pp 669-677
10. Cherniack RM, Hodson A (1963) Compliance of the chest wall in chronic bronchitis and emphysema. J Appl Physiol 18:707-711
11. Cherniack RM (1959) The oxygen consumption and efficiency of the respiratory muscles in health and emphysema. J Clin Invest 35:494-499
12. Haluszka J, Chartrand DA, Grassino AE, Milic-Emili J (1990) Intrinsic PEEP and arterial $PaCO_2$ in stable patients with chronic obstructive pulmonary disease. Am Rev Respir Dis 141:1194-1197
13. De Troyer A, Pride NB (1995) The chest wall and respiratory muscles in chronic obstructive pulmonary disease. In: Roussos C (ed) Thorax. Marcel Dekker, New York, pp 1975-2001
14. Celli BR (1996) Pathophysiology of chronic obstructive pulmonary disease. Chest Surg Clin North Am 5: 623-634
15. Cooper J, Trulock E, Triantafillou A et al (1995) Bilateral pneumonectomy for chronic obstrctive pulmonary disease. J Thor Cardiovasc Sur 109:106-119
16. Sciurba F, Rogers R, Keenan R et al (1996) Improvement function and elastic recoil after lung reduction surgery for diffuse emphysema. New Engl J Med 334:1095-1099
17. Daniel TM, Chan BB, Blaskar V et al (1996) Lung volume reduction surgery: case selection, operative technique, clinical results. Ann Surg 523:526-531
18. McIlroy MB, Bates DV (1956) Respiratory function after pneumonectomy. Thorax 11: 303-311
19. Cook CD, Med J, Schreiner GI et al (1959) Pulmonary mechanics induced in anesthetized dogs. J Appl Physiol 14:177-186
20. Katz JA, Zinn SE, Ozanne GM, Fairley HB (1981) Pulmonary, chest wall, and lung thorax elastances in acute respiratory failure. Chest 80:304-311
21. Broseghini C, Brandolese R, Poggi R, Polese G, Milic-Emili J, Rossi A (1988) Respiratory mechanics during first day of mechanical ventilation in patients with pulmonary edema and chronic airway obstruction. Am Rev Respir Dis 138:355-361
22. Bone RC (1983) Monitoring ventilatory mechanics in acute respiratory failure. Respiratory Care 28: 597-603
23. Rossi A, Gottfried SB, Zocchi L et al (1985) Measurement of static compliance of respiratory system in patients with acute respiratory failure during mechanical ventilation. Am Rev Respir Dis 131:672-678

24. Bates JHT, Rossi A, Milic-Emili J (1985) Analysis of behaviour of respiratory system with constant inspiratory flow. J Appl Physiol 58:1840-1848
25. Polese G, Rossi A, Brandi G, Bates JHT, Brandolese R, (1991) Partitioning of respiratory mechanics in mechanically ventilated patients. J Appl Physiol 71(6):2425-2433
26. Behrakis PK, Higgs BD, Bevan DR, Milic-Emili J (1985) Partitioning of respiratory mechanics in halothane anesthetized humans. J Appl Physiol 58:285-289
27. Robatto FM, D'Angelo E, Calderini E, Torri D, Bono D, Milic-Emili J (1990) Lung and chest wall mechanics in anesthetized-paralyzed humans. Am Rev Respir Dis 141: A850
28. Venegas JG, Scott Harris R, Simon BA (1998) A comprehensive equation for the pulmonary pressure-volume curve. J Appl Physiol 84(1):389-395
29. Roupie E, D'Ambrosio M, Servillo G et al (1995) Titration of tidal volume and induced hypercapnia in acute respiratory distress syndrome. Am J Respir Crit Care Med 152:121-128

Chapter 18

Intrinsic PEEP

A. Rossi

In mechanically ventilated patients, alveolar pressure can remain positive if the time available to breathe out is shorter than the time required for lung volume to return to V_r [1]. This can be the consequence of: a) reduced lung elastic recoil; b) increased flow resistance; c) expiratory flow limaation; d) excessive tidal volume (VT); and e) short duration of expiration (TE) (due, for instance, to high breathing frequency or shorter duty cycle). Under these circumstances, expiration is not completed before the onset of the next mechanical lung inflation and the end-expiratory lung volume (EELV) will stabilize above relaxed functional residual capacity (FRC) or V_r [1-4]. The end-expiratory elastic recoil (Pel,rs), due to incomplete expiration has been termed auto PEEP, occult PEEP [5], inadverted PEEP, endogenous PEEP, internal PEEP, and intrinsic PEEP [6]. Basically, in mechanically ventilated patients, factors causing the elevation of EELV and intrinsic PEEP (PEEPi) and determining its magnitude are:

- abnormal Patient resDiratory mechanics, i.e. high resistance and compliance, and expiratory flow limaation;
- added flow resistance, i.e. endotracheal tube and ventilator circuas and valves;
- ventilatory pattern, with large Vt, high frequency, short Te (due to the ventilator setting, a patient's own ventilatory pattern and demand, or both), and the end-inspiratory pause.

In other words, mechanisms that eaher decrease expiratory flow or shorten TE promote PEEPi in ventilator-dependent patients. Recently, it has been shown that another factor promoting PEEPi is the brief end-inspiratory pause (<0.5 S), which is often set to improve gas exchange. An end-inspiratory pause not only increases inspiratory time, and hence decreases TE at any given frequency, but also decreases the driving pressure available to produce expiratory flow, due to the decrease in Pel,rs as a result of stress relaxation [7].

PEEPi has important implications for all ventilator-dependent patients. Among other adverse effects, PEEPi can depress cardiac output, and a poses an inspiratory threshold load for inspiration. The latter consequence is relevant only wah assisted modes, whereas the fommer has to be taken into account regardless of the ventilator mode. From a monitoring standpoint, PEEPi can be suspected, though not quantified, from the shape of the expired flow-time or flow-volume relationship: if flow does not become nil toward the end of expiration and at the onset of inspiration or if flow increases abruptly from expiration to inspiration, then there may be PEEPi unless expiratory muscle activity is present. Dynamic hyperinflation is almost systematically associated with PEEPi [3, 5].

Dynamic pulmonary hyperinflation

During controlled ventilation, and often during assisted ventilation, the presence of PEEPi implies dynamic pulmonary hyperinflation (DPH), i.e. an increase in end-expiratory lung volume (EELV) above V_r, the difference between EELV and V_r being defined as ΔFRC. The measurement of ΔFRC has been used by William et al. [8] in asthmatic patients to quantify the degree of pulmonary hyperinflation; they termed this quality V_{EI}, i.e. V_T plus DFRC. These authors recommended monitoring V_{EI} in patients with acute asthma to prevent excessive alveolar overdistension and barotrauma. They have shown that keeping V_{EI} <20 ml/kg can improve survival in asthma. This manoeuvre is simple and suaable for bedside monaoring in relaxed patients. However, with extreme airway obstruction even 30 s may not be suffficient to reach V_r, particularly in presence of patient's inspiratory efforts or because of the need to reinstitute ventilation to prevent deterioration in arterial blood gases. The contribution of chest wall recoil to PEEPi is rather small.

Implications of PEEPi

Measurement of PEEPi is important during both controlled and assisted ventilation. During controlled ventilation, detecting PEEPi may help explain an unexpected drop in cardiac output, prevent fluid overload, and make ventilator settings more appropriate. During assisted ventilation, PEEPi is an inspiratory threshold load which has to be fully counferbalanced by increasing inspiratory muscle effort in order to generate a negative pressure in the central airway and trigger the ventilator. Therefore, PEEPi adds to the triggering pressure such that the total inspiratory effort needed to trigger the ventilator is the set trigger sensitivity, usually -1 to -2 cm H_2O, plus PEEPi. With high levels of PEEPi, the effort to trigger a mechanical breath can be substantial and a supported breath can require virtually the same energy expenditure as an unsupported breath, with PEEPi accounting for most of the load. Furthermore, the negative pleural pressure (Ppl) swing generated by some inspiratory efforts can be smaller than PEEPi and not sufficient to trigger the ventilator, resulting in ineffective efforts [9, 10]. Under these circumstances, a patient's respiratory muscles continue to contract under load and cannot recover from fatigue, with the result that the weaning process gets inexplicably hampered in a patient who had apparently adapted to the ventilator.

In summary, the major adverse effects of PEEPi in ventilator-dependent patients are:
- impaired cardiac filling;
- increased effort to trigger the ventilator;
- ineffective inspiratory effort.

All the mechanical characteristics of the respiratory system, i.e. compliance, resistance, and PEEPi, have important implications for the dynamics of breathing.

Dynamics of breathing

During unsupported spontaneous breathing, the pressure to inflate the respiratory system is provided by the contracting inspiratory muscles (Pmus). In mechanically ventilated patients, inflation pressure is provided either by the ventilator alone (i.e. controlled mechanical ventilation (CMV)) or by a combination of the patient's respiratory muscle activity and ventilator positive pressure; examples include assist-control ventilation (AMV), syncronised intermittent mandatory ventilation (SIMV), pressure support ventilation (PSV), and proportional assist ventilation (PAV). According to the simplest model of the respiratory system, i.e. a pipe-ballon system, lung inflation can be described by the equation of motion:

$$Pappl_{(t)} = PEEPi + (\Delta V_{(t)}/Crs) + Rt + (K_1 \dot{V}_{(t)} + K_2 \dot{V}^2_{(t)}) \qquad (1)$$

where Pappl is the applied pressure, Crs is the compliance of the total respiratory system and Rt is the thoracic tissue resistance. Clearly, the pressure neededto inflate the respiratory system increases with increasing ventilatory load, i.e. increasing PEEPi, decreasing compliance, and increasing total flow resistance. This may be irrelevant when the ventilator is performing the entire task, for instance during CMV in a well-adapted patient, but it must be borne in mind when the patient shares inspiration during assisted modes. In a patient poorly adapted to the ventilator setting, because of problems within the patien (pain, anxiety, fever) or because of inappropriate ventilator settings-giving rise to the patient "fighting the ventilator"- the burden provided by abnormal respiratory muscles rather than the ventilator. Under these circumstances, mechanical ventilation may fail one of its major goals, namely to rest the respiratory muscles.

Work of breathing

Work of breathing (WOB) is the machanical work performed to expand the respiratory system either by the subject's contractinginspiratory muscles, by the ventilator, or by a variable contribution from each. Mechanical work implies that that the applied force or pressure (i.e. Pappl in Eq. 1) produces some displacement of the system, i.e. volume (V), according to the formula:

$$W = Pappl \cdot V = \int_0^2 Pappl \cdot dV \qquad (2)$$

which represents the area subtented by the volume-pressure (VP) curve. A commonly accepted unit to express WOB per breath is the joule, which has the units of 1 liter per 10 cm H_2O. The WOB per unit of time is power (W), obtained by multiplying work per breath by frequency (1 watt=1 J/s). WOB can be also expressed per liter of ventilation (J/I) In spontaneously breathing subjects, WOB is commonly measured using an oesophageal ballon-catheter system to estimate changes in pleural pressure (Ppl). However, that technique measures the work done in expanding the lungs, and hence does not represent the work done on the total respiratory system including the chest wall. The work needed to expand the total respiratory system, including the chest wall, can be measured non-invasively during machanical ventilation by plotting inflation volume vs. the transrespiratory pressure.

During spontaneous breathing, WOB is usually increased in critically ill patients due to abnormal respiratory mechanics. The increased workload is usually associated with a reduced pressure-generating capability of the respiratory muscles due to several factors, such as pulmonary hyperinflation, malnutrition, sepsis, or shock. Under these conditions, the load-capacity balance can deteriorate to the point that WOB becomes excessive and the ventilatory pump eventually fails [11, 12]. Unloading the inspiratory muscles is a primary goal of mechanical ventilation. Accordingly, a variable portion of the ventilatory workload is assumed by the ventilator, such thatb the inspiratory muscles are relieved by an amount that should be proportional to the degree of mechanical support. Although it is commonly believed that a ventilator puts a patient's respiratory muscles almost to rest, it has been shown that the degree of patient inspiratory effort may be little dfflerent between unassisted and ventilator-assisted breaths with almost any method of mechanical ventilation. Sometimes even during CMV, a patient without sedation or neuromuscular paralysis may adapt poorly to ventilator settings and maintain significant respiratory muscle activity-either fghting the ventilator or sharing unduly in the inspiratory work.

The same may occur with modes that provide partial support. If a patient's WOB is excessive, the respiratory muscles cannot recover from fatigue, with the result that the progressive reduction and eventual discontinuation of mechanical ventilation becomes arduous. Moreover, an additional load results from the narrow bore endotracheal tube plus the ventilator valves and circuits. This added workload increases disproportionally with decreasing endotracheal-tube diameter and with sinusoidal and decelerating flow waveforms. Furthermore, flow resistance of the endotracheal tube is higher as a patient's ventilatory demands increase, due to the concomitant increase in flow, and can vary considerably among devices from different manufacturers. A patient's WOB during mechanical ventilation can be greater than expected due to poor patient-ventilator interaction and ineffective efforts. In this connection it has to be mentioned that flow-triggering systems seem to offer less impediment to breathing than pressure-triggering systems and can decrease a patient's WOB [13].

During the early phase of acute respiratory failure (ARF), even accurate adjustment of the ventilator settings may not be sufficient to attain satisfactory patient-ventilator interaction, and sedation and occasionally muscle paralysis may be needed to achieve adequate alveolar ventilation and respiratory muscle rest. In particular, sedation and paralysis are needed with some modes which are uncomfortable for the awake patient, such as pressure-control ventilation (PCV), controlled hypoventilation, inverse-ratio ventilation, high levels of PEEP, as well as the prone position [14]. Due to the potential for adverse effects, the duration of sedation and especially paralysis should be as short as possible.

During CMV, in the relaxed patients, all the pressure needed to inflate the respiratory system is provided by the ventilator. In these circumstances, measurement of WOB can provide useful information about a patient's passive respiratory mechanics [15]. Passive work during CMV has been used also to estimate a patient's WOB by mimicking a spontaneous breathing pattem.

This computation, which can be done for each possible breathing pattern, might be useful in predicting whether a ventilatory workload is compatible with unsupported breathing after the patient has been disconnected from the ventilator.

References

1. Rossi A, Ranieri VM (1994) Positive end-expiratory pressure. In: Tobin MJ (ed) Principles and practice of mechanical ventilation. McGraw Hill, New York, pp 259-303
2. Kimball WR, Leith DE, Robins AG (1982) Dynamic hyperinflation and ventilator dependence in chronic obstructive pulmonary disease. Am Rev Respir Dis 126:991-995
3. Tuxen DV, Lane S (1987) The effects of ventilatory pattern on hyperinflation airway pressures and circulation in mechanical ventilation of patients with severe airflow obstruction. Am Rev Respir Dis 136:872-879
4. Rossi A, Ganassini A, Polese G, Grassi (1997) Pulmonary hyperinflation and ventilator-dependent patients. Eur Respir J 10:1663-1674
5. Pepe PE, Marini JJ (1982) Occult positive end-expiratory pressure in mechanically ventilated patients with airflow obstruction. Am Rev Resp Dis 126:166-170
6. Rossi A, Polese G, Brandi G, Conti G (1995) The intrinsic positive end expiratory pressure (PEEPi): physiology, implications, measurement and treatment. Intensive Care Med 21:522-536
7. Georgopoulos D, Mistrouska I, Markopoulou, Patakas D, Anthoninsen NR (1995) Effects of breathing pattern on mechanically ventilated patients with chronic obstructive pulmonary disease and dynamic hyperinflation. Intensive Care Med 21:880-886
8. William TJ, Tuxen DV, Scheinkestel CD, et al (1992) Risk factors morbidity in mechanically ventilated patients with acute severe asthma. Am Rev Respir Dis; 146:607-615
9. Rossi A, Appendini L (1995) Wasted efforts and dyssynchrony: the patien-ventilator battle is back? Intensive Care Med 21:867-870
10. Nava S, Bruschi C, Rubini F, et al (1995) Respiratory response and inspiratory effort during pressure support ventilation in COPD patients. Intensive Care Med 21:871-879
11. Rossi A, Polese G, De Sandre G (1992) Respiratory failure in chronic airflow obstrudion: Rercent advances and therapeutic implications in the critically ill patient. Eur J Med 1:349-357
12. Appendini L, Purro A, Patessio A, et al. (1996) Partitioning of inspiratory muscle workload and pressure assistance in ventilator-dependent COPD patients. Am J Respir Crit Care Med 154:1301-1309
13. Polese G, Lubli P, Poggi R, Luzani A, Milic-Emili J, Rossi A (1997) Effects of inspiratory flow waveforms on arterial blood gases and respiratory mechanics after open heart surgery. Eur Respir J 10:2820-2824
14. Rossi A, Polese G, Milic-Emili J (1998) Monitoring respiratory mechanics in ventila-

tor-dependent patients. In: Tobin MJ, (ed) Principle and practice of intensive care monitoring. McGraw Hill, New York, pp 553-596

15. Derenne JP, Simlowsky T, Whitelaw WA (1996) Definition and clinical presentation. In: Derenne JP, Similowsky T, Whitelaw WA (eds) Acute respiratory failure in chronic obstructive pulmonary disease. Marcel Dekker, New York, pp 1-12

Chapter 19

Gas-exchange in mechanically ventilated patients

J. Roca

Adequate management of patients with respiratory failure requires proper assessment of pulmonary gas exchange. Partial pressures of arterial blood gases (PaO_2 and $PaCO_2$) and pH are the directly measurable variables used by most clinicians for this purpose. Although arterial blood gases have become increasingly easy to obtain in both intensive care and medical care settings, often the interpretation of the pathophysiologic determinants of abnormal PaO_2 and/or $PaCO_2$ in the clinical arena is not straightforward. This is because arterial blood gases reflect not only the functional conditions of the lung as a gas exchanger, thereby their intrapulmonary determinants (i.e. ventilation-perfusion heterogeneities, intrapulmonary shunt and alveolar to end-capillary diffusion limitation for oxygen), but also the conditions under which the lung operates, namely the composition of inspired gas and mixed venous blood (i.e. extrapulmonary factors) [1-6].

The present review first addresses the interplay between the factors determining arterial blood gases (PaO_2 and $PaCO_2$). Then, the effects of different ventilatory strategies on gas exchange are considered.

Pulmonary and systemic factors

The chief function of the lung is pulmonary gas exchange, which requires adequate levels of ventilation and perfusion of the alveoli. The lung must match pulmonary O_2 uptake ($\dot{V}O_2$) and elimination of CO_2 ($\dot{V}CO_2$) to the whole body metabolic O_2 consumption and CO_2 production, whatever the O_2 and CO_2 partial pressures are in the arterial blood. Tables 1 and 2 show the intrapulmonary factors that may contribute individually or in combination to hypoxemia and hypercapnia as well as the extrapulmonary factors that can also influence arterial PO_2 and PCO_2.

We will focus essentially on the determinants of arterial PO_2 and PCO_2 in the light of the results obtained with the multiple inert gas elimination technique-(MIGET) [3, 7]. MIGET was developed in the early 1970s [8-12] as a robust tool to obtain more information about the entire spectrum of ventilation-perfusion ($\dot{V}_A/\dot{Q}$) distribution in the lung by measuring the exchange of six inert gases of different solubility in trace concentrations. It is based on the principle that the retention (or excretion) of any gas is dependent on the solubility (λ) of that gas and the $\dot{V}_A/\dot{Q}$ distribution. During the last 20 years a substantial amount of clinical data using the MIGET has been generated by several research groups around the

Table 1. Factors determining arterial hypoxemia

Intrapulmonary		Extrapulmonary
$\dot{V}A/\dot{Q}$ mismatching Shunt Alveolar-end capillary O_2 diffusion limitation	**Primary Factors**	Decreased Ventilation Decreased Cardiac output Decreased Inspired PO_2 Increased O_2 uptake
	Secondary Factors	Decreased P_{50} Decreased Hb concentration Increased pH

$\dot{V}A/\dot{Q}$, ventilation-perfusion; *Hb*, haemoglobin; *P_{50}*, PO_2 that corresponds to 50% oxyhaemoglobin saturation

Table 2. Factors determining hypercapnia

Intrapulmonary	Extrapulmonary
$\dot{V}A/\dot{Q}$ mismatching	Decreased Ventilation Increased CO_2 production Metabolic alkalosis

$\dot{V}A/\dot{Q}$, ventilation-perfusion

world. The technique has been shown to be adequate for understanding the basic mechanisms of PaO_2 and $PaCO_2$ abnormalities and the effects of therapeutic interventions.

Intrapulmonary factors

The highest efficiency of the lung as O_2 and CO_2 exchanger should be achieved when ventilation and blood flow to each individual alveolar unit are adequately balanced ($\dot{V}_A/\dot{Q}$=1.0) and, consequently, homogeneity of $\dot{V}_A/\dot{Q}$ ratios among alveolar units is present. This so-called "perfect lung" is not seen in normal subjects because mild heterogeneities of pulmonary $\dot{V}_A/\dot{Q}$ ratios are present due to gravity and a slight amount of physiologic post-pulmonary shunt (approximately 1%) due to the Thebesian veins [13] draining blood flow from the coronary veins directly to the left atrium and the bronchial venous blood going to pulmonary veins. Figure 1 illustrates the characteristic $\dot{V}_A/\dot{Q}$ distribution in normal individuals obtained with MIGET which consists of narrow perfusion and ventilation distributions (2nd moment) centered around a $\dot{V}_A/\dot{Q}$ ratio of 1.0 (1st moment). Mean values for the second moment of both blood flow and ventilation distributions range from 0.35-0.43 [12]. At age 20, the upper 95% confidence limit for dispersion of perfusion distribution is 0.60 and for dispersion of ventilation distribution is 0.65 [14-17] but at age 70, these are 0.70 and 0.75, respectively [18]. No (or virtually no) perfusion to ratios <0.005 (shunt) is present [12]. Likewise, the amount of ventilation to $\dot{V}_A/\dot{Q}$ ratios >100 (dead space) (including instrumen-

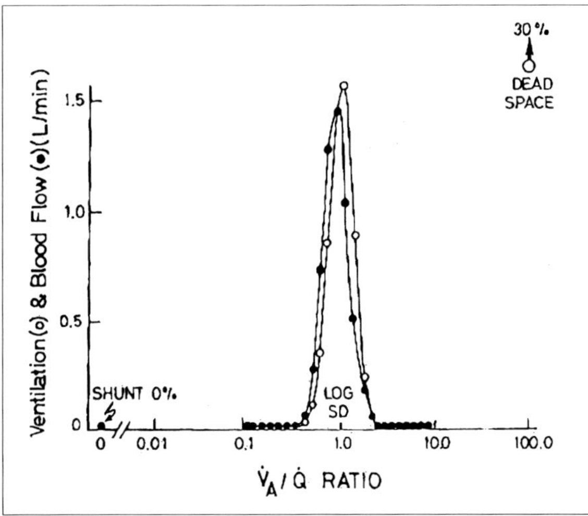

Fig. 1. Ventilation-perfusion distributions. Ventilation (open symbols) and perfusion (closed symbols) are plotted against ventilation-perfusion ($\dot{V}A/\dot{Q}$) ratio on a logarithmic scale in a resting young healthy subject, breathing room air

tal, anatomical and physiological dead space) is approximately 30%. No perfusion to lung units with $\dot{V}_A/\dot{Q}$ ratios <0.1 (low $\dot{V}_A/\dot{Q}$) is observed; similarly, ventilation to lung units with $\dot{V}_A/\dot{Q}$ ratios >10 (high $\dot{V}_A/\dot{Q}$) is not present. In most instances, $\dot{V}_A/\dot{Q}$ mismatch is the predominant factor disturbing both pulmonary O_2 uptake and CO_2 output and consequently inducing hypoxemia and hypercapnia [19, 20]. It should be noted, however, that patients with $\dot{V}_A/\dot{Q}$ inequality usually present hypoxemia but not hypercapnia. This is because increased activity of central chemoreceptors provokes a rise in total ventilation (extrapulmonary factor) that returns $PaCO_2$ back to normal values but it is not as effective on PaO_2, due to the different shape of the oxygen and carbon dioxide dissociation curves [2, 13]. Particular features of uneven $\dot{V}_A/\dot{Q}$ distributions in different disease states are described below.

The amount of $\dot{V}_A/\dot{Q}$ inequality observed in a given patient is essentially the combined end-result of three distinct factors: 1) the functional consequences of pulmonary impairment caused by the underlying disease, 2) the efficiency of the ventilatory pattern (for a given minute ventilation, the combination of high tidal volume and low respiratory rate improves $\dot{V}_A/\dot{Q}$ matching), and 3) the magnitude of hypoxic pulmonary vasoconstriction (increased arteriolar tone in low $\dot{V}_A/\dot{Q}$ areas constitutes a well known compensatory phenomenon that reduces $\dot{V}_A/\dot{Q}$ inequality). Increased intrapulmonary shunt is the foremost factor causing hypoxemia in ARDS. Since it refers to perfusion to unventilated alveolar units ($\dot{V}_A/\dot{Q}$ <0.005), it should be considered as a particular condition of $\dot{V}_A/\dot{Q}$ inequality. However, because of its pathophysiologic and therapeutic implications (hypoxemia refractory with O_2 therapy), it is considered to be a separate entity. Alveolar to end-capillary O_2 diffusion limitation is a rather uncommon cause of hypoxemia in patients. In practice it has only been demonstrated in idiopathic pulmonary fibrosis [21], particularly during exercise, and in the hepatopulmonary syndrome [22].

Primary extrapulmonary factors

Of primary importance are: 1) inspired O_2 fraction (F_IO_2); 2) total ventilation ($\dot{V}_E$); 3) cardiac output ($\dot{Q}_T$); and 4) metabolic rate ($\dot{V}O_2$). The importance of F_IO_2 as a key determinant of alveolar PO_2 (P_AO_2), and in turn of PaO_2, is indicated by the components of the ideal alveolar gas equation [2, 13]:

$$P_AO_2 = [(Pb - PH_2O) \cdot F_IO_2] - (PaCO_2/R) + [PaCO_2 \cdot F_IO_2 \cdot ((1-R)/R)]$$

where, Pb is the barometric pressure, PH_2O corresponds to the partial pressure of water vapor at 37°C and R is the respiratory exchange ratio. However, the relationships between F_IO_2 and PaO_2 are also modulated by the degree of pulmonary $\dot{V}_A/Q$ inequality, as described in [1, 2, 4]. Total ventilation is considered an extrapulmonary factor because it is essentially set by the respiratory centers (central drive). The impact of $\dot{V}_E$ on respiratory blood gases (PaO_2 and $PaCO_2$) also varies with the degree of $\dot{V}_A/\dot{Q}$ mismatch (Fig. 2) [1, 2, 4]. However, as mentioned above, an increase in $\dot{V}_E$ is always more efficient in removing CO_2 from the blood than increasing O_2 uptake. Because the CO_2 dissociation curve is almost linear in its working range, an increase in $\dot{V}_E$ to a lung with substantial $\dot{V}_A/\dot{Q}$ inequality continues to be effective in eliminating more CO_2. This is why arterial PCO_2 is so sensitive to changes in $\dot{V}_E$ [19, 20]. It should be noted that the equation:

$$P_ACO_2 = K \cdot \dot{V}CO_2/\dot{V}_A$$

where P_ACO_2 is alveolar PO_2, K is a constant term, $\dot{V}CO_2$ is CO_2 output and $\dot{V}_A$ is alveolar ventilation can be meaningfully applied only to a single alveolar unit or to homogeneous healthy lung. But the above equation does not hold accurately to describe the relationships between $PaCO_2$ and $\dot{V}_E$ in diseased lungs because it is assumed that the mixed alveolar gas equals to the mixed arterial PCO_2. Yet, the latter two variables may be quite different when $\dot{V}_A/\dot{Q}$ abnormalities are present. Under these circumstances, hypercapnia does not necessarily imply a decrease in "effective" alveolar ventilation since there is no way of determining the latter other than by measuring $PaCO_2$ [19]. By contrast, because of the nonlinear O_2 dissociation curve an increase in $\dot{V}_E$ typically results in a modest gain in PaO_2 (Fig. 2). This is because the high $\dot{V}_A/\dot{Q}$ units that are operating on the "plateau" of the oxyhemoglobin dissociation curve are unable to compensate for the hypoxic blood associated with the presence of low $\dot{V}_A/\dot{Q}$ units.

It is important to emphasize the role of mixed venous PO_2 ($P\bar{v}O_2$) and how extrapulmonary factors (other than inspired PO_2 and total ventilation) may contribute to reduce PaO_2 through the effects on $P\bar{v}O_2$. In this regard, a diminished $P\bar{v}O_2$ may result from: 1) a low cardiac output; 2) an increased oxygen uptake; and/or 3) a decreased blood oxygen content due to several alterations in the principal factors modulating the oxyhemoglobin dissociation curve. It should be noted that the impact of $P\bar{v}O_2$ on arterial PO_2 also varies with the pattern of $\dot{V}_A/\dot{Q}$mismatch [1, 2, 5, 23] (Fig. 3).

In addition to the four primary extrapulmonary factors, secondary variables

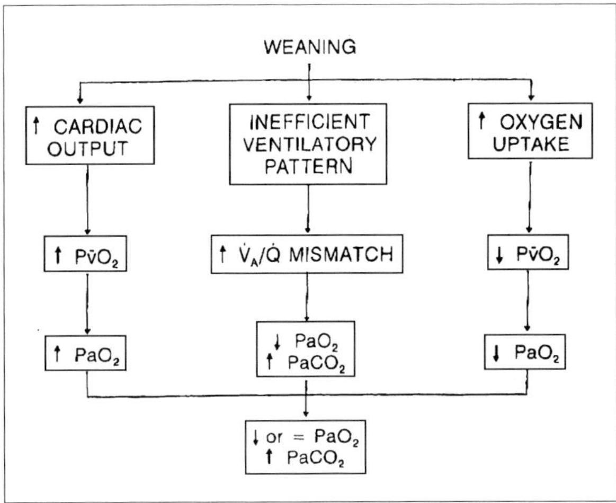

Fig. 2. Interplay between intrapulmonary and extrapulmonary factors influencing arterial PO_2, during ventilator weaning

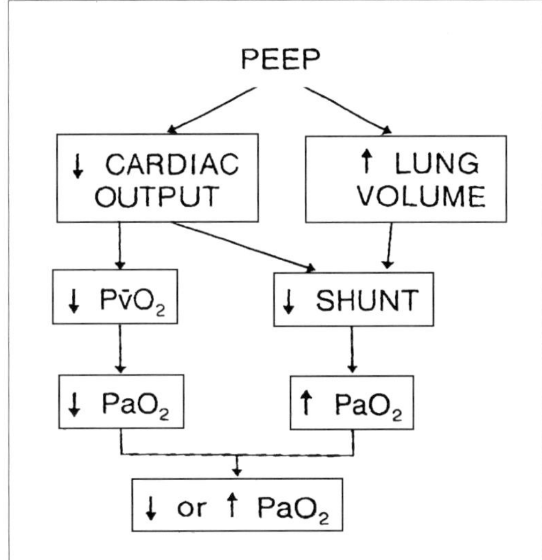

Fig.3. Application of external PEEP may reduce cardiac output and increases pulmonary functional residual capacity. The impact of the intrapulmonary and systemic factors ultimately determines Pao_2

such as hemoglobin concentration, hemoglobin P_{50}, body temperature, and blood acid-base status together play a secondary role in the clinical setting. Metabolic alkalosis deteriorates, in critically sick patients with more severe respiratory failure needing mechanical support, both intrapulmonary shunt and $\dot{V}_A/\dot{Q}$ imbalance, whereas its correction by hydrochloric acid improves overall pulmonary gas exchange [24]. The most likely mechanism is that acidosis ameliorates the intrapulmonary determinants of hypoxemia, possibly causing an enhancement of hypoxic pulmonary vasoconstriction, so that blood flow away is redistributed from the hypoxic areas of the lung; in contrast, shifts of the oxyhemoglobin dissociation curve related to the Bohr effect account for a marginal improvement in arterial oxygenation [24]. In a canine model of permeability pulmonary edema [25], metabolic acidosis improved arterial oxygenation; and *viceversa*, metabolic acidosis deteriorated it. Because cardiac output and minute ventilation remained unchanged, changes in intrapulmonary shunt and $\dot{V}_A/\dot{Q}$ mismatch, either enhancing or releasing hypoxic pulmonary vasoconstriction respectively, mostly influenced pulmonary gas exchange.

As described by West and Wagner [4], it is possible to predict the arterial PO_2 expected from the measured $\dot{V}_A/\dot{Q}$ inequality and the particular combination of extrapulmonary factors that existed at the time of measure. The MIGET algorithm, however, allows the observer to change any or all of the extrapulmonary factors (primary and/or secondary), and then to compute the expected value of arterial PO_2. Such a flexibility is useful to understand not only potential expected effects of therapeutic interventions, but also to separately determine the quantitative role of each extrapulmonary factor when they change between two conditions of MIGET measurement. This can be particularly useful to analyze the underlying physiologic effects of different ventilatory settings on arterial PO_2. For example, if weaning is initiated in a patient with chronic ostructive pulmonary disease (COPD), the change from mechanical ventilation to spontaneous breathing may increase cardiac output [26, 27] due to the increase in the pre-load of the right ventricle secondary to the marked increase of venous return. However, the $\dot{V}_A/\dot{Q}$ distribution may simultaneously change for the worse due to a less efficient ventilatory pattern. The latter will be due to a fall in tidal volume together with a simultaneous increase in respiratory rate (rapid and shallow breathing) while total $\dot{V}_E$ does not change [26, 27]. Arterial PO_2 will reflect the integrated effect of both phenomena (Fig. 2). To separately analyze the effect of the increase in cardiac output, it is a simple matter to execute the MIGET algorithm: a) with the data during mechanical ventilation; b) using the spontaneous breathing data with the cardiac output measured during mechanical ventilation; and c) using all spontaneous breathing data to assess the individual influences on arterial PO_2 of each factor. It is possible to use the $\dot{V}_A/\dot{Q}$ algorithm to differentiate separately, for example, the effect of increased intrapulmonary shunt versus that of $\dot{V}_A/\dot{Q}$ inequality on arterial PO_2.

Spontaneous versus mechanical ventilation

Gravity plays a key role in adjusting alveolar ventilation and pulmonary blood flow during spontaneously breathing and both mechanical ventilation. In the awake, spontaneously breathing individual, gravity establishes a vertical gradient of pleural pressure that augments the degree of ventilation at the lung bases provided that lung volumes remain unchanged. Similarly, gravity induces hydrostatic pressure differences from the top to the bottom of the lungs so that a vertical gradient of pulmonary perfusion facilitating the lower regions is created. As a consequence, the $\dot{V}_A/\dot{Q}$ ratio decreases down the lung because it is abnormally high at the top where the blood is minimal and much lower at the bottom [2].

It is important to note, however, that during mechanical ventilation this pattern is reversed such that regional ventilation is distributed preferentially to the nondependent regions, although the distribution of regional perfusion remains essentially unchanged. During positive-pressure ventilation, diaphragmatic movement is passive and has greater displacement in the nondependent areas, whereas the dependent zones are less compliant [28]. With mechanical ventilation, in the supine position an equal pressure is applied throughout the lung and is opposed by the hydrostatic pressure gradient of the abdomen. Yet, larger mechanical breaths facilitate an evener distribution of tidal volume with a diaphragm more evenly displaced, thus resulting in more ventilation and recruitment of the dependent regions of the lung [28].

Ventilatory strategy approaches

This section examines the gas exchange responses to different ventilatory modalities. Although assisted breaths during controlled mechanical ventilation are usually delivered via constant flow or a square wave flow waveform, other contours (accelerating or decelerating) of the inspiratory flow waveforms can be available in some ventilators. The effects of external positive end-expiratory pressure (PEEP) both in acute respiratory distress syndrome (ARDS) and chronic obstructive airway disease are analyzed as well as the comparison between application of equal levels of external PEEP and intrinsic PEEP (PEEPi) on arterial blood gases. External PEEP is also compared with alternative modes of mechanical ventilation in ARDS, such as inverse ratio ventilation and permissive hypercapnia. Modalities of partial ventilatory support and changes during weaning are also explored. Finally, potential mechanisms to explain the effects of non invasive positive pressure ventilation on arterial blood gases are described. Other ventilatory modalities with no information available using the MIGET (i.e. high frequency ventilation) will not be discussed.

Effects of inspiratory flow pattern

In a study by Modell and Cheney [29], in animals with normal lungs, the accelerating and decelerating patterns had no effect on gas exchange; in contrast, the decelerating waveform contour resulted, in oleic acid-injured lungs, in a rise in PaO_2 without differences in $PaCO_2$ or hemodynamics. It is suggested that the decelerating profile ventilated more efficiently those alveolar units with low $\dot{V}_A/\dot{Q}$ ratios, hence facilitating a better intrapulmonary gas mixing. If no significant $\dot{V}_A/\dot{Q}$ imbalance exists, oxygenation in all regions would be adequate without need for additional gas mixing time. When ventilatory parameters (tidal volume, inspiratory time, inspiratory-expiratory ratio and respiratory frequency) were kept constant, in patients with respiratory insufficiency needing mechanical support, the decelerating waveform profile improved overall gas exchange, as assessed by arterial blood gases, and lung mechanics [30]. This amelioration of gas exchange supports the view that the decelerating waveform improves both gas distribution and uptake within the lung without detrimental effects on hemodynamics. In a methacholine porcine lung model, no inspiratoy flow pattern studied offered a unique advantage for gas exchange, although peak tracheal pressure was significantly lower with decelerating flow [31].

Application of external PEEP in ARDS patients, in whom increased intrapulmonary shunt is the key factor disturbing pulmonary gas exchange, has been demonstrated to be an effective tool to manage refractory hypoxemia [32-35]. External PEEP increases functional residual capacity but two different responses in terms of lung mechanics have been reported [36]. When the static volume-pressure curve at zero PEEP exhibits a concave shape with a progressive increase in slope with increasing volume, application of PEEP results in alveolar recruitment (reopening of collapsed alveoli). In contrast, in those patients exhibiting a convex volume-pressure curve at baseline (PEEP=0), application of PEEP only enhances overdistension of the functional alveolar units but no alveolar recruitment is observed. Parallel findings of PEEP application are a reduction in cardiac output, due to the increase in intrathoracic pressure, and a redistribution of extravascular lung water from alveoli to peribronchial and perivascular spaces [37].

The effects of PEEP on $\dot{V}_A/\dot{Q}$ distributions in ARDS are, as illustrated in Figure 3, reduction in intrapulmonary shunt, broadening of the dispersion of ventilation distribution, and increase in dead space. The decrease in intrapulmonary shunt can be explained by:

1. reopening of collapsed alveoli with redistribution of pulmonary blood flow from severely injured (shunt) areas to poorly or normally ventilated alveolar units;
2. fall in cardiac output;
3. the combined effect of these two mechanisms.

Recruitment of alveolar units and redistribution of pulmonary blood flow within the lung is the main beneficial effect of PEEP that, in some instances, may give rise to an increase in low $\dot{V}_A/\dot{Q}$ areas. If we apply the PEEP, the lung is more efficient in terms of O_2 uptake and slightly less efficient as a CO_2 exchanger. A fundamental clinical benefit of PEEP is that the changes in $\dot{V}_A/\dot{Q}$ distribution allow O_2 therapy to be effective.

Moreover, since PEEP decreases the number of "critical" lung units [32, 38], high F_IO_2 can be used more safely with less likelihood of reabsorption atelectasis. However, a potential negative effect to be taken into account is that the fall in cardiac output with PEEP may facilitate a decrease in systemic O_2 delivery. It is of note that the different studies [32-35] have shown some degree of individual variation in terms of the beneficial response to PEEP which cannot be predicted by the etiology of ARDS or the underlying severity of abnormal gas exchange. However, an acceptable correlation seems to exist between the characteristics of the static volume pressure curve measured at zero PEEP and the gas exchange response to different levels of PEEP [36].

Application of PEEP in ARDS patients illustrates a good example of the interactions between intrapulmonary and extrapulmonary determinants of arterial blood gases. Arterial PO_2 increases during PEEP if beneficial effects on gas exchange, essentially the reduction of intrapulmonary shunt (intrapulmonary factor), are not offset by the simultaneous deleterious effect on PaO_2 secondary to decreased cardiac output (extrapulmonary factor), which would cause mixed venous PO_2 to decrease, other factors being equal. However, it should be noted that the interactions among the factors determining mixed venous PO_2 (cardiac output, tissue O_2 extraction and arteria O_2 content) can be particularly complex in ARDS patients [5, 6, 39].

Traditionally, the use of external PEEP has been discouraged in chronic airway disease to prevent the risk of barotrauma due to excessive pulmonary hyperinflation. However, alveolar pressure in patients with acute or chronic airway disease may remain positive throughout the ventilatory cycle without any PEEP set by the ventilator, because expiratory flow limitation prevents complete expiration within the time available to, so that both dynamic hyperinflation and intrinsic PEEP (PEEPi) occur [40-42]. It has been shown that, in these patients, application of low values of PEEP does not increase intrathoracic pressure and lung volumes, because PEEP replaces PEEPi; until a critical value slightly lower than the initial PEEPi (approximately 75%-80%) is achieved [43-46]. Under these circumstances, PEEP counterbalances PEEPi, and reduces the magnitude of the inspiratory effort required either to trigger the ventilator or to resume spontaneous breathing. The effects of two levels of PEEP, 50% and 100% of PEEPi, on $\dot{V}_A/\dot{Q}$ distributions were recently examined by Rossi et al. [47] in mechanically ventilated patients with chronic airway disease during acute exacerbation. It was shown that moderate values of PEEP (50% of PEEPi) did not provoke significant changes in airway pressure, pulmonary hemodynamics nor in mixed venous PO_2, whereas when PEEP equaled PEEPi (100% PEEPi) airway pressure increased slightly but significantly. More importantly, application of PEEP amounting to 50% of PEEPi caused the highest improvement in overall gas exchange. A slight but significant increase in the first moment of both perfusion and ventilation distributions was observed, resulting in a mild but significant increase in PaO_2 and in a trend to reduce $PaCO_2$. Therefore, in contrast to the traditional view, these results provide further support to the use of low levels of external PEEP in mechanically ventilated patients with chronic obstructive airway disease, although caution and close adequate monitoring of the patient's condition are mandatory.

Inverse ratio ventilation (IRV) has been proposed as an alternative ventilatory strategy in patients with ARDS to improve gas exchange at lower than conventional lung peak distending pressure and PEEP, thereby decreasing the risk of barotrauma [48]. Three different potential mechanisms have been invoked to explain improvement of PaO_2 with IRV: 1) higher mean airway pressure [49], 2) PEEPi elicited by the short expiratory time [50-53], and 3) improved distribution of inspired gas due to the low mean inspiratory flow [54-56]. However, the discrepant results obtained in clinical studies [51, 55, 57-64] do not suggest a predominant mechanism for IRV to improve gas exchange nor provide evidence whether IRV offers any real, even short-term, benefit over conventional controlled mechanical ventilation with PEEP. This is particularly true when comparison is made at similar levels of both end-expiratory pressure [52, 63] and volume [65], while the ventilatory variables are adequately controlled [64]. Recently, we assessed the effects of short-term application of four different ventilatory conditions on $\dot{V}_A/\dot{Q}$ inequality [66]: 1) controlled mechanical ventilation without PEEP (CMV); 2) volume-controlled mechanical ventilation with PEEP (CMV-PEEP); 3) volume-controlled IRV (VC-IRV); and, 4) pressure-controlled IRV (PC-IRV). The comparison among the CMV-PEEP, VC-IRV and PC-IRV settings was done at the same level of total end expiratory pressure (on average 8 cm H_2O), the other ventilatory settings being kept constant. As expected, CMV-PEEP significantly increased PaO_2 due to a significant fall in the amount of intrapulmonary shunt. Since cardiac output did not change and lung elastance showed a tendency to increase, the improvement in intrapulmonary shunt during CMV-PEEP could be attributed to recruitment of previously non-ventilated alveolar units [67]. Similar to the results reported by Brandolese [52], improvement in PaO_2 with VC-IRV was lower than that seen with CMV-PEEP. Such a rise in PaO_2 during VC-IRV was caused by a small fall in intrapulmonary shunt together with a moderate increase to PEEP after acute oleic acid lung injury.

Noninvasive positive pressure ventilation

The clinical interest of using non invasive positive pressure ventilation to prevent orotracheal intubation in patients with acute respiratory failure [68-71], as well as to manage clinically stable patients with severe restrictive ventilatory diseases is a relatively new modality of ventilatory support rapidly and positively accepted by both the chest and intensive care community. Future applications of this ventilatory modality as a weaning strategy and its usefulness in clinically stable patients with severe obstructive ventilatory limitation are under analysis. However, the underlying mechanisms by which non invasive ventilation reduces arterial PCO_2 and increases PaO_2 are still controversial. Historically, three different hypotheses [72] have been suggested to this respect. The rest theory proposes that hypercapnic chronic respiratory failure is associated with chronic respiratory fatigue [73]. However, the existence of the latter has been never clearly demonstrated nor has any study shown that respiratory muscle rest is necessary for improving daytime gas exchange or symptoms [16, 25, 34]. A second hypothesis postulates that non-invasive ventilation increases lung compliance, hence reopening alveolar units. Thirdly, it also has been proposed that respiratory center sensitivity to CO_2 is blunted in these patients. Intermittent non-invasive ventilation, by preventing nocturnal hypoventilation, would allow the resetting of respiratory center sensitivity to CO_2 and daytime gas exchange improvement [72]. These two last contentions are not mutually exclusive and can contribute more or less depending upon individual clinical conditions of the patient. However, preliminary data [77] collected in patients with COPD during an acute episode of respiratory failure indicate that alternative explanations for the beneficial effect of non-invasive ventilation on respiratory blood gases should be taken into account. These data show that increase in total ventilation and its two components (decrease in respiratory rate and higher tidal volume) with no changes in inert gas dead space were key factors to provoke a right-shift of the ventilation distribution and an reduction in its dispersion. Both changes may improve alveolar PCO_2, hence, increasing PaO_2 and reducing $PaCO_2$.

Both, intrapulmonary shunt and low $\dot{V}_A/\dot{Q}$ areas remained essentially unchanged during this ventilatory approach. It is of note that cardiac output significantly fell but its deleterious effect on mixed venous PO_2 was fully counterbalanced by: 1) an increase in both the first moment of the perfusion and ventilation distributions (this would increase alveolar PO_2 and decreased alveolar PCO_2, other things being equal); and 2) a trend to decreased respiratory muscle O_2 uptake.

In summary, arterial respiratory blood gases significantly improved by the concomitant effect of their intrapulmonary ($\dot{V}_A/\dot{Q}$ distributions) and extrapulmonary (overall ventilation, cardiac output, O_2 uptake) factors. Short-term application of non invasive mechanical ventilation in these patients did not show evidence of alveolar recruitment. Further examination of the effects of non-invasive positive pressure ventilation on pulmonary gas exchange needs to be done in longer serial studies in this type of COPD patients and, also, in clinically stable subjects with a restrictive ventilatory defects namely neuromuscular diseases, thoracic wall deformities, and hypoventilation-obesity syndrome.

References

1. West JB (1969) Ventilation-perfusion inequality and overall gas exchange in computer models of the lung. Respir Physiol 7:88-110
2. West JB (1977) Ventilation-perfusion relationships. Am Rev Respir Dis 116:919-943
3. Roca J, Wagner PD (1993) Contribution of multiple inert gas elimination technique to pulmonary medicine (1): principles and information content of the multiple inert gas elimination technique. Thorax 49:815-824
4. West JB, Wagner PD (1977) Pulmonary gas exchange. In: West JB (ed) Bioengineering aspects of the lung, 1st ed. Marcel Dekker, New York, pp 361-457
5. Dantzker DR (1983) The influence of cardiovascular function on gas exchange. Clin Chest Med 4:149-159
6. Wagner PD (1982) Ventilation-perfusion inequality in catastrophic lung disease. In: O Prakash (ed) Applied physiology in clinical respiratory care. Martinus Nijhoff, The Hague, pp 363-379
7. Light RB (1988) Intrapulmonary oxygen consumption in experimental pneumococcal pneumonia. J Appl Physiol 64:2490-2495
8 Wagner PD, Saltzman HA, West JB (1974) Measurements of continuous distributions of ventilation-perfusion ratios: theory. J Appl Physiol 36:588-599
9. Wagner PD, Naumann PF, Laravuso RB, West JB (1974) Simultaneous measurement of eight foreign gases in blood by gas chromatography. J Appl Physiol 36:600-605
10. Evans IW, Wagner PD (1977) Limits on VA/Q distributions from analysis of experimental inert gas elimination. J Appl Physiol 36:600-605
11. Wagner PD (1979) Susceptibility of different gases to ventilation-perfusion inequality. J Appl Physiol 46:372-386
12. Wagner PD, Laravuso RB, Uhl RR, West JB (1974) Continuous distributions of ventilation-perfusion ratios in normal subjects breathing air and 100% O_2. J Clin Invest 54:54-68
13. West JB (1985) Ventilation-blood flow and gas exchange, 4th ed. Blackwell Scientific Publications, Oxford
14. Gale GE, Torre-Bueno J, Moon RE, Salzman HA, Wagner PD (1985) Ventilation-perfusion inequality in normal humans during exercise. J Appl Physiol 58:978-988
15. Wagner PD, Gale GE, Torre-Bueno JE, Stoip BW, Saltzman HA (1986) Pulmonary gas

exchange in humans exercising at sea level and simulated altitude. J Appl Physlol 61:260-270
16. Hammond MD, Gale GE, Kapitan KS, Ries A, Wagner PD (1986) Pulmonary gas exchange in humans during normobaric hypoxic exercise. J Appl Physiol 60:1590-1598
17. Hammond MD, Gale GE, Kapitan KS, Ries A, Wagner PD (1985) Pulmonary gas exchange in humans during normobaric hypoxic exercise. J Appl Physiol. 58:978-988
18. Cardús J, Burgos F, Diaz O, Roca J, Barberà JA, Marrades RM, Rodriguez-Roisin R, Wagner PD (1997) Increase in pulmonary ventilation-perfusion inequality with age in healthy individuals. Am J Resp Crit Care Med 156(2):648-653
19. West JB (1971) Causes of carbon dioxide retention in lung disease. New Engl J Med 284:1232-1236
20. Weinberger SE, Wchwartzstein RM, Weis JW (1989) Hypercapnia. New Engl J Med 321:1223-1231
21. Agustí AG, Roca J, Rodriguez-Roisin R, Gea J, Xaubet A, Wagner PD (1991) Mechanisms of gas exchange impairment in idiopathic pulmonary fibrosis. Am Rev Respir Dis 143:219-225
22. Rodriguez-Roisin R, Agustí AG, Roca J (1992) The hepatopulmonary syndrome: new name, old complexities (Editorial). Thorax 47:897-902
23. Hansen JE, Clausen JL, Levy SE, Mohler IG, Van Kessel AL (1986) Proficiency testing materials for pH and blood gases. The California Thoracic Society Experience. Chest 89:214-217
24. Brimouille S, Kahn RJ (1990) Effects of metabolic acidosis on pulmonary gas exchange. Am Rev Respir Dis 141:1185-1189
25. Brimouille S, Vachiery JL, Lejeune P, Leeman M, Melot C, Naeije R (1991) Acid-base status affects gas exchange in canine oleic acid pulmonary edema. Am J Physiol 260:H1080-H1086.
26. Torres A, Reyes A, Roca J, Wagner PD, Rodriguez-Roisin R (1989) Ventilation-perfusion mismatching in chronic obstructive pulmonary disease during ventilator weaning. Am Rev Respir Dis. 140:1246-1250
27. Lemaire F, Teboul JL, Cinotti L et al (1988) Acute left ventricular dysfunction during unsuccessful weaning from mechanical ventilation. Anesthesiology 69:171-179
28. Froese AB, Bryan AB (1974) Effect of anesthesia and paralysis on diaphragmatic mechanics in man. Anesthesiology 41:242-245
29. Modell HI, Cheney FW (1979) Effects of inspiratory flow pattern on gas exchange in normal and abnormal lung. J Appl Physiol 46:1103-1107
30. Al-Saad N, Bennet ED (1985) Decelerating inspiratory flow waveform improves lung mechanics and gas exchange in patients on intermittent positive-pressure ventilation. Intensive Care Med 11:68-75
31. Smith RA, Venus B (1988) Cardiopulmonary effect of various inspiratory flow profiles during controlled mechanical ventilation in a porcine lung model. Crit Care Med 16:769-772
32. Dantzker DR, Brook L, DeHart P, Lynch J, Weg J (1979) Ventilation-perfusion distribution in the adult respiratory distress syndrome. Am Rev Respir Dis 120:1039-1052
33. Matamis D, Lemaire F, Harf A, et al (1984) Redistribution of pulmonary blood flow induced by positive end-expiratory pressure and dopamine infusion in acute respiratory failure. Am Rev Respir Dis 129:39-44
34. Ralph DD, Robertson HT, Weaver LJ et al (1985) Distribution of ventilation and perfusion during positive end-expiratory pressure in the adult respiratory distress syndrome. Am Rev Respir Dis 131:54-60

35. Coffey RL, Albert RK, Robertson HT (1983) Mechanism of physiological dead space response to PEEP after acute oleic acid lung injury. J Appl Physiol Respir Environ Exer Physiol 55:1550-1557
36. Ranieri MV, Giuliani R, Fiore T, Dambrosio M, Milic-Emili J (1994) Volume-pressure curve of the respiratory system predicts effects of PEEP in ARDS: "occlusion" versus "constant flow" technique. Am J Respir Crit Care Med 149:19-27
37. Hopewell PC, Murray JF (1975) Effects of continuous positive-pressure ventilation in experimental pulmonary edema. J Appl Physiol 39:672-679
38. Dantzker DR, Wagner PD, West JB (1975) Instability of lung units with low VA/Q ratios during O_2 breathing. J Appl Physiol 38:886
39. Rodriguez-Roisin R (1994) Effect of mechanical ventilation on gas exchange. In: Tobin MJ (ed) Principles and practice of mechanical ventilation, 1st ed. McGraw-Hill, New York, pp 673-693
40. Pepe PP, Marini JJ (1982) Occult positive end-expiratory pressure in mechanically ventilated patients with airflow obstruction. Am Rev Respir Dis 126:166-170
41 Rossi A, Gottfried SB, Zocchi L, Higgs BD, Lennox S, Calverley PMA, Begin P, Grassino A, Milic-Emili J (1982) Measurement of static compliance of the total respiratory system in patients with acute respiritory failure during mechanical ventilation. Am Rev Respir Dis 131:672-677
42. Kimball WR, Leith DE, Robins AG (1982) Dynamic hyperinflation and ventilator dependence in chronic obstructive pulmonary disease. Am Rev Respir Dis. 126:991-995
43. Guy PC, Rodarte JR, and Hubmayr RD (1987) The effect of positive-expiratory pressure on isovolume and dynamic hyperinflation in patients receiving mechanical ventilation. Am Rev Respir Dis 139:621-626
44. Tuxen DV (1989) Detrimental effects of positive end expiratory pressure during controlled mechanical ventilation. Am Rev Respir Dis 140:5-9
45. Rossi A, Brandolese R, Milic-Emili J, Gottfried SB (1990) The role of PEEP in patients with chronic obstructive pulmonary disease during assisted ventilation. Eur Respir J 3:818-822
46. Ranieri VM, Giuliani R, Cinnella G, Pesce C, Brienza N, Ippolito EL, Pomo Y, Fiore T, Gottfried SB, Brienza A (1993) Physiologic effects of positive end-expiratory pressure in patients with chronic obstructive pulmonary disease during acute ventilatory failure and controlled mechanical ventilation. Am Rev Respir Dis 177:5-13
47. Ross A, Santos C, Roca J, Torres A, Félez MA, Rodriguez-Roisin R (1994) Effects of PEEP on (VA/Q) mismatching in ventilated patients with chronic airflow obstruction. Am J Respir Crit Care Med 149:1077-1084
48. Marcy TW (1994) Inverse ratio ventilation. In: Tobin MJ (ed) Principles and practice of mechanical ventilation, 1st ed. McGraw-Hill, New York, pp 319-331
49. Gattinoni L, Marcolin R, Caspani M, Fumagali R, Mascheroni D, Pesenti A (1985) Constant mean airway pressure with different patterns of positive pressure breathing during the adult respiratory distress syndrome. Bull Eur Physiopathol Respir 21:275-279
50. Duncan S, Rizk N, Raffin T (1987) Inverse ratio ventilation. PEEP in disguise? Chest 92:390-391
51. East T, Bohm S, Wallace J, Clemmer T, Weaver L, Orme J, Morris A (1992) A successful computerized protocol for clinical management of pressure control inverse ratio ventilation in ARDS patients. Chest 101:697-710
52. Brandolese RC, Broseghini C, Polese G, Bernasconi M, Brandi G, Milic-Emili J, Rossi A (1992) Effects of intrinsic PEEP on pulmonary gas exchange in mechanically-ventilated patients. Eur Respir J 6:358-363

53. Bernard G, Artigas A, Brighman K, Carlet J, Falke K, Hudson L, Lamy M, Legall J, Morris A, Spragg R (1994) The American-European Consensus Conference on ARDS. Definitions, mechanisms, relevant outcomes, and clinical trial coordination. Am J Respir Crit Care Med 149:818-824
54. Hubmayr R, Abel M, Rehder K (1990) Physiologic approach to mechanical ventilation. Crit Care Med 18:103-113
55. Manthous C, Schimidt G (1993) Inverse ratio ventilation in ARDS. Improved oxygenation without AutoPEEP. Chest 103:953-954
56. Marini JJ (1994) Ventilation of the acute respiratory distress syndrome. Looking for Mr. Goodmode. Anesthesiology 80:972-975
57. Gurevitch M, Van Dyke J, Young E, Jackson K (1986) Improved oxygenation and lower peak airway pressure in severe adult respiratory distress syndrome. Treatment with inverse ratio ventilation. Chest 89:211-213
58. Tharratt R, Allen R, Albertson T (1988) Pressure controlled inverse ratio ventilation in severe adult respiratory failure. Chest 94:755-762
59. Lain D, Di Benedetto R, Morris S, Van Nguyen A, Saulters R, Causey D (1989) Pressure control inverse ratio ventilation as a method to reduce peak inspiratory pressure and provide adequate ventilation and oxygenation. Chest 95:1081-1088
60. Abraham E, Yoshihara G (1989) Cardiorespiratory effects of pressure controlled inverse ratio ventilation in severe respiratory failure. Chest 96:1356-1359
61. Poelaert J, Vogelaers D, Colardyn F (1991) Evaluation of the hemodynamic and respiratory effects of inverse ratio ventilation with a right ventricular ejection fraction catheter. Chest 99:1444-1450
62. Chan K, Abraham E (1992) Effects of inverse ratio ventilation on cardiorespiratory parameters in severe respiratory failure. Chest 102:1556-1561
63. Mercat A, Graïni L, Teboul J, Lenique F, Richard C (1993) Cardiorespiratory effects of pressure-controlled ventilation with and without inverse ratio in the adult respiratory distress syndrome. Chest 104:871-875
64. Lessard M, Guérot E, Lorino H, Lemaire F, Brochard L (1994) Effects of pressure-controled with different I:E ratios versus volume-controlled ventilation on respiratory mechanics, gas exchange, and hemodynamics in patients with adult respiratory distress syndrome. Anesthesiology 80:972-975
65. Cole A, Weller S, Sykes M (1984) Inverse ratio ventilation compared with PEEP in adult respiratory failure. Intensive Care Med 10:227-232
66. Zavala E, Ferrer M, Polese G, Masclans JR, Planas M, Milic-Emili J, Rodriguez-Roisin R, Roca J, Rossi A (1996) Effects of PEEPi generated by inverse I:E ratio ventilation on pulmonary gas exchange in ARDS. Am J Respir Crit Care Med 153:A374
67. Rossi A, Ranieri M (1994) Positive End-Expiratory Pressure. In: Tobin M (ed) Principles and practice of mechanical ventilation, 1st ed. Mc Graw-Hill, New York, pp 259-303
68. Brochard L, Isabey D, Piquet I, Amaro P, Mancebo J, Messadi AA, Brun-Buisson C, Rauss A, Lemaire F, Harf A (1990) Reversal of acute exacerbations of chronic obstructive lung disease by inspiratory assistance with a face mask. New Engl Med 323:1523-1530
69. Kramer N, Meyer TJ, Meharg J, Cece RD, Hill NS (1995) Randomized, prospective trial of noninvasive positive pressure ventilation in acute respiratory failure. Am J Respir Crit Care Med 151:1799-1806
70. Appendini L, Patessio A, Zanaboni S, Carone M, Gukov B, Donner CF, Rossi A (1994) Physiologic effects of positive end-expiratory pressure and mask pressure support during exacerbations of chronic obstructive pulmonary disease. Am J Respir Crit Care Med 149:1069-1076

71. Bott J, Carroll MP, Conway JH, Keilty SEJ, Ward EM, Brown AM, Paul EA, Elliott MW, Godfrey RC, Wedzicha JA, Moxham J (1993) Randomised controlled trial of nasal ventilation in acute ventilatory failure due to chronic obstructive airways disease. Lancet 341:1555-1557
72. Hill NS (1993) Noninvasive ventilation. Does it work, for whom, and how? Am Rev Respir Dis 147:1050-1055
73. Roussos C (1985) Function and fatigue of respiratory muscles. Chest 88:1245-1315
74. Gay PC, Patel AM, Viggiano RW, Hubmayr RD (1991) Nocturnal nasal ventilation for treatment of patients with hypercapneic respiratory failure. Mayo Clin Proc 66:695-703
75. Mohr CH, Hill NS (1990) Long-term follow-up of nocturnal ventilatory assistance in patients with respiratory failure due to Duchenne-type muscular dystrophy. Chest 97:91-96
76. Elliot MW, Mulvey DA, Moxham J, Green M, Bronthwaite MA (1991) Domiciliary nocturnal nasal intermittent positive pressure ventilation in COPD: mechanisms underlying changes in arterial blood gas tensions. Eur Respir J 4:1044-1052
77. Ferrer M, Iglesia R, Roca J, Escarrabil J, Farrero E, Gómez FP, Farré R, Barberà JA, Rodriguez-Roisin R (1998) Factors determining PaO_2 during noninvasive ventilation in clinically stable chronic respiratory failure. Am J Respir Crit Care Med 157(3): A370

Chapter 20

Effects of anaesthesia on respiratory mechanics

G. Hedenstierna

Anaesthesia has effects on both the mechanics of the respiratory system and pulmonary gas exchange. Thus, the respiratory system appears to be stiffer, i.e. the compliance is reduced, than in the awake state and the resistance to breathing is increased. The effects on gas exchange result in impairment of blood oxygenation and sometimes also in less efficient elimination of CO_2. Several of the pioneering studies in this field were published in the 1950s [1-3]. During the forty years that have elapsed after these initial reports, there is increasing evidence that the changes in respiratory mechanics are the cause of gas exchange impairment. Thus, understanding respiratory mechanics during anaesthesia may guide in the understanding impaired gas exchange as well as in promoting techniques that counter the deterioration in gas exchange. This review will analyse the effects of anaesthesia on respiratory mechanics and the corresponding morphological correlates, and then relate gas exchange impairment to the anaesthesia-induced mechanical and morphological changes.

Compliance and resistance of the respiratory system

In 1955, Nims and co-workers [1] found that the static compliance in the total respiratory system (lungs and chest wall) was reduced from 95 to 60 ml/cm H_2O during anaesthesia.

Several studies have since then confirmed this observation (for a review, see Don [4]). The vast majority of studies on lung compliance carried out during anaesthesia indicates a decrease compared to the awake state (i.e. static compliance fell from mean 187 ml/cm H_2O awake to 149 ml/cm H_2O during anaesthesia in the review by Don [4]). Westbrook and co-workers [5] found a marked right-shift of the pressure-volume curve of the lung (more recoil pressure or force to decrease lung volume at a given volume) during anaesthesia. There was also a minor right shift at low lung volume of the curve of the chest wall (reduced "expansion pressure"), both of which contribute to the reduction of functional residual capacity (FRC) (Fig. 1). Westbrook and coworkers found no further effect on the pressure-volume curve by muscle paralysis [5]. This supports the hypothesis, initially put forward by Nims et al. [1], that the anaesthetic per se reduces the respiratory muscle tone, "decreases the "expansion pressure" and lowers FRC. If so, paralysis of muscles should cause no further change in the pressure-volume curves and no further decrease in FRC. Rehder and co-workers analysed possible sources of reduced compliance during anaesthesia

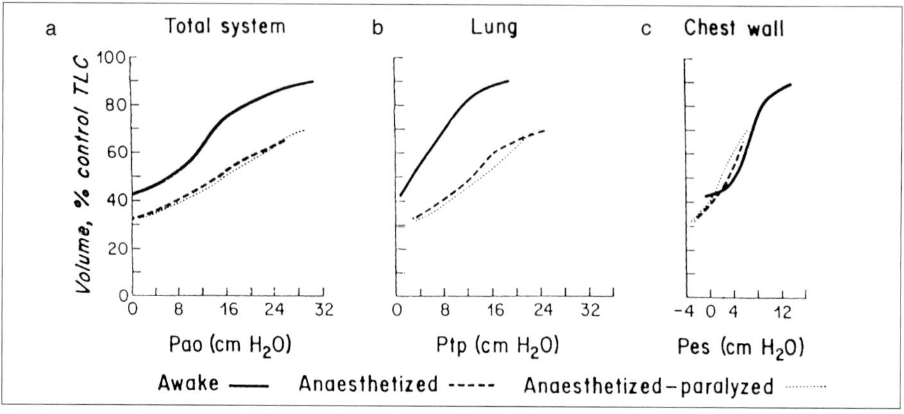

Fig. 1 a-c. Pressure-volume curves of the total respiratory system (left panel), the lung (mid panel) and the chest wall (right panel) awake and during anaesthesia without and with muscle paralysis. Note the right shift and flatter slope of the curves of the total system and of the lung (reduced compliance) during anaesthesia and the minor effect of adding muscle paralysis. The pressure-volume curve of the chest wall remains much the same awake and anaesthetised. *Pao*, airways opening (wouth) pressure; *Ptp*, transpulmonary (Pao-Pes) pressure; *Pes*, esophageal pressure. (From [5] with permission)

[6]. They considered direct anaesthetic effects on the lung tissue rather unlikely, but were unable at that time to evaluate possible effects of airway closure and atelectasis. These two phenomena will be discussed in more detail in the following sections. Here, it will just be mentioned that it is common opinion that formation of atelectasis or consolidation of lung tissue, i.e., in ARDS, lower compliance. That the compliance reflects the amount of normally aerated lung tissue in ARDS, has led Gattinoni and co-workers to coin the expression "baby lung" [7]. When atelectasis during anaesthesia (see the section on Atelectasis) is reopened by a large inflation of the lung, compliance is mostly increased [8]. Interestingly, compliance decreased over time after such an inflation, whether atelectasis reappeared or not (Fig. 2). This suggests that additional factors, besides atelectasis and amount of aerated lung tissue, determine compliance during anaesthesia. One possible contributor may be changes in the amount or effect of surfactant [9]. It is thus obvious that work still remains to be done to clarify why compliance is reduced during anaesthesia.

There are also studies on the resistance of the total respiratory system and the lungs during anaesthesia, most showing a considerable increase during both spontaneous breathing and mechanical ventilation [4, 6]. However, studies on resistance during anaesthesia have been hampered by different experimental conditions during the awake and anaesthetised situations. Thus, a study that enables comparison of resistance under both isovolume and isoflow conditions is still missing. The possibility remains that the increased lung resistance merely reflects a reduced FRC during anaesthesia which will be discussed in the next paragraphs.

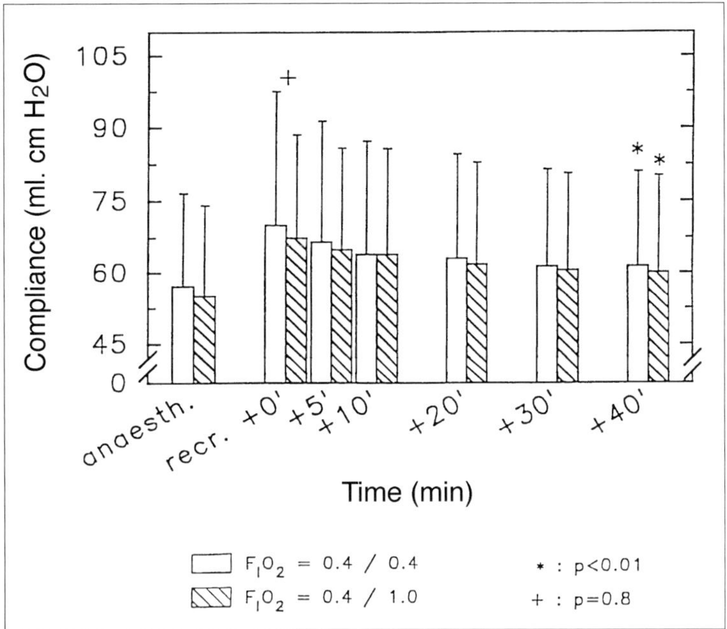

Fig. 2. Compliance of the total respiratory system before and after a so-called vital capacity manoeuvre that opens up atelectatic lung tissue (mean and SD). The x-axis shows events and time in minutes. Open columns, results from 6 patients ventilated with 40% O_2 in nitrogen before and after the recruitment manoeuvre. Dashed columns, results from another 6 patients ventilated with 40% O_2 before and 100% O_2 after the recruitment manoeuvre. Note that compliance is increased by the vital capacity manoeuvre (Time 0), but that it decreases slowly thereafter in both groups. This was unexpected since the patients ventilated with 40% O_2 all the time did not show much atelectasis after the vital capacity manoeuvre, whereas the patients on 100% O_2 after the manoeuvre rapidly developped atelectasis (compare with Fig. 6). Anaesth, anaesthesia; recr, recruitment manueuvre. (From [8] with permission)

Diaphragm shape and position

Several studies suggest that the diaphragm moves cephalad during anaesthesia which contributes to the decrease in functional residual capacity (FRC) [10, 11] (Fig. 3). A cephalad displacement of the diaphragm may be explained by loss of respiratory muscle tone, allowing the abdominal content to push the diaphragm cranially. The major findings of a study by my colleagues and I were that the whole diaphragm dome moved cephalad during anaesthesia and muscle paralysis, and less so when the diaphragm was not paralysed [12]. In addition, mechanical ventilation decreased the inspiratory displacement of the dependent part of the diaphragm compared with its movement during conscious, spontaneous breathing.

However, other groups have obtained different results. In studies by Krayer and co-workers [13] the diaphragm, on an average, did not move cephalad during anaesthesia in the supine patient (Fig. 3). Warner and co-workers [14]

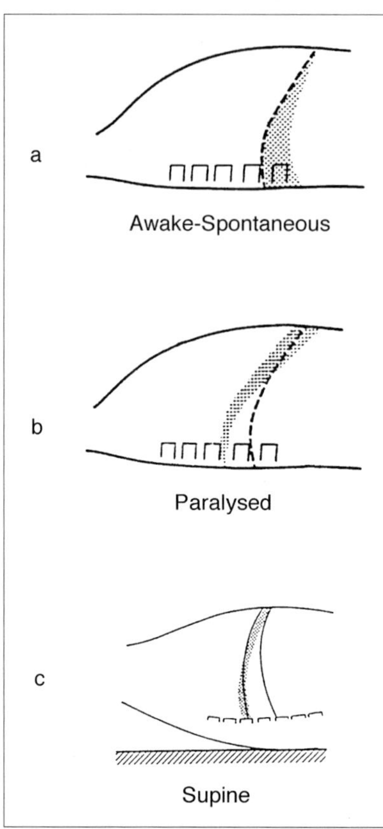

Fig. 3 a-c. Diaphragm position and movement. (a) awake, during spontaneous breathing; (b) during anaesthesia with muscle paralysis and mechanical ventilation; (c) also during anaesthesia and mechanical ventilation but from another study with a different result. Dashed curve (a and b) and left-most continuous curve (c) show the position of the diaphragm at FRC awake. Stippled area shows the displacement of the diaphragm during tidal ventilation. Note the cranial shift of the diaphragm during anaesthesia in b and less so in c. Note also the different excursions while awake vs. anaesthetised. (Panels a and b from [11] and panel c from [13] with permission)

observed regional differences in diaphragm displacement with cephalad movement of the posterior region and caudal movement of the anterior region.

In the cited studies, different techniques have been used, although all have been based on radiological principles. Thus, in the pioneering work of Froese and Bryan from 1974, cineradiography was used [11]. Warner and co-workers used a specially designed X-ray computed tomography (CT) scanner that enabled a large number of exposures simultaneously [14]. In the study from my group, spiral CT was used [12]. Spiral CT seems to offer the highest resolution of the three techniques, but requires a prolonged apnea time that may allow movement of the diaphragm during exposure, in particular in the awake subject. The multiexposure technique that has been used by the Mayo Clinic group [13, 14] does not suffer from any significant influence of time, but the resolution was not clearly described in their papers. Finally, the cineradiography used by Froese and Bryan [11] has the advantage of a good time resolution but is two-dimensional and requires exposures in two planes to enable a three-dimensional reconstruction.

Lung volume

The resting lung volume, or functional residual capacity (FRC), is reduced during anaesthesia. The supine body position by itself reduces FRC by 0.7-0.8 l compared with the upright position, so that the further decrease of 0.4-0.5 l caused by the anaesthesia decreases the FRC to close to the awake residual volume. The reduction in FRC occurs with spontaneous breathing and whether the anaesthetic is inhaled or given intravenously [15]. Muscle paralysis and mechanical ventilation cause no further decrease in FRC. The average reduction corresponds to around 20% of the awake FRC and may contribute to an altered distribution of ventilation and impaired oxygenation of blood, as will be discussed later.

Using computed tomography (CT) a decrease in the chest area has been demonstrated during anaesthesia whereas reports on the shape and position of the diaphragm differ, as discussed above. Many studies, including that of my colleagues and me, suggest that the diaphragm is moved cephalad during anaesthesia, and so contributes to the decrease in FRC. By combining computed tomography, lung volume measurement by gas dilution and recording of central blood volume and extravascular lung water by double indicator dilution technique, a comprehensive analysis of chest dimensions and structure was made [16]. The fall in FRC by 0.4 was accompanied by a small blood volume shift from the thorax to the abdomen during anaesthesia and positive pressure ventilation, and a cranial shift of the diaphragm corresponding to the net change in gas and blood in the lung, of approximately 0.8.

Airway closure

In awake, healthy human volunteers, airways in dependent lung regions close during a deep expiration [17]. Gas can be trapped in the lungs during anaesthesia and can be released by deep inflations [18]. This suggests that airway closure occurs during ordinary breathing in the anaesthetised patient although conflicting results have also been obtained [19, 20]. It has also been shown that a decrease of FRC during anaesthesia below the awake closing capacity (CC) (the lung volume at which airways close) was accompanied by a significantly larger shunt (mean 11%) than when FRC during anaesthesia was larger than awake CC (mean 2%) [21]. In a recent study by Rothen et al. [22], airway closure was studied by the helium bolus technique in subjects with healthy lungs who were to undergo scheduled surgery. The bolus technique consists of a maximum expiration to residual volume (RV) and the inhalation of the bolus of a tracer gas (i.e., helium) that will not reach alveoli behind occluded airways. During the ongoing inspiration to total lung capacity all airways will open and the corresponding alveoli will be filled with air without the tracer gas. During the succeeding expiration down to RV the tracer gas is diluted by the air coming from alveoli that have not received the tracer. When airways begin to close during the ongoing expiration the tracer gas concentration will increase as measured at the airway opening since air with no tracer contributes less to the expiration.

Measurements were made with the subject awake and then after approximately one hour of anaesthesia and mechanical ventilation in a study group of 35 patients with a mean age of 45 years. Closing volume (CV, i.e. the lung volume above residual volume where airway closure begins during an expiration) was 980 ml awake, and the difference between CV and the expiratory reserve volume (CV-ERV) was 330 ml [20]. During anaesthesia CV was 870 ml and CV-ERV was 570 ml, an increase of 250 ml that was significant (p=0.002). Thus, airway closure occurred more frequently above FRC and covered a larger part of the tidal volume during anaesthesia than in the awake state. Moreover, simultaneous measurements of the ventilation/perfusion matching ($\dot{V}A/\dot{Q}$) by multiple inert gas elimination technique showed a correlation between CV-ERV and the amount of poor ventilation in relation to perfusion (low $\dot{V}A/\dot{Q}$) [22]. The corresponding regression equation was:

$$\text{low } \dot{V}A/\dot{Q}\,[\%\ CO] = 0.68 + 0.006 \cdot (CV\text{-}ERV)[ml];\ R = 0.57,\ p=0.001.$$

There was also a linear correlation between arterial oxygen tension (PaO_2) and airway closure, expressed as CV-ERV (R=0.59, p=0.001).

These findings suggest that airway closure is more frequent in anaesthetised than awake subjects, has an effect on the $\dot{V}A/\dot{Q}$ matching, and contributes to the impairment of oxygenation regularly seen during anaesthesia. However, it is not the sole cause of gas exchange impairment during anaesthesia. Other morphological and mechanical changes can also be seen and may play an even more important role for the oxygenation of blood, as will be discussed in the next paragraph.

Atelectasis

Approximately 15 years ago, atelectasis was demonstrated in anaesthetised patients: neonates as well as adults [23, 24]. The atelectasis can be demonstrated by computed X-ray tomography but is invisible on conventional chest X-ray (Fig. 4). It is located in the most dependent parts of both lungs and appears in almost 90% of all patients who are anaesthetised [25]. It develops whether the anaesthesia is intravenous or inhalant and whether the patient is breathing spontaneously or is paralysed and ventilated mechanically [26]. The atelectasis is largest near the diaphragm in the supine patient and decreases in size towards the apex [27]. A three-dimensional reconstruction of the atelectasis is shown in Figure 5. The atelectasis covers approximately 5% of the transverse pulmonary area near the diaphragm, with a large variation from 0 to 10%-15%. In the average patient, the atelectasis may not look too impressive. However, it should be remembered that the collapsed area comprises four times more lung tissue than the aerated regions. Thus, in the average patient the atelectasis comprises about 15%-20% of the lung tissue near the diaphragm and about 10% of

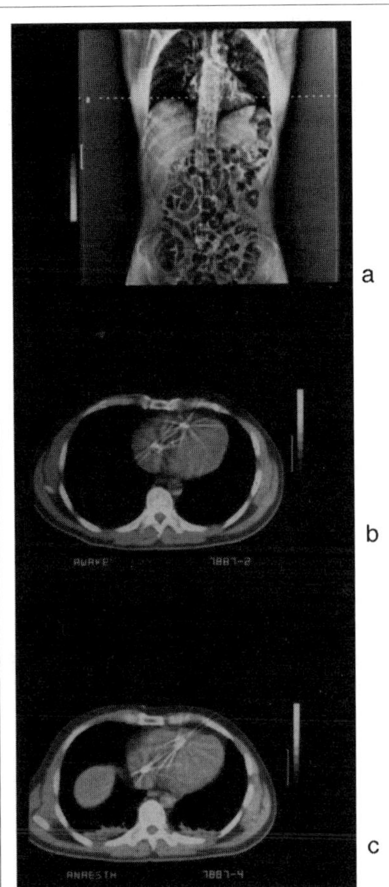

Fig. 4 a-c. A computed tomogram (CT) in a 50-year-old man. (a) scout view with the dotted line indicating the level of the transverse CT cut; (b) chest CT while awake; (c) chest CT during anaesthesia. Note the appearance of densities in the dependent region of both lungs, interpreted as atelectasis. The white area in the middle of the right lung (seen to the left) is the diaphragm (and liver) that has been displaced cranially during anaesthesia

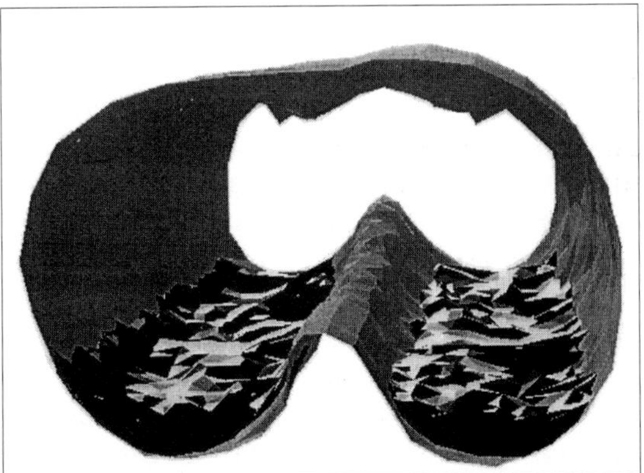

Fig. 5. Three-dimensional reconstruction of the chest wall and the atelectatic regions from apex to base in an anaesthetised patient. Note the irregular appearance of the atelectasis and the slight decrease in atelectasis from base to apex. (From [43] with permission)

the total lung tissue [27]. In extreme cases almost half the lung can be collapsed during anaesthesia, before any surgery has taken place.

Almost all anaesthetics that have been studied cause atelectasis during standard anaesthesia. Anaesthetic agents that have been studied are inhalational agents such as halothane, enflurane, isoflurane and desflurane, neuroleptic drugs as well as intravenous agents like barbiturates and propofol. The only exception so far is ketamine, when used alone or together with a sedative [28]. Interestingly, ketamine preserves respiratory muscle tone and does not lower FRC, contrary to the other anaesthetics [29]. However, if muscle relaxation is required, atelectasis will appear as with other anaesthetics [28].

Positive end-expiratory pressure (PEEP) of 10 cm H_2O consistently reopens collapsed lung tissue [24]. However, some atelectasis persists in most patients at this PEEP level. It is likely that a further increase in PEEP may reopen this tissue. Moreover, the lung re-collapses rapidly after discontinuation of PEEP. Within one minute after the cessation of PEEP, the collapse is as large as it was before the application of PEEP [24]. This means that in order to bring the patient over the perioperative period without lung collapse, the PEEP must be maintained without interruption, also during the wake-up and early postoperative periods.

The use of a sigh manoeuvre, or a double tidal volume, has been advocated to reopen any collapsed lung tissue [30]. However, the atelectasis is not affected by an ordinary tidal volume, to an end-inspiratory airway pressure of 10 cm H_2O, nor by a deep sigh with an airway pressure to +20 cm H_2O [31]. Not until an airway pressure of 30 cm H_2O was reached did the atelectasis decrease to approximately half the initial value. For a complete reopening of all collapsed lung tissue an inflation pressure of 40 cm H_2O was required and the breath was held for 15 s [31]. Such a large inflation and subsequent expiration down to -20 cm H_2O corresponded to a vital capacity measured during spontaneous breathing with the patient awake.

Causes of atelectasis

The rapid formation of atelectasis after induction of anaesthesia and discontinuation of PEEP may suggest that a major cause of atelectasis is compression of lung tissue rather than slow absorption of gas behind occluded airways. A similar conclusion was drawn by Morimoto et al. [32] in a study of anaesthetised, mechanically ventilated rabbits. They injected air into the abdomen (pneumopenditoneum) in order to displace the diaphragm cranially and to reduce lung volume. This caused atelectasis in dependent lung regions which the authors called "gravity dependent atelectasis". As mentioned earlier, humans anaesthetised with ketamine that allowed the maintenance of respiratory muscle tone did not show any atelectasis unless the patient was paralysed and mechanically ventilated [28]. Tensing the diaphragm by phrenic nerve stimulation reduced the atelectasis in anaesthetised patients [33]. These findings fit with the concept of compression or gravity-dependent atelectasis.

However, recent observations have made the explanation of atelectasis formation during anaesthesia more complex. First, collapsed lung tissue can be re-expanded by a vital capacity manoeuvre (as mentioned above), but if the lungs are ventilated with pure oxygen they rapidly re-collapse within five minutes after the vital capacity manoeuvre [8]. If, on the other hand, the lungs are ventilated with 40% O_2 in nitrogen after the re-expansion, the lungs remain open with no or only little atelectasis formation for half an hour or longer (Fig. 6). Second, if anaesthesia is induced without "preoxygenation" and ventilation is given with 30% O_2 in nitrogen, no or little atelectasis is formed [34, 35]. These observations underscore the importance of the inspired oxygen fraction which suggests that the rate of absorption of gas from the alveoli may play an important role in the formation of atelectasis. However, the breathing of oxygen alone for more than half an hour does not promote atelectasis [24]. If the oxygen breathing is done at a reduced lung volume atelectasis may ensue, as suggested by the reduction in compliance and oxygenation in healthy volunteers during chest strapping [36]. Thus, for atelectasis to occur during anaesthesia, there must be both a reduced respiratory muscle tone with lowered FRC and ventilation with high fractions of oxygen, at least for a period of time. Atelectasis is thus an effect of both compression of lung tissue and resorption of gas.

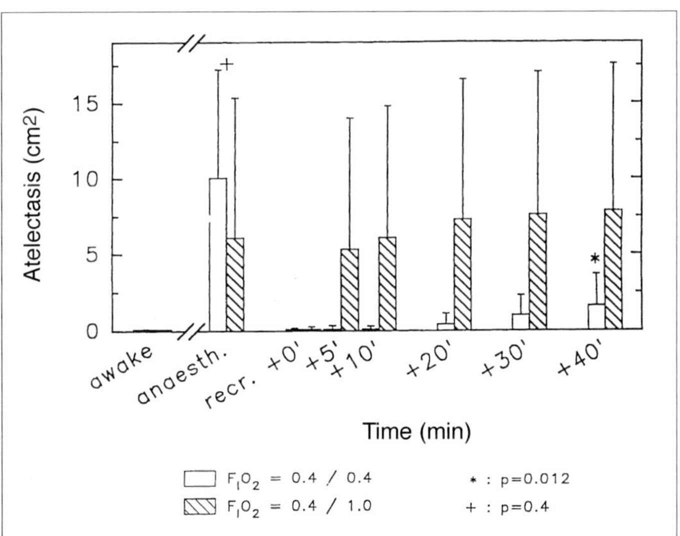

Fig. 6. Atelectasis before and after a so-called vital capacity manoeuvre that opens up essentially all atelectatic lung tissue (mean and SD). The x-axis shows events and time in minutes. *Open columns*, results from 6 patients ventilated with 40% O_2 in nitrogen before and after the recruitment manoeuvre; *dashed columns*, results from another 6 patients ventilated with 40% O_2 before and 100% O_2 after the recruitment manoeuvre. Note the elimination of atelectasis after the manoeuvre (Time 0) and the slow re-appearance of atelectasis if ventilation is by 40% O_2 in nitrogen, and the rapid re-formation of atelectasis if ventilation is by 100% O_2. Compare with data in Fig. 2. anaesth; *rect*, recruitment manoeuvre. (From [8] with permission)

Atelectasis and gas exchange

The magnitude of shunt correlates well with the size of the atelectasis [37]. That the shunt is located in dependent lung regions, corresponding to the location of atelectasis, has also been demonstrated by single photon emission computed tomography (SPECT) [38]. An interesting finding is that the atelectasis does not increase with the age of the patient, nor does shunt increase with age [39]. This may appear surprising since gas exchange impairment mostly worsens when patients get older [40]. However, perfusion of poorly ventilated lung regions (low $\dot{V}A/\dot{Q}$) increases with age [39]. The dependence of shunt and low $\dot{V}A/\dot{Q}$ on age is shown in Figure 4. It can also be seen that venous admixture increases with age, since it will be affected both by shunt and low $\dot{V}A/\dot{Q}$.

As said earlier both airway closure and atelectasis impair the oxygenation of blood. In the above mentioned study on 35 patients where airway closure was assessed by the helium bolus technique, atelectasis was simultaneously assessed by computed tomography [22]. A highly significant correlation between atelectasis and airway closure on one hand and arterial oxygenation on the other was found according to the equation:

$$PaO_2\ (kPa) = 29 - 2.9 \cdot \ln\ (atelectasis\ [cm^2]) - 0.0085\ (CV - ERV)\ [ml];$$
$$R = 0.86,\ p<0.001$$

where PaO_2 is the arterial partial pressure of oxygen measured at FIO_2=0.40, ln (atelectasis)=natural logarithm of atelectasis. Thus, the coefficient of determination (R^2) was as high as 0.74. In other words, as much as three-quartes of the impairment in oxygenation can be explained by atelectasis and airway closure leaving only little to be explained by other mechanisms during uneventful anaesthesia.

The effect of PEEP on gas exchange deserves a paragraph by its own. This is because atelectasis is reduced, as said above, but shunt is not reduced and the arterial oxygenation is not improved, on an average. This was demonstrated already in 1974 by Hewlett et al. who warned about the "indiscriminate use of PEEP in routine anaesthesia" [41]. The maintenance of shunt may be explained by the redistribution of blood flow towards the most dependent parts when intrathoracic pressure is increased, so that any persisting atelectasis in the bottom of the lung receives a larger share of the pulmonary blood flow than without PEEP [42]. The increased intrathoracic pressure will also impede venous return and lower cardiac output. This results in a lower venous oxygen tension for a given oxygen uptake which will augment the desaturating effect of shunted blood and perfusion of poorly ventilated regions on the arterial oxygenation [43].

Conclusions

Lung function, both the mechanics of the respiratory system and the gas exchange, is affected during anaesthesia. Changes in the mechanics contribute to the impaired gas exchange. Thus, FRC is reduced during anaesthesia which is accompanied by atelectasis formation and, most likely, airway closure. The resistance to breathing is also increased, possibly an effect of reduced lung volume that decreases the caliber of the airways, but other mechanisms may also contribute or predominate. The decrease in lung volume is reasonably explained by loss of respiratory muscle tone but, again, other mechanisms may also contribute, e.g. loss of or impeded function of surfactant. Resorption atelectasis may be considered an effect of reduced lung volume but will also by itself contribute to lung volume reduction. The atelectasis, whether it has been caused by compression of tissue or gas resorbtion, causes shunt; airway closure and airway narrowing cause reduced ventilation in proportion to the blood flow (low $\dot{V}A/\dot{Q}$). Finally, the shunt and the low $\dot{V}A/\dot{Q}$ are the causes of the impairment of blood oxygenation that is regularly seen during anaesthesia.

References

1. Nims RG, Conner EH, Comroe JH (1955) The compliance of the human thorax in anesthetized patients. J Clin Invest 34:744-750
2. Campbell RJM, Nunn JF, Peckett BW (1958) A comparison of artificial ventilation and spontaneous respiration with particular reference to ventilation-blood flow relationships. Br J Anaesth 30:166-175
3. Severinghaus JW, Stupfel M (1957) Alveolar dead space as an index of distribution of blood flow in pulmonary capillaries. J Appl Physiol 10:335-348
4. Don H (1977) The mechanical properties of the respiratory system during anesthesia. Int Anesthesiol Clin 15:113-136
5. Westbrook PR, Stubbs SE, Sessler AD et al (1973) Effects of anesthesia and muscle paralysis on respiratory mechanics in normal man. J Appl Physiol 34:81-86
6. Rehder K, Sessler AD, Marsh HM (1975-1976) General anesthesia and the lung. In: Murray JF (ed) Lung disease state of the art. American Lung Association, New York, pp 367-389
7. Gattinoni L, Pesenti A, Avalli L et al (1987) Pressure volume curve of the total respiratory system in acute respiratory failure. Am Rev Respir Dis 136:730-736
8. Rothen HU, Sporre B, Engberg G, Wegenius G, Hogman M, Hedenstierna G (1995) Influence of gas composition on recurrence of atelectasis after a reexpansion maneuver during general anesthesia. Anesthesiology 82:832-842
9. Wirtz H, Schmidt M (1992) Ventilation and secretion of pulmonary surfactant. Clin Invest Med 70:3-13
10. Don HF, Wahba M, Cuadrado L, Kelkar H (1970) The effect of anesthesia and 100% oxygen on the functional residual capacity of the lungs. Anesthesiology 32:521-529
11. Froese AB, Bryan CH (1974) Effects of anesthesia and paralysis on diaphragmatic mechanics in man. Anesthesiology 41:242-255
12. Reber A, Nylund U, Hedenstierna G (1998) Position and shape of the diaphragm: Implications for atelectasis formation. Anaesthesia (in press)
13. Krayer S, Rehder K, Vettermann J, Didier EP, Ritman EL (1989) Position and motion of the human diaphragm during anesthesia-paralysis. Anesthesiology 70:891-898
14. Warner DO, Warner MA, Ritman EL (1995) Human chest wall function while awake and during halothane anesthesia. I. Quiet breathing. Anesthesiology 82:6-19

15. Wahba RWM (1991) Perioperative functional residual capacity. Can J Anaesth 38: 384-400
16. Hedenstierna G, Strandberg Å, Brismar B, Lundquist H, Svensson L, Tokics L (1985) Functional residual capacity, thoracoabdominal dimensions, and central blood volume during general anesthesia with muscle paralysis and mechanical ventilation. Anesthesiology 62:247-254
17. Milic-Emili J, Henderson JAM, Dolovich MB et al (1966) Regional distribution of inspired gas in the lung. J Appl Physiol 21:749-759
18. Don HF, Wahba WM, Craig DB (1972) Airway closure, gas trapping and the functional residual capacity during anesthesia. Anesthesiology 36:533-539
19. Juno P, Marsh M, Knopp TJ et al (1977) Closing capacity in awake and anesthetized-paralyzed man. J Appl Physiol 44:238-244
20. Bergman NA, Tien YK (1983) Contribution of the closure of pulmonary units to impaired oxygenation during anesthesia. Anesthesiology 59:395-401
21. Dueck R, Prutow RJ, Davies NJ, Clausen JL, Davidson TM (1988) The lung volume at which shunting occurs with inhalation anesthesia. Anesthesiology 69:854-861
22. Rothen HU, Sporre B, Engberg G, Wegenius G, Hedenstierna G (1988) Airway closure, atelectasis and gas exchange during general anaesthesia. Brit J Anaesth (in press)
23. Damgaard Pedersen K, Qvist T (1980) Pediatric pulmonary CT-scanning Anaesthesia-induced changes. Pediatr Radiol 9:145-148
24. Brismar B, Hedenstierna G, Lundquist H, Strandberg A, Svensson L, Tokics L (1985) Pulmonary densities during anesthesia with muscular relaxation: a proposal of atelectasis. Anesthesiology 62:422-428
25. Lundquist H, Hedenstierna G, Strandberg A, Tokics L, Brismar B (1995) CT-assessment of dependent lung densities in man during general anaesthesia. Acta Radiol 36:626-632
26. Strandberg A, Tokics L, Brismar B, Lundquist H, Hedenstierna G (1986) Atelectasis during anaesthesia and in the postoperative period. Acta Anaesthesiol Scand 30:154-158
27. Reber A, Engberg G, Sporre B, Kviele L, Rothen HU, Wegenius G, Nylund U, Hedenstierna G (1996) Volumetric analysis of aeration in the lungs during general anaesthesia. Br J Anaesth 76:760-766
28. Tokics L, Strandberg A, Brismar B, Lundquist H, Hedenstierna G (1987) Computerized tomography of the chest and gas exchange measurements during ketamine anaesthesia. Acta Anaesthesiol Scand 31:684-692
29. Shulman D, Beardsmore CS, Aronson HB, Godfrey S (1985) The effect of ketamine on the functional residual capacity in young children. Anesthesiology 62:551-556
30. Nunn JF (1993) Applied respiratory physiology, 4th edn. Butterworths, Oxford, p 43-44
31. Rothen HU, Sporre B, Engberg G, Wegenius G, Hedenstierna G (1993) Re-expansion of atelectasis during general anaesthesia: a computed tomography study. Br J Anaesth 71:788-795
32. Morimoto S, Takeuchi N, Imanaka H, Nishimura M, Takezawa J, Taenaka N, Matsuura N, Tomoda K, Ikezoe J, Arisawa J et al (1989) Gravity-dependent atelectasis. Radiologic, physiologic and pathologic correlation in rabbits on high-frequency oscillation ventilation. Invest Radiol 24:522-530
33. Hedenstierna G, Tokics L, Lundquist H, Andersson T, Strandberg A, Brismar B (1994) Phrenic nerve stimulation during halothane anesthesia. Effects of atelectasis. Anesthesiology 80:751-760
34. Rothen HU, Sporre B, Engberg G, Wegenius G, Reber A, Hedenstierna G (1995) Prevention of atelectasis during general anaesthesia. Lancet 345:1387-1391
35. Reber A, Engberg G, Wegenius G, Hedenstierna G (1996) Lung aeration. The effect of

pre-oxygenation and hyperoxygenation during total intravenous anaesthesia. Anaesthesia 51:733-737

36. Burger EJ, Macklem P (1986) Airway closure: demonstration by breathing 100% O_2 at low lung volumes and by N_2 washout. J Appl Physiol 25:139-148
37. Tokics L, Hedenstierna G, Strandberg A, Brismar B, Lundquist H (1987) Lung collapse and gas exchange during general anesthesia: effects of spontaneous breathing, muscle paralysis, and positive end-expiratory pressure. Anesthesiology 66:157-167
38. Tokics L, Hedenstierna G, Svensson L, Brismar B, Cederlund T, Lundquist H, Strandberg Å (1996) V/Q distribution and correlation to atelectasis in anesthetized paralyzed humans. J Appl Physiol 81:1822-1833
39. Gunnarsson L, Tokics L, Gustavsson H, Hedenstierna G (1991) Influence of age on atelectasis formation and gas exchange impairment during general anaesthesia. Br J Anaesth 66:423-432
40. Nunn JF, Bergman NA, Coleman AJ (1965) Factors influencing the arterial oxygen tension during anaesthesia with artificial ventilation. Br J Anaesth 37:898-914
41. Hewlett AM, Hulands GH, Nunn JF, Milledge JS (1974) Functional residual capacity during anaesthesia III: artificial ventilation. Br J Anaesth 46:495-503
42. West JB (1977) State of the art: ventilation-perfusion relationships. Am Rev Respir Dis 116:919-943
43. Reber A (1998) Lung aeration and pulmonary gas exchange during general and epidural anaesthesia. Acta Universitatis Upsaliensis 756:18

Chapter 21

Respiratory mechanics during the long-term artificial ventilation

M. Cereda, A. Pesenti

Respiratory mechanics alterations during acute lung injury (ALI) are mainly ascribed to changes in pulmonary tissue structure. In the initial stages, interstitial edema and alveolar collapse predominate [1]. Tissue healing and a relatively rapid clinical improvement may follow in some patients. A subpopulation of ALI patients does not improve and needs mechanical ventilatory support for an extended time. In these patients, the pathological picture may evolve, and lung tissue reorganization phenomena may prevail over edema and atelectasis [2].

Although respiratory mechanics in ALI have been extensively investigated, relatively few studies addressed the issue of their evolution with time. Available data suggest that, in the course of long-term ventilation in ALI, changes in respiratory mechanics occur that may be associated with specific changes in morphology and histopathology [3, 4].

Respiratory mechanics during the early ALI

Initial stages of ALI are characterized by disruption of the alveolar capillary membrane and by interstitial edema and alveolar flooding [1]. The resulting increase in lung tissue weight and high alveolar surface tension are probably the cause of a tendency to alveolar collapse. Atelectasis occurs in the most dependent lung areas and can be observed by computed tomography (CT) analysis as a gravity dependent increase in tissue density [5]. Inspired gas volumes are redistributed to the non-dependent portions of the lungs [6]. In this stage of the injury process, the characteristic decrease in lung compliance can be ascribed to a reduction in the number of patent alveolar units, rather than to increased tissue stiffness. In fact, the total static lung compliance is related to the amount of normally aerated tissue [7]. Other features of the volume-pressure curve can be related to alveolar instability phenomena. The inflection point visible on the inflation arm of the curve and the hysteresis area between the inflation and the deflation arms are probably due to the recruitment of previously collapsed alveoli with increasing airway pressure [3, 7]. The application of positive end-expiratory pressure (PEEP) increases the number of open alveolar units [8] and effects a more homogeneous distribution of inspired gas [6].

Respiratory mechanics in late ALI

In a retrospective study [4], patients with severe ALI were divided into three different groups according to the duration of mechanical ventilation: late ALI (more than 2 weeks from onset), intermediate ALI (1-2 weeks), and early ALI (less than 1 week). Patients with late and intermediate ALI showed lower respiratory compliance compared with patients from the early ALI group. Moreover, late ALI patients had decreased PEEP requirements, compared to the early patients.

Duration of ALI has been associated to changes in the volume-pressure curve morphology. In an early study by Matamis et al. [3], patients with late ALI, i.e. 2-3 weeks from onset, showed no inflection point and no increase in hysteresis on the volume-pressure curve. On the contrary, an inflection point and hysteresis were present in patients studied in the early phases of their diseases. Besides, the volume-pressure curve in late ALI patients was flatter than those of, the early patients. In the same study, changes in respiratory mechanics corresponded to an evolution in the radiological appearence of the lungs. In patients with late acute respiratory distress syndrome (ARDS), opacities on X-ray were mostly classified as "alveolar", while "interstitial" opacities prevailed in the late ALI group.

These findings suggest different lung pathology pictures in patients at different stages of the ALI process. In patients who do not improve early, lung anatomy alterations may progress over time. Autoptic series showed an evolution from interstitial and alveolar edema to scar formation and fibrosis [2]. The evolution into late pulmonary fibrosis seems to be due to a protracted release of inflammatory mediators, which result in abnormal and exaggerated activation of the normal tissue repair mechanisms. Liberation of cytokines enhances fibroblast proliferation and collagen deposition [9]. At the same time, edema fluid is reabsorbed, leading to a decrease in alveolar collapse. Therefore, it is the increased interstitial collagen content that, causing intrinsic tissue stiffness, probably results in the low lung compliance in late ALI. Reduced alveolar collapse accounts for the loss of hysteresis and of the inflection point on the volume-pressure curve and explains why PEEP is less effective on oxygenation in this stage [10]. Probably, increasing airway pressures in late ALI does not recruit alveoli but distends open units, due to a numerical decrease of collapsed or collapsable alveoli.

Effects of mechanical ventilation on respiratory mechanics and lung structure

Published experimental data suggest that mechanical ventilation may worsen the picture of ALI and affect outcome. High inflation volumes in animal models, in fact, generate lung injury that resembles human ALI, with edema and reduced lung compliance [11, 12]. Cyclic closure and reopening of unstable alveoli is thought to be associated with lung tissue damage and worsening lung mechanics [13]. The mechanism of lung injury due to mechanical ventilation seems to involve physical damage of the interstitial structure, with disruption of alveolar-capillary membrane integrity at both the epithelial and endothelial levels [14, 15]. It is therefore possible that the ventilatory treatment itself contributes to the progression of lung pathology and of lung mechanics observed in ALI of long duration. Another typical pathologic finding in ARDS is the presence of airspace enlargement, which seems to occur more frequently in late ALI. Patients observed in late stages of ALI show an increased number of bullae on CT, compared to patients in earlier stages [4]. Although other factors could be responsible for the formation of bullae, mechanical ventilation may play at least a contributory role. In fact, the presence of airspace enlargements has been associated to high peak distending pressures [16].

Awareness of ventilator-associated lung injury led to the proposal of a "lung protective strategy" to minimize iatrogenic damage [17]. This approach includes both the optimization of alveolar recruitment, with relatively high levels of PEEP, and the limitation of peak distending pressures, achieved by low tidal volume ventilation. Whether the adoption of this ventilatory strategy in ARDS results in improved outcome is still controversial [18, 19]. However, the use of this approach seems to improve the evolution over time of respiratory compliance [19], suggesting a favorable effect on lung pathology.

Conclusions

Respiratory mechanics measurements could be useful in the ventilatory management of patients with ALI. It is currently suggested that alveolar recruitment should be optimized and the common thought is that information obtained from the volume-pressure curve should be used to select PEEP. However, the progression of lung pathology occuring in long-term ventilated ALI patients results in changes in respiratory mechanics. More importantly, the pathophysiology of late stages of ALI seems to be different from early stages. In late ALI, PEEP is probably less effective and mechanisms other than alveolar recruitment could underlie its action. Therefore, the response to ventilatory treatment could be affected by the duration of ALI, and the time from onset should be considered an important variable in selecting the ventilatory strategy.

References

1. Tomashefski JF (1990) Pulmonary pathology of the adult respiratory distress syndrome. Clin Chest Med 11:581-592
2. Pratt PC, Vollmer RT, Shellburne JD, Crapo JD (1979) Pulmonary morphology in a multihospital collaborative extracorporeal membrane oxygenation project:1. Light microscopy. Am J Pathol 95:191-214
3. Matamis D, Lemaire F, Harf A, Brun-Buisson C, Ansquer JC, Atlan G (1984) The total respiratory pressure-volume curves in the adult respiratory distress syndrome. Chest 86:58-66

4. Gattinoni L, Bombino M, Lissoni A, Pesenti A, Fumagalli R, Tagliabue M (1994) Lung structure and function in different stages of severe adult respiratory distress syndrome. JAMA 271:1772-1779
5. Gattinoni L, Pesenti A, Bombino M, Baglioni S, Rivolta M, Rossi F, Rossi G, Fumagalli R, Marcolin R, Mascheroni D, Torresin A (1988) Relationships between lung computed tomographic densities, gas exchange, and PEEP in adult respiratory failure. Anesthesiology 69:824-832
6. Gattinoni L, Pelosi P, Crotti S, Valenza F (1995) Effects of positive end-expiratory pressure on regional distribution of tidal volume and recruitment in adult respiratory distress syndrome. Am J Respir Crit Care Med 151:1807-1814
7. Gattinoni L, Pesenti A, Avalli L, Rossi F, Bombino M (1987) Pressure/volume curve of total respiratory system in acute respiratory failure: computerized tomographic scan study. Am Rev Respir Dis 136:730-736
8. Gattinoni L, D'Andrea L, Pelosi P, Vitale G, Pesenti A, Fumagalli R (1993) Regional effects and mechanism of positive end-expiratory pressure in early adult respiratory distress syndrome. JAMA 269:2122-2127
9. Meduri GU, Kohler G, Headley S, Tolley E, Stentz F, Postlethwaite A (1995) Inflammatory cytokines in the BAL of patients with ARDS. Persistent elevation over time predicts poor outcome. Chest 108:1303-1314
10. Holzapfel L, Robert D, Perrin F, Blanc PL, Palmier B, Guerin C (1983) Static pressure-volume curves and effect of positive end-expiratory pressure on gas exchange in adult respiratory distress syndrome. Crit Care Med 11:591-597
11. Kolobow T, Moretti MP, Fumagalli R, Mascheroni D, Prato P, Chen V, Joris M (1987) Severe impairment in lung function induced by by high peak airway pressure during mechanical ventilation. An experimental study. Am Rev Respir Dis 135:312-315
12. Dreyfuss D, Soler P, Basset G, Saumon G (1988) High inflation pressure pulmonary edema. Respective effects of high airway pressure, high tidal volume, and positive end-expiratory airway pressure. Am Rev Respir Dis 137:1159-1164
13. Muscedere JG, Mullen JBM, Gan K, Slutsky AS (1994) Tidal ventilation at low airway pressures can augment lung injury. Am J Respir Crit Care Med 149:1327-1334
14. West JB, Tsukimoto K, Matieu-Costello O, Prediletto R (1991) Stress failure in pulmonary capillaries. J Appl Physiol 70:1731-1742
15. Parker JC, Townsley MI, Rippe B, Taylor AE, Thigpen J (1984) Increased microvascular permeability in dog lungs due to high airway pressures. J Appl Physiol 57:1809-1816
16. Rouby JJ, Lherm T, Martin de Lassale E, Poete P, Bodin L, Finet JF, Callard P, Viars P (1993) Histologic aspects of pulmonary barotrauma in critically ill patients with acute respiratory failure. Intensive Care Med 19:383-389
17. Lachmann B (1992) Open up the lung and keep the lung open. Intensive Care Med 18:319-321
18. Stewart TE, Meade MO, Cook DJ, Granton JT, Hodder RV, Lapinsky SE, Mazer DC, McLean RF, Rogovein TS, Schouten BD, Todd TRJ, Slutsky AS (1998) Evaluation of a ventilation strategy to prevent barotrauma in patients at high risk for acute respiratory distress syndrome. Pressure and Volume-limited Ventilation Strategy Group. N Engl J Med 338:355-361
19. Amato MBP, Barbas CSV, Medeiros DM, Magaldi RB, Schettino GPP, Lorenzi-Filho G, Kairalla RA, Deheinzelin D, Munoz C, Oliveira R, Takagaki TY, Carvalho CRR (1998) Effect of a protective-ventilation strategy on mortality in the acute respiratory distress syndrome. N Engl J Med 338:347-354

Chapter 22

Closed-loop control mechanical ventilation

G. Iotti, M.C. Olivei, C. Galbusera, A. Braschi

Closed-loop control mechanical ventilation includes any ventilation mode that is specifically designed to maintain the constancy of a given physiological respiratory parameter, continuously monitored (the controlled variable), by means of automatic adjustments of one or more ventilator settings (the control variables).

The first example of closed-loop control ventilation dates back to the beginning of modern mechanical ventilation [1]. In the experimental system designed by Frumin et al., and tidal CO_2 ($ETCO_2$) was continuously monitored and served as controlled variable, while tidal volume was the control variable. The value for the respiratory rate was constant, and user-set. Tidal volume was automatically increased when $ETCO_2$ was higher than the $ETCO_2$ target set by the user. On the contrary, tidal volume was automatically decreased when $ETCO_2$ was lower than the target. Such system proved to be effective in stabilizing the $ETCO_2$ and, in subjects with normal lungs, the $PaCO_2$ at the set targets.

Closed-loop control mechanical ventilation offers potential advantages over the conventional ventilation modes, such as more precise control of physiological respiratory parameters, and greater simplicity of use. The conventional ventilation modes are poorly sensitive to changes in patient's respiratory mechanics, as well as to changes in spontaneous respiratory activity. Pressure support ventilation (PSV) is the most adaptable among the conventional modes, since the cycling from exhalation to inspiration and vice versa is controlled by the patient, and the instantaneous flow delivery is not fixed. However, even in PSV, the level of mechanical support does not vary over time, unless the control settings of the ventilator are manually changed by the user. PSV is also the simplest among the conventional ventilation modes, since the only ventilator parameters set by the user are inspiratory pressure, PEEP and FiO_2. However, PSV is not suitable for all kinds of patients, and not suitable for any step of the management of a given patient.

Many different modes based on closed-loop control have been developed in the past years. Some of these modes remained confined in the field of experimental medicine, while other ones were implemented in commercial ventilators. So far, all these modes have shown evident limits, and none of them has become of widespread clinical use. However, the research and the development in the field of closed-loop control mechanical ventilation did not stop, and the most recent solutions seem promising.

According to the most modern approach, a closed-loop mode of ventilation should satisfy the following requirements:

- applicability to any patient;
- applicability during any step of the ventilatory management of a given patient;
- simplicity of use, which means few manual controls;
- self-adaptability to changes in patient's conditions and requirements.

Theoretically, these goals can be achieved by means of systems based on:

- few user-set controls, defining:
  - the physiological target(s);
  - the limits within which the closed-loop control is free to play;
- automatic, breath-by-breath analysis of the patient's respiratory function;
- automatic adaptation of the system, based on:
  - continuous check of the agreement between the respiratory function of the patient and the target(s) set by the user;
  - automatic, breath-by-breath adjustment of the mechanical support, based on the information provided by the monitoring system. The algorithms used for this purpose should be in line with the latest achievements of mechanical ventilation.

Evidently, such a system is more than a mere closed-loop control system, and can be considered as a simple kind of application of artificial intelligence to mechanical ventilation.

On the basis of the general principles outlined above, a family of closed-loop control modes of ventilation has been developed, including:

- the experimental mode adaptive lung ventilation (ALV);
- a simplified variant of ALV, represented by the adaptive support ventilation (ASV), presently available on the new Hamilton® Galileo ventilator;
- a more complex variant of ALV, still experimental, the P0.1-controller. The main feature of this mode is the control of the patient's respiratory drive and inspiratory effort.

The principles of these modes will be described in next paragraphs.

Adaptive lung ventilation

The basic ventilation mode for ALV is pressure-controlled synchronized intermittent mandatory ventilation (P-SIMV) combined with PSV. In other words, the basic mode for ALV is an SIMV in which the mandatory breaths are pressure-controlled and the spontaneous breaths are pressure-supported. The level of the inspiratory pressure delivered by the ventilator is the same for both mandatory breaths and spontaneous breaths. The adjustment of inspiratory pressure as well as mandatory respiratory rate is done automatically. The inspiratory phase of all ventilator-initiated breaths is terminated according to a time-based criterion, automatically adapted by the system. In contrast, the inspiratory phase of all patient-initiated breaths is terminated according to a flow-based criterion, exactly as it usually happens during PSV. Therefore, the inspiratory time of any breath started by the patient is controlled by the patient.

ALV can work both as total ventilatory support (as a kind of pressure control ventilation, PCV) and as partial ventilatory support (as a kind of PSV). The mode of working depends on the relationship between the respiratory rate automatically selected by the system, and the respiratory rate driven by the respiratory center of the patient. When the system respiratory rate is higher than the patient respiratory rate, the ventilator overcomes the patient and works as total ventilatory support, like a kind of PCV. On the contrary, when the system respiratory rate is lower than the patient respiratory rate, all cycles are started by the patient (by means of the trigger), and the ventilator works as partial ventilatory support, like a kind of PSV. Also in this case, however, the ventilator will resume the complete control of the ventilation as soon as the respiratory rate of the patient becomes inadequate.

ALV is designed to warrant a user-set minimal minute ventilation [2, 3]. In order to warrant that ventilation is really effective in terms of gas exchange, ALV uses a setting of minimal alveolar ventilation ($\dot{V}a$), instead of the commonly used setting of total minute ventilation. ALV is based on just four manual controls:

- minimal $\dot{V}a$ (i.e. the minimal $\dot{V}a$ guaranteed by the automatic controller);
- maximal inspiratory pressure (i.e. the upper pressure limit for the working of the automatic controller);
- PEEP;
- FiO_2.

In order to work as a $\dot{V}a$ controller, ALV uses a continuous measurement of series dead space (Vds); this latter is obtained by means of capnometry and airflow measurement.

ALV is designed to prevent the delivery of too small, or too large, tidal volumes (Vt). Vt includes a component that does not participate to the gas exchange; this component is represented by the Vds of the patient-ventilator unit. The second component of Vt reaches the alveoli, and is defined as alveolar volume (Va). An efficacious Vt must necessarily be higher than the Vds. In order to avoid a too low Vt, ALV calculates for each breath a minimum Vt to be delivered of twice the Vds. On the other hand, ALV defines a maximum Vt, in order to avoid any potential volo-trauma. This upper limit is calculated on the basis of the automatic, breath-by-breath measurement of the ratio between Vt and inspiratory pressure (above PEEP) delivered by the ventilator. This ratio is an estimate of the apparent dynamic compliance of the respiratory system, and together with the maximum inspiratory pressure set by the user, allows to calculate the maximum safe Vt that the system can select. In other words, ALV uses the measurements of Vds and dynamic compliance to obtain an estimate of the size of the lungs, and thus identifies the lower and the upper boundaries for the automatic selection of Vt.

After the identification of the lower and upper boundaries for Vt, ALV calculates, on a breath-by-breath basis, the best values for Vt and respiratory rate (Fr). This choice is performed according to a criterion of energetic optimization. The pioneering work by Otis and Wallace on the respiratory mechanics of spontaneous breathing demonstrated that, for any given couple of values of $\dot{V}a$ and Vds, there is an optimal Fr that corresponds to the minimal total work of breathing [4]. Otis, and more clearly, Mead demonstrated that the optimal Fr depends on the time constant of the respiratory system [5]. When the time constant is higher than normal, as in patients with obstructive lung disease, the optimal Fr will be lower than normal. Conversely, in patients with restrictive lung disease, with a low time constant, the optimal Fr will be higher than normal. According to these principles, at each breath the system fulfils the following tasks:

- calculation of the optimal Fr, based on minimal $\dot{V}a$ setting, measured Vds, and measured time constant;
- calculation of the Va target for the next breath, as minimal $\dot{V}a$ setting divided by optimal Fr;
- calculation of the Vt target for the next breath, as sum of Va target and Vds.

The criterion of energetic optimization will ensure that the ventilator will work by using the lowest possible level of inspiratory pressure. The breath-by-breath measurement of the expiratory time constant (RCe) of the patient-ventilator unit is one of the basis of the procedure described above. RCe is obtained according to a simplified method, based on the calculation of the ratio between expiratory tidal volume and expiratory peak flow [6].

According to the above described procedure, the ALV controller divides the minimal $\dot{V}$ a set by the user into a target value for Fr and a target value for Vt. These targets are updated at each breath. At this point, the simplest and most typical part of a closed-loop control system is involved. For each breath the system compares the actual Vt with the target Vt, and programs whether to increase, decrease or keep unchanged the inspiratory pressure that will be delivered in the next cycle. Simultaneously, the system compares the actual Fr with the target Fr, and programs the start of the next mandatory cycle. When the actual Fr is lower than the target, the start of the next cycle is anticipated, i.e. the mandatory rate is increased. When the actual Fr is higher than the target, the start of the next cycle is delayed, i.e. the mandatory rate is decreased. When the actual Fr is higher than the target due to spontaneous patient's activity, this makes that any mandatory breath is anticipated and hence inhibited by a patient-initiated breath. This will result in a progressive reduction of the mandatory rate, while ASV will behave like a kind of PSV.

The last aspect of the ALV principles is the definition of the inspiratory time (Ti) of the mandatory breaths. This aspect is very important when ALV works as total ventilatory support. The selection of Ti is aimed at giving an expiratory time (Te) long enough to prevent autoPEEP and dynamic hyperinflation. These phenomena depend on the balance between the RCe and the available Te. A minimum Te to be always guaranteed is calculated as three times the RCe value. Since the selected duration of an entire respiratory cycle (Ttot) depends on the target for Fr, Ti can be calculated as difference between Ttot and minimum Te. The system will then readjust the value for Ti, in order to fulfil the criterion of a maximum I/E ratio of 1:1. As a final result, when ALV works as total ventilatory support, the I/E ratio is automatically adapted on the basis of respiratory mechanics. A low I/E ratio is selected in patients with obstructive lung disease, and an I/E ratio close to 1:1 is selected in patients with restrictive lung disease.

In summary, the main distinctive features of ALV are the following.

- The user sets a single main control, the minimal $\dot{V}$ a to be warranted by the system.
- The ventilatory support is automatically adapted (in terms of mandatory frequency, inspiratory pressure, and times) in order to achieve the $\dot{V}$a target with an optimal respiratory pattern. This latter is automatically selected on the basis of measurements of capnometry, ventilation, and respiratory mechanics. When the setting of minimal $\dot{V}$ a is equal or greater than the ventilatory demand of the patient, the ventilator tends to overcome the patient, and to work as a total support mode. When the clinical goal is to promote the spontaneous activity of the patient, it is necessary to set the minimal $\dot{V}$ a target below the ventilatory demand of the patient. In this case, the system responds to the respiratory activity of the patient by working as a partial ventilatory support mode. Nonetheless, even in this case the system continues to warrant the minimal $\dot{V}$a that has been set, and to control the ventilatory pattern of the patient. In particular, the system continues to provide an adequate Vt, and to prevent inefficient ventilation. The adequacy of Vt will, in turn, prevent the development of rapid shallow breathing. In all cases, ALV is a mode in which any single breath can be greatly influenced by the patient, who can control start and stop of inspiration, as well as the instantaneous flow inspired and exhaled. The targets are never abruptly forced. They are rather achieved by small, continuous adjustments of the mechanical support delivered by the ventilator. The patient is never forced into a given condition of ventilation, but rather driven towards the optimal condition.

Adaptive support ventilation

ASV and ALV are based essentially on the same algorithms. The main difference between these two modes is that ASV works without CO_2 monitoring, and hence without measurement of the patient's Vds. To compensate for this lack, ASV is provided with an additional manual control, that allows the user to set the ideal body weight of the patient. ASV assumes that the Vds of the patient equals to 2.2 ml/kg of body weight. The main manual control of ASV is a setting for minimal minute ventilation, that corresponds to the minimal alveolar ventilation control of ALV.

ASV is available on the new Hamilton® Galileo ventilator. The first clinical trials have given satisfactory results: ASV has shown to be effective in patients affected by severe respiratory diseases (both restrictive and obstructive), and to allow a progressive weaning process by means of manual adjustments of the minimal minute ventilation control. In this regard, we report data on the preliminary experience of use of ASV in our ICU. In the period between January and May 1998 we treated 43 patients (age 64±13 years, 26 males, 17 females) with ASV. Of these patients, 12 were free from lung diseases, while 19 were affected by a restrictive lung disease, and 12 by an obstructive lung disease. The control group consisted of 37 patients (age 59±17 years, 25 males, 12 females), including 11 patients free from lung diseases, 22 affected by a restrictive lung disease, and 4 affected by an obstructive lung disease. The following modes were used to ventilate the control patients: CMV (3 patients), PCV (17 patients), PSV (28 patients) and SIMV (5 patients). Different modes (two or more) were sequentially used on 18 patients of the control group. Ventilation was delivered by means of the same ventilator in both groups (ASV and control). The conventional ventilatory treatment and the ASV did not differ in terms of duration of ventilation and (controlled mechanical ventilation) patient outcome. In no patient of both groups we could observe complications that could be specifically referred to mechanical ventilation. During weaning, the operation of ASV, based on a single main control, appeared to be simpler than the operation of the conventional modes. The weaning process could be managed just by playing with the minimal minute ventilation setting. However, it appeared clearly that ASV is designed for maintaining a stable condition, rather than for promoting automatic weaning. The weaning of patients could be achieved only by manual adjustments of ASV.

P0.1-controller

ALV and ASV are not designed for allowing a fine tuning of the inspiratory effort performed by the patient, when used as partial ventilatory support modes. This does not mean that the user has not the opportunity of modifying the degree of patient effort. Actually, the respiratory effort is reflected by the respiratory pattern, which is closed-loop controlled by both ALV and ASV. A decrease in the minimal alveolar ventilation target for ALV, or in the minimal minute ventilation target for ASV, leads to a decrease in the Vt target. The patient will respond to these changes with an increase in its spontaneous respiratory activity. However, it is difficult to predict how much the patient will be loaded by a given setting of minimal alveolar ventilation, or of minimal minute ventilation.

In order to achieve an easier and more precise control of the respiratory effort performed by the patient, we have developed an additional controller, that closes the loop by using information concerning the respiratory effort performed by the patient. This information is obtained by means of breath-by-breath monitoring of P0.1. In principle, this parameter is just an index of respiratory drive [7]. However, it has been shown that, in mechanically ventilated patients, P0.1 is also well correlated with the inspiratory work performed by the patient [8–10]. The P0.1-controller is based on the observation that, during PSV, it is possible to titrate the patient's inspiratory work by means of adjustments of the pressure support level. Provided that the respiratory center is not depressed, the patient rapidly responds to a given change in the pressure support level, with an opposite change in his inspiratory work.

In practice, with the P0.1-controller the user has a manual control by which he can set a target for P0.1, and hence a desired level of inspiratory activity performed by the patient. At each cycle, the system compares the actual P0.1, which is continuously monitored, with the target P0.1. When the actual P0.1 is above the target, the system increases the pressure support level in the next cycle. Conversely, when the actual P0.1 is below the target, the system decreases the pressure support level in the next cycle.

In an experimental study, we have shown that the P0.1-controller is able to bring P0.1 to a given desired level, and to stabilize it at that level [11]. In the same study, the P0.1-controller was combined with ALV, in order to provide both the ability of control of the patient's inspiratory effort, typical of the P0.1-controller, and the ability of control of effective ventilation, typical of ALV. For similar purposes, the P0.1-controller could be combined with ASV.

References

1. Frumin MJ, Bergman NA, Holadat DA (1959) Carbon dioxyde and oxygen blood levels with a CO_2 controlled ventilator. Anesthesiology 20:313-320
2. Laubscher TP, Heinrichs W, Weiler N, Hartmann G, Brunner JX (1994) An adaptive lung ventilation controller. IEEE Trans Biomed Eng 41:51-59
3. Veronesi R, Galbusera C, Olivei M, Palo A, Comelli A et al (1997) Adaptive lung ventilation (ALV): a new method of closed-loop controlled ventilation. Am J Respir Crit Care Med 155:A526
4. Otis AB, Wallace O (1950) Mechanics of breathing in man. J Appl Phys 2:592-607
5. Mead J (1960) Control of respiratory frequency. J Appl Phys 15:325-336
6. Brunner JX, Laubscher T, Banner M, Iotti G, Braschi A (1995) Simple method to measure total expiratory time constant based on the passive flow-volume curve. Crit Care Med 23:1117-1122
7. Milic-Emili J, Whitelaw WA, Derenne JP (1975) Occlusion pressure: a simple measurement of respiratory's center output. N Engl J Med 292:1029-1030
8. Galbusera C, Iotti G, Palo A, Olivei M et al (1993) Relationship between P0.1 and inspiratory work of breathing during pressure support ventilation (PSV). Am Rev Respir Dis 147:A876
9. Foti G, Cereda M, Banfi G, Pelosi P, D'Andrea L, Pesenti A (1993) Simple estimate of patient inspiratory effort (PE) at different levels of pressure support (PS). Am Rev Respir Dis 147:A876
10. Alberti A, Gallo F, Fongaro A, Valenti S, Rossi A (1995) P0.1 is a useful parameter in setting the level of pressure support ventilation. Intensive Care Med 21:547-553
11. Iotti G, Brunner JX, Braschi A, Laubscher T, Olivei M, Palo A, Galbusera C, Comelli A (1996) Closed loop control of airway occlusion pressure at 0.1 second (P0.1) applied to pressure support ventilation: algorithm and application in intubated patients. Crit Care Med 5:771-779

Main symbols

ab, w	Abdominal Wall
ALI	Acute Lung Injury
ALL	Alveolar Lining Layer
ALV	Adaptive Lung Ventilation
ARDS	Adult Respiratory Distress Syndrome
BMI	Body Mass Index
C	Capacitor
CMRR	Common Mode Rejection Ratio
CMV	Controlled Mechanical Ventilation
COPD	Chronic Obstructive Pulmonary Disease
Crs	Compliance of the Respiratory System
Cst,L	Static Lung Compliance
Cst,rs	Compliance Static Respiratory System
Cst,w	Chest Wall
CT	Computed Tomography
CV	Closing Volume
CV-ERV	Closing Volume-Expiratory Reserve Volume
DPH	Dynamic Pulmonary Hyperinflaction
DVw	Volume Changes of the Chest Wall
E	Elastance
Edyn	Dynamic Elastance
EL	Elastance
EMG	Electromyogram
F	Farad
FFT	Fast Fourier Transform
FO	Forced Oscillation
FOT	Forced Oscillation Technique
FRC	Functional Residual Capacity
FVC	Forced Vital Capacity
HIC	Hyperpnea-Induced Constriction
Irs	Inertance of the Respiratory System
L	Lung
LVRS	Lung Volume Reduction Surgery
MEFV	Maximal Expiratory Flow Volume
MIGET	Multiple Inert Gas Elimination Technique
MRR	Maximum Relaxion Rate
MVV	Maximum Voluntary Ventilation
P-SIMV	Pressure Synchronized Intermittent Mandatory Ventilation

P-V	Pressure Volume
PA	Alveolar Pressure
Pab	Abdominal Pressure
Pao	Airway Pressure
PAV	Proportional Assist Ventilation
Paw	Airway Pressure
Pbs	Body Surface Pressure
PCV	Pressure-Control Ventilation
Pdi	Transdiaphragmatic Pressure
$PECO_2$	Expiratory Carbon Dioxide
PEF	Peak Expiratory Flow
Pel,L	Pressure of the Lung
Pes	Esophageal Pressure
Pflex	Inflection Point
Pimax	Maximum Expiratory Effort
Pmo	Mouth Pressure
Poes	Oesophageal Pressure
Ppl	Pleural Pressure
Ppt	Transpulmonary Pressure
Prs	Pressure Respiratory System
PS	Pressure Support
Ps	Surface Pressure
PSV	Pressure Support Ventilation
R	Resistence
Raw	Airway Resistance
rc	Rib Cage
RCe	Expiratory Time Constant
RCW	Chest Wall Resistance
Ref	Effective Resistance
RL	Lung Resistance
Rmax,rs	Total Resistance of the Respiratory System
Rti	Tissue Resistance
RTL	Tissue Resistance of the Lung
RW	Wall Resistance
S	Sinusoidal flow
SIMV	Syncronised Intermittent Mandatory Ventilation
SPECT	Single Photon Emission Computed Tomography
τ	Time Constant
t2,L	Time Constants of the Lung
τ2,w	Time Constant Chest Wall
Te	Expiratory Time
Ti	Inspiratory Time
TLC	Total Lung Capacity
TTdi	Tension-time product of the Diaphragm
V	Volume
$\dot{V}$	Volume Acceleration
$\ddot{V}$	Volume Flow
V max	Magnitude of the Maximal Flow
Va	Alveolar Volume
VC	Vital Capacity

VC	Vital Capacity
VT	Tidal Volume
W	Wall
W	Work
Waw	Airway resistive work
Wdyn,L	Dynamic Work per Breath
Wi, st	Static Inspiratory Work
Wi, visc	Viscoelastic Inspiratory Work
Wi,res	Resistive Inspiratory Work
WOB	Work of Breathing
Xc	Capacitive Reactance
xL	Inductive Reactance
ZL	Lung-Dependent
Zrs	Impedance of the Respiratory System
Ztr	Respiratory Transfer Impedance

Subject index